Fundamentals of IMMUNOLOGY AND ALLERGY

Please do not trim pages!

RICHARD F. LOCKEY, M.D.

Professor of Medicine and Pediatrics
Director, Division of Allergy and Immunology
University of South Florida, College of Medicine
Chief, Section of Allergy and Immunology
James A. Haley Veterans Hospital
Tampa, Florida

SAMUEL C. BUKANTZ, M.D.

Professor of Medicine
Director Emeritus, Division of Allergy and Immunology
University of South Florida, College of Medicine
Chief Emeritus, Section of Allergy and Immunology
James A. Haley Veterans Hospital
Tampa, Florida

A Companion Text of
Principles of Immunology and Allergy,
also by Richard F. Lockey, M.D., and Samuel C. Bukantz, M.D.

1987
W. B. SAUNDERS COMPANY
Philadelphia □ London □ Toronto □ Mexico City
Rio de Janeiro □ Sydney □ Tokyo □ Hong Kong

W. B. Saunders Company: West Washington Square
Philadelphia, PA 19105

Library of Congress Cataloging-in-Publication Data

Lockey, Richard F.

Fundamentals of immunology and allergy.

1. Allergy.   2. Immunology.   I. Bukantz, Samuel C.
II. Title.   [DNLM: 1. Allergy and Immunology. 2. Hypersensitivity. 3. Immunologic Diseases. WD 300 L815f]

RC584.L63 1987   616.97   85–31786

ISBN 0–7216–2054–X

Editor: W. B. Saunders Staff
Designer: Karen O'Keefe
Production Manager: Bill Preston
Manuscript Editor: Erika Shapiro
Illustration Coordinator: Walt Verbitski
Indexer: George Vilk

Cover Illustration: Reprinted, with permission, from Austen, K. F.: Tissue mast
cells in immediate hypersensitivity. Hospital Practice, Vol.
17, No. 11, p. 106. Illustration by Bunji Tagawa.

Fundamentals of Immunology and Allergy   ISBN   0–7216–2054–X

Last digit is the print number: 9   8   7   6   5   4   3   2   1

Dedicated to Anna F. Lockey and in loving memory of her husband, pioneer allergist Stephen Daniel Lockey, M.D., 1904–1985.

Contributors

K. FRANK AUSTEN, M.D.
Theodore B. Bayles Professor of Medicine, Harvard Medical School, Boston, Massachusetts; Chairman, Department of Rheumatology and Immunology, Brigham and Women's Hospital, Boston, Massachusetts
The Biology of the Mast Cell

FRITZ H. BACH, M.D.
Harry Kay Chair Professor of Immunobiology, Departments of Laboratory Medicine/Pathology and Surgery, and Director, Immunobiology Research Center, University of Minnesota Medical School, Minneapolis, Minnesota
HLA: The Major Histocompatibility Complex in Man

REBECCA H. BUCKLEY, M.D.
J. Buren Sidbury Professor of Pediatrics and Professor of Immunology, Duke University School of Medicine, Durham, North Carolina; Chief, Division of Allergy and Immunology, Department of Pediatrics, Duke University Medical Center, Durham, North Carolina
Primary and Acquired Immunodeficiency Diseases

JOSEPH H. BUTTERFIELD, M.D.
Assistant Professor of Internal Medicine, Mayo Medical School, Rochester, Minnesota; Consultant, Division of Allergic Diseases and Internal Medicine, Mayo Clinic and Mayo Foundation, Rochester, Minnesota
Eosinophilia

HENRY N. CLAMAN, M.D.
Professor of Medicine and Microbiology/Immunology, University of Colorado School of Medicine, Denver, Colorado
The Biology of the Immune Response

PETER DENSEN, M.D.
Associate Professor of Medicine, University of Iowa School of Medicine, Iowa City, Iowa; Attending Physician, University of Iowa Hospitals and Clinics, and Veterans Administration Medical Center, Iowa City, Iowa
Phagocytosis

DAVID W. FISHER
Editorial Director, *Hospital Practice*, New York, New York
The Biology of the Mast Cell

MICHAEL M. FRANK, M.D.
Clinical Director, National Institute of Allergy and Infectious Diseases, Bethesda, Maryland
The Complement System

RAMA GANGULY, Ph.D.
Associate Professor, University of South Florida College of Medicine, Tampa, Florida; Department of Internal Medicine, James A. Haley Veterans Hospital, Tampa, Florida
Active and Passive Immunization

GERALD J. GLEICH, M.D.
Professor of Immunology and Internal Medicine, Mayo Medical School, Rochester, Minnesota; Chairman, Department of Immunology, Mayo Clinic and Mayo Foundation, Rochester, Minnesota
Eosinophilia

ROBERT A. GOOD, M.D., Ph.D.
Professor and Chairman, Department of Pediatrics, University of South Florida College of Medicine, St. Petersburg, Florida; Physician-in-Chief, All Children's Hospital, St. Petersburg, Florida
Bone Marrow Transplantation

MICHAEL H. GRIECO, M.D., J.D.

Professor of Clinical Medicine, College of Physicians and Surgeons, Columbia University, New York, New York; Chief, Division of Allergy, Clinical Immunology and Infectious Diseases, St. Luke's/Roosevelt Hospital Center, New York, New York
Hypersensitivity in Infectious Diseases

JOHN W. HADDEN, M.D.

Professor of Medicine, Medical Microbiology and Immunology, and Director, Program of Immunopharmacology, University of South Florida College of Medicine, Tampa, Florida
Immunopharmacology: Immunosuppression and Immunopotentiation

KIMISHIGE ISHIZAKA, M.D., Ph.D.

O'Neill Professor of Immunology and Medicine, and Director of the Subdepartment of Immunology, The Johns Hopkins University School of Medicine, Baltimore, Maryland
Mechanisms Involved in the Regulation of IgE Synthesis

MICHAEL A. KALINER, M.D.

Head, Allergic Diseases Section, National Institutes of Allergy and Infectious Diseases, Bethesda, Maryland
Anaphylaxis

CHARLES H. KIRKPATRICK, M.D.

Professor of Medicine and Co-Director, Division of Allergy and Clinical Immunology, University of Colorado School of Medicine, Denver, Colorado; Director, Division of Allergy & Clinical Immunology, National Jewish Center for Immunology & Respiratory Medicine, Denver, Colorado
Mechanisms of Allergic Injury

FRANCISCO G. LA ROSA, M.D.

Instructor, Department of Microbiology and Immunology, University of Colorado School of Medicine, Denver, Colorado
Transplantation Immunity

MANUEL LOPEZ, M.D.
Associate Professor of Medicine, Tulane Medical School, New Orleans, Louisiana; Director, Clinical Immunology Laboratories, and Attending Physician, Tulane Medical Center Hospital, New Orleans, Louisiana
Climate, Weather, Air Pollution, and Environmental Control

GERALD L. MANDELL, M.D.
Professor of Medicine, Head of Division of Infectious Diseases, and Owen R. Cheathem Professor of the Sciences, University of Virginia School of Medicine, Charlottesville, Virginia; Physician, University of Virginia Medical Center Hospital, Charlottesville, Virginia
Phagocytosis

LYNNE KESKINER MERRIAM, R.N., M.S.M.S.
Instructor, St. Petersburg Junior College, St. Petersburg, Florida; Teacher, Countryside High School, Clearwater, Florida
Immunopharmacology: Immunosuppression and Immunopotentiation

RALPH A. REISFELD, Ph.D.
Head, Laboratory of Tumor Cell Biology, Scripps Clinic and Research Foundation, La Jolla, California
Tumor Antigens

DAVID T. ROWLANDS, Jr., M.D.
Professor and Chairman, Department of Pathology and Laboratory Medicine, University of South Florida, College of Medicine, Tampa, Florida
Diagnostic Tests for Assessment of Immunity

JOHN E. SALVAGGIO, M.D.
Henderson Professor and Chairman, Department of Medicine, Tulane Medical School, New Orleans, Louisiana; Attending Physician, Tulane Medical Center Hospital, New Orleans, Louisiana
Climate, Weather, Air Pollution, and Environmental Control

MAX SAMTER, M.D.
Professor of Medicine Emeritus, University of Illinois College of Medicine at Chicago, Chicago, Illinois; Senior Consultant, Max Samter Institute of Allergy and Clinical Immunology, Grant Hospital of Chicago, Chicago, Illinois
Historical Notes

DAVID W. TALMAGE, M.D.
Professor of Microbiology and Immunology, University of Colorado School of Medicine, Denver, Colorado
Transplantation Immunity

ROBERT H. WALDMAN, M.D.
Dean, College of Medicine, and Professor, Department of Internal Medicine, University of Nebraska Medical Center, Omaha, Nebraska
Active and Passive Immunization

WILLIAM O. WEIGLE, Ph.D.
Head, Division of Cellular Immunology, and Member and Chairman, Department of Immunology, Scripps Clinic and Research Foundation, La Jolla, California
Immunologic Tolerance

Preface

The remarkable increase in knowledge of the allergic and immunologic processes results from many ingenious biologic investigations. These have unraveled the cellular and molecular events responsible for the exquisitely sensitive and specific two-system process resulting in immunity. The practical application of the knowledge of basic immunity to clinical medicine has been described in the companion volume, *Principles of Immunology and Allergy*. Presentation of the fundamental biologic basis for these acquired clinical skills has been the task of this volume, *Fundamentals of Immunology and Allergy*. The scientific contributions are themselves intriguing to review, and the contributors to this volume are exceptionally qualified to describe them by virtue of their laboratory expertise and broad clinical experience. Their subjects have been lucidly, concisely, and readably presented for comprehension of fundamental immunologic processes. It is thus possible to understand the development of diagnostic and therapeutic capabilities to deal with natural and induced disease states resulting from an incompetent or abnormal immune process, or both.

Each chapter is written with style and content suitable for medical students, house officers, and primary care physicians, as well as for the specialty-oriented student, to serve as a guide to more intensive study of all scientific aspects of immunology and allergy.

Our editing task was greatly eased by the broad knowledge and communication skills of the contributing authors and by the planning and editing of the W. B. Saunders staff. We are, indeed, grateful to all of them. We also are indebted to many other individuals for their assistance in completing these books, especially our wives and families, who excused us for the time needed to complete this task. We are particularly grateful to Mrs. Deborah Serbousek, who assisted us with editing manuscripts, obtaining permission slips, corresponding with authors, and carrying out other activities.

RICHARD F. LOCKEY, M.D.
SAMUEL C. BUKANTZ, M.D.
Editors

Contents

1

Historical Notes

MAX SAMTER, M.D.,
and SAMUEL C. BUKANTZ, M.D.

The "historical notes" that introduce this text reflect a
dialogue that began more than 30 years ago. At that time, Robert
C. Cooke felt that clinical allergy was standing on safe and
reproducible foundations, while Harry L. Alexander, Cooke's
contemporary, felt that we were just at the beginning.

During the recent past, the major associations of allergists—
national and international—have changed their label; they have
become, almost worldwide, societies of allergy *and* immunology.
The urge to add immunology is understandable, but the sequence
is misleading, since immunology has existed longer than allergy.
The German Journal of Immunology—die "Zeitschrift für Im-
munitätsforschung"—was founded during the last quarter of the
last century. We tried to trace the origin of the term, but were
not successful. It is an inspired term: "Immunis" is the Latin
word applied to the senators in Rome who were exempt from
paying taxes. To be immune, then, is to be exempt from disease.
The introduction and ready acceptance of the term reflects the
fact that the immunologic system was generally considered to be
a system of protection.

Classic immunologists must have been shocked when Portier
and Richet demonstrated in casual, but careful, experiments, in
1902, that the injection of foreign proteins might not, as expected,
induce protection, but instead might predispose the injected
animals to severe, occasionally fatal reactions (anaphylaxis).

1

The term "allergy" was introduced by von Pirquet in 1906. It is interesting to analyze von Pirquet's reasoning. He introduced the term "allergy" to describe altered reactivity that protects as well as altered reactivity that causes clinical symptoms. Protection equals immunity—achieved by "alexins" (natural immunity), by antitoxins (as in diphtheria and tetanus), and by adaptation to poison. Strangely enough, he attributed the altered reactivity caused by "allergens" (in other words, what we call "allergy" [or "atopy"] today) to the absence of antibodies. Since "reagins"—the antibodies that mediate "atopy"—had not been identified, von Pirquet's predicament is understandable, but he firmly established the concept of altered reactivity—diminished or heightened—in medical terminology.

The early development of immunology is distinguished by significant observations for which rational explanations were not available. Bordet discovered complement in 1894. He observed that specific "immune serum" that was incubated with a culture of cholera bacilli killed the bacilli effectively but lost its bactericidal activity after it had been heated. The bactericidal power could be restored by adding one drop of normal guinea pig serum. Bordet reasoned that the heating had destroyed a substance that he called "alexin"—present in normal serum—and that alexin, i.e., normal serum, added to the heated culture, restored its bactericidal effect. Portier and Richet, Theobald Smith (who observed anaphylactic shock in guinea pigs, but never published his findings), Sir Henry Dale (who described "H-substance," the mediator of anaphylaxis, before histamine was identified), and Prausnitz and Küstner (who showed that specific sensitivities could be transferred from one human to another by the transfer of serum) all made significant observations even though they could only speculate about the physiologic meaning of what they had observed. Yet it is fair to say that even in the absence of immediate or eventual proof, the philosophers of immunology have shaped the long-term growth of the discipline. The ability to distinguish "self" from "non-self" was recognized as the primary instrument for the preservation of the species. In 1959, Burnet published "The Clonal Selection Theory of Acquired Immunity." During the same year, Lewis Thomas, in a discussion of Peter Medawar's paper on the mechanism of homograft rejection, stressed the need of the body to maintain uniform cell types—to reject mutations in order to defeat malignancies. Thomas extended his remarks to the miracle of pregnancy—i.e., how does the mother prevent the rejection of the fetus?—a miracle that is still unexplained.

Meanwhile, immunology concentrated its efforts on unraveling the cellular mechanics for such a multipurpose system of defense.

Scientific progress is slow. Eosinophils were discovered in 1878, but we are still uncertain as to their function: i.e., whether they are modulating controls of excessive edema in anaphylaxis or killer cells that are attracted to parasites by antibody-carrying mast cells, or perhaps a combination of both plus something else.

The mast cell was discovered by Ehrlich in 1878. It took 57 years before it was established that mast cell granules contain heparin; another 10 years before Riley and West found histamine in human mast cells; and yet another 10 years before Benditt demonstrated that the mast cells of rats contain serotonin. Only the discovery that early "reagins"—thought to be mediators of atopic disease—were found to be IgE made it possible to identify specific receptors for the Fc fraction of IgE in the walls of mast cells and basophils.

It is difficult to believe that fifty years ago it was not known that lymphocytes are antibody producers. Yet, their acceptance was delayed by fascinating detours. In the late 1950s, Gowans drained the thoracic duct of rats until lymphocytes could no longer be detected. Reexamined after an interval, lymphocytes had returned, but, Gowans noted, those that had reappeared were uniformly small. Gowans felt that there might be two classes of lymphocytes, large and small, but his colleagues laughed: Small lymphocytes, they reasoned, were young lymphocytes and would grow up. Gowans, of course, was right.

Once it became apparent that lymphocytes—derived in humans from a stem cell in the bone marrow (not, as in birds, from the bursa of Fabricius)—are transformed by the nonpassage or passage through the thymus, the fate and function of lymphocytes became the area of major impact in allergy: Allergy became transformed from an in vivo endeavor to an in vitro science. With this breakthrough, the patient became the source for experimental cells, and teams of investigators rather than individual observers controlled conclusions.

It is probably fair to say that the current era of immunology began with our skill in placing unmistakable labels on cells and cell-related products that participate in immunologic reactions. Radioactive isotopes initiated this era, with Coons and Kaplan encouraging in vitro identification by fluorescent labels; and our startling technical ability to separate cells and components of cells, serum and secretions has given rise to the spectacular development of laboratories that identify and count B lymphocytes and T lymphocytes, "null cells," "natural killer cells," as well as "innocent bystanders" that might have been trapped by immunologic events. Kohler and Milstein's inspired creation of a hybridoma that transformed short-lived B lymphocytes into an immortal source of monoclonal antibodies has been the major recent addition to the armamentarium of immunology.

"Progress" is a difficult term. None of us would care to practice without access to the glucocorticosteroids, which were discovered as the result of one man's perception. During the late 1930s, Philip S. Hench observed that rheumatic diseases showed a spectacular improvement in patients who had jaundice, and in pregnant women. He reasoned that these two conditions must have biochemical changes in common and encouraged Edward C. Kendall to isolate and synthesize adrenal hormones. Compound E became available in September, 1948. Yet, it is conceivable that our understanding of immunologic controls would have grown more rapidly had glucocorticosteroids not made it possible for us to treat immunologic diseases without particular attention to underlying causes. The excitement of new discoveries often exaggerates their significance. This was true for histamine—once considered *the* chemical mediator of allergy—but it is also true for Sutherland's second messenger, cyclic AMP, which leaves us with unanswered questions. It might also apply to the derivatives of arachidonic acid, which are still under intense investigation.

What does the future hold? The joys of the laboratory are real, but not without risk. In "atopy"—the peculiar term adopted by Cooke and Coca for the inherited trait to form "reagins" after exposure to "allergens"—the patient's history is often a better guide to the diagnosis and, even more so, to the prognosis of the disease than are skin tests, RIST (radioimmunosorbent test), or RAST (radioallergosorbent test). Hereditary angioedema was first described by Osler in 1888, but it was not until 1963 that Donaldson and Evans demonstrated the absence of the inhibitor of the activated first component of complement in patients with this disorder. Even now, we do not know how children manage to survive in spite of this genetic defect, or why attenuated androgens like danazol are able to restore normal levels of $C\overline{1}$ INH and C4. Most spectacularly, bronchial asthma—a condition that was known and dreaded for centuries—has during the past generation become controllable. Unlike Marcel Proust and Theodore Roosevelt, most asthmatic patients today can be medically managed to live normal lives, in spite of the fact that we still do not know what bronchial asthma is.

To end with a prediction: The recognition of the "network" that operates the immunologic system has been one of the most provocative examples of the need for integration of basic sciences into clinical medicine. Its meaning for the development and course of immunologic behavior and disease will most likely be established by the clinicians of immunology.

Bibliography

Samter, M. (ed.): Excerpts from Classics in Allergy. Edited for the 25th anniversary committee on the American Academy of Allergy. Columbus, OH, Ross Laboratories, 1969, pp. 1–117.

2

The Biology of the Immune Response

HENRY N. CLAMAN, M.D.

THE IMMUNE SYSTEM AS A WHOLE—SPECIFIC AND NONSPECIFIC

The immune system is a large and complex series of elements widely distributed throughout the body. It has many functions, including protection against pathogens and reactions against foreign substances while not reacting against self components. The immune system, as one of its primary abilities, accomplishes the distinction between self and non-self through an elaborate *specific recognition system* inherent in T and B lymphocytes. The immune system also contains *nonspecific effector systems,* which include the complement system and cells such as mononuclear phagocytes and polymorphonuclear leukocytes (PMN), which are often part of inflammatory responses.

The immune system has a number of interesting properties. These include:

Specificity. The immune system will respond to antigen A without responding to antigen B (if the antigens do not cross-react immunologically). The specificity of immune reactions is mediated by specific receptors on the surfaces of lymphocytes and on immunoglobulin molecules.

Memory. The immune response to antigen A leaves the immune system changed; the system is usually "primed" so that a second exposure to antigen A results in a faster, more efficient, and more powerful response, i.e., the anamnestic response, which is the basis for booster immunizations. In more sophisticated terms, the phenomenon would be called an instance of "positive" immunologic memory. The converse of this is "negative" immunologic memory, in which exposure to antigen A prepares the immune system so that a second exposure to antigen A gives *no* response. This is an example of acquired immunologic tolerance, or unresponsiveness (see Chapter 7).

Specificity and memory are such important characteristics of immune processes that they are often used as criteria for identification of a clinical reaction as an immunologic one. For example, the adverse reactions to aspirin experienced by certain asthmatics are considered to be nonimmunologic, at least in part, because they exhibit neither specificity nor memory (see Chapter 3 in *Principles of Immunology and Allergy*).

Mobility. The elements of the immune system can travel around the body. For instance, sensitization via the respiratory mucosa can lead to sensitization of the entire body. This is true of lymphocytes and immunoglobulins, but it is not true, for example, for the musculoskeletal system.

Replicability. The cellular elements of the immune system, lymphocytes, frequently replicate when activated. They may replicate many times, perhaps indefinitely. Replicability is not a feature of cells in other systems, such as the central nervous system. The normal replicability of lymphocytes requires regulatory control mechanisms, the absence of which can lead to lymphoid malignancy.

Cooperation. This is not a unique property of the immune system, but it is an essential one. The specific cellular elements (lymphocytes), the specific humoral elements (antibodies), and the nonspecific cells and molecules of the immune system do not work effectively in isolation. There is constant interaction among lymphoid cells, immunoglobulins, non-lymphoid cells, and cytokines (soluble cellular secretory products).

Lymphocytes—Specific Immunologic Elements

The basis of immunologic specificity resides in the interaction with antigens of a series of specific receptors on the surfaces of both thymus-derived (T) and bone marrow–derived (B) lymphocytes. These are called antigen-specific receptors, or *idiotopes*.

The Clonal Selection Theory. This theory was independently set forth in 1957 by Nobel laureate Sir MacFarlane Burnet of Australia and David W. Talmage of the United States as a revolutionary (and evolutionary) hypothesis to explain immunologic specificity and memory (both positive and negative). The theory was based on the ability of lymphocytes to make antibodies, as the distinction between T and B lymphocytes had not yet been recognized. A major tenet of the clonal selection theory was that there existed a small number of identical lymphoid cells (a "clone") that could respond to a limited number of antigens (that number probably being 1) by producing the corresponding antibody (or antibodies). The lymphoid system, then, was considered to be composed of a large number of sets or clones of cells, each clone restricted to a specific antigen. The antigen *selected* the appropriate clone of cells (hence, the phrase, clonal *selection*), and the cells from other clones were unaffected. This was an unexpected view of the immune system, but a second major tenet was even more surprising, i.e., that each clone of cells was *predetermined* to respond to its own distinctive antigen *before* the antigen was introduced, and that the clonal individuality was genetically inherent in each cell of the clone. This feature of the theory was slow to gain acceptance. The recognition that B lymphocytes able to secrete specific antibodies carried the same specific antibody on their surfaces made it easy to accept that immunoglobulin surface receptors could serve as specific recognition receptors for antigen. The phenotypic expression of the clonal selection theory, at least for B cells, was clearly surface immunoglobulin. This molecule was both the antigen recognition unit for that particular clone and a sample of the immunologically specific protein (antibody) destined to be produced by that clone, when activated. Identification of clonal specificity as also inherent in the T-cell system created a problem concerning the structure (or structures) of the T-cell receptor for antigen, because conventional immunoglobulin was not demonstrable on the T-cell surface. Either the T cell used an "immunoglobulin-like" molecule for its specific antigen receptor, or there was another immunologic library of specificities, entirely different from immunoglobulins! This controversy, which had been going on for almost two decades, has now been resolved, and the answer resembles most closely the first possibility.

The clonal selection theory provided some interesting concepts. The absence of immunologic reactivity to self could be explained by the absence of autoreactive clones of cells. The development of autoimmunity could result from mutant clones able to recognize self-antigens as foreign. The development of acquired immunologic unresponsiveness (tolerance) to a specific antigen, e.g., antigen A, could be explained by the elimination of the particular clones reacting to that antigen.

Two Theories for the Origin of Diversity. A question that remained until recently was how an individual came to be equipped with, perhaps, 10^6 clones of lymphocytes, each committed to a different antigen. The first theory conceived of a *germ line* that contained all the DNA sequences for all the specific antigen-combining receptors for all the clones of specific T and B cells. During proliferation and differentiation to the mature lymphoid system, genetic material to make one antigen receptor was randomly distributed to each lymphocyte descendant of the original lymphoid precursor. A second theory explained diversity as arising from a few primordial germ line genes by *somatic mutation* occurring during lymphoid development. The final explanation (sometimes called the Generation Of Diversity,

G.O.D.) appears to contain aspects of both theories—germ line and somatic mutation (see the section on B-Cell Biology, p. 30).

Nonspecific Aspects of the Immune System

Lymphocytes, via their antigen receptors, are the unique bearers of immunologic specificity, but they and their products are critically dependent upon other cellular and humoral elements in order to express full immunologic ability. These additional elements, listed below, should be considered as *amplifiers* and *effectors* for the immune system.

Antigen-Presenting Cells. Many lymphoid cells will be activated, even by their "own" antigen, only if that antigen is presented via "the proper diplomatic channels." These antigen-presenting cells are generally considered to be non-lymphoid, not clonally selected, and to be derived from the mononuclear phagocyte system.

Polymorphonuclear Leukocytes (PMNs) and Mast Cells. Many immunologic reactions, triggered by immunologically-specific antigens, lymphocytes, and antibodies, also involved PMNs for amplification and effectiveness. Immediate (Type I) hypersensitivities, involving IgE, are mediated by basophil and mast cell activation (Chapters 10, 11, and 12). Opsonization of bacteria by immunoglobulin and the inflammation produced by deposition of antigen-antibody complexes require neutrophils (Chapters 4 and 10).

Complement. Activation of the classic complement pathway by a small number of IgM or IgG antibodies and antigen promotes a cascade of reactions ultimately involving a large number of complement components responsible for chemotaxis, phagocytosis, and liberation of mediators of inflammation (Chapter 3).

Phagocytic Cells. Immunologic activation of T cells or production of IgM and IgG promotes activation of phagocytic cells of the PMN and mononuclear phagocyte systems. These phagocytic cells are the ultimate effectors of some forms of antimicrobial and, perhaps, antitumor activity (Chapter 4).

Some Immunologic Definitions

The study of immunology is replete with terms, some of which are ambiguous.

Antigen—a substance capable of interacting specifically with an antigen receptor on the appropriate T or B lymphocyte or secreted antibody. The binding of an antigen to such a receptor occurs because the antigen "shape" fits the receptor ("lock and key"), and the binding may be of high or low affinity. The binding of an antigen may or may not lead to further events, i.e., cell triggering or immune complex lattice formation.

Immunogen—an antigen capable of inducing an immunologic response in vivo or in vitro. Immunogens are generally complex antigens such as proteins, complex polysaccharides, or haptens complexed to carriers.

Hapten—a low-molecular-weight, "simple" antigen, such as a drug (e.g., penicillin). Classically, haptens will bind to specific anti-hapten cells or antibodies, but they are considered "incomplete antigens" (i.e., not immunogens) unless complexed to a carrier molecule (usually a protein).

Tolerogen—the inverse of immunogen. Tolerogens are antigens that, because of the way they are "presented" to the immune system, do not induce a positive immune response, but instead alter the system so that it will not respond to that specific antigen when given later. Tolerogens may work in various ways, e.g., by blocking immunocompetent cells or by inducing suppressive mechanisms (Chapter 7).

LYMPHOID ORGANS AND TISSUES

Lymphatic channels exist in all tissues of the body, except for the central nervous system and cornea. The CNS, however, has a rich blood supply, so lymphocytes are constantly traversing it.

For purposes of discussing ontogeny, the lymphoid organs are divided into *primary* and *secondary* (or *central* and *peripheral*) organs.

Primary Lymphoid Organs—Thymus and Bone Marrow

Thymus. This is one of the two primary lymphoid organs. Peripheral immunocompetent T lymphocytes develop in the thymus, and the absence or developmental defects of the thymus lead to severe immunodeficiency states, such as the DiGeorge syndrome (Chapter 6).

Development. The thymus develops from endodermal tissue of the third and fourth pharyngeal pouches. This tissue supplies the thymic epithelial cells, which are macrophage-like cells and are essential for the proper development of T lymphocytes and their MHC (major histocompatibility complex) restriction (see Chapter 5 and section on T-cell activation, later in this chapter). Small numbers of lymphoid cell precursors (stem cells) arise from the yolk sac, fetal liver, and bone marrow and colonize the thymus. This colonization begins early in embryonic life so that, by birth, the individual is equipped with a fully formed (but small) thymus, including cortex and medulla.

Traffic Within the Thymus. The "stem cells" are small, immunologically incompetent, basophilic-staining cells carried by the bloodstream into the outer cortex of the thymus, where they divide rapidly and populate the cortex with still immature thymocytes. The cells move toward the thymic medulla as they divide, gradually develop more mature attributes, and slow their division rate.

Lymphocyte division is far less rapid in the thymic medulla, and medullary cells have more of the characteristics of mature peripheral T lymphocytes. There is not complete agreement about the pathways of thymocyte development or migration; a general consensus is that thymic cortical cells divide rapidly and have surface markers such as receptors for OKT3, OKT6 and OKT10 monoclonal antibodies (in man) and TL (thymus-leukemia) and Thy-1 antigens in the mouse. Most thymocytes born in the cortex die in the cortex, thus accounting for the high rate of cell division there. Surviving thymocytes move toward the medulla, at the same time losing some immature cell markers and gaining increased density of some MHC antigens. Not yet agreed upon is whether an important route of exit of cortical thymocytes to the peripheral lymphoid tissue can bypass the thymic medulla. A number of cortical cells do reach the medulla, where they behave as mature immunocompetent T lymphocytes and then migrate to the periphery.

Thymic Inflow and Outflow. The rate of inflow of stem cells into the thymus is not well understood, but it is known to be low, even in fetal life. Thymic inflow *may* continue into maturity, in which case thymic function requires an input from stem cells throughout life.

The bulk of cells born in the thymus also die in the thymus. (It is not known whether the dying ones are defective, or autoreactive.) About 1 percent of thymocytes migrate to the periphery daily in the young mouse, and this rate slows to 0.1 percent in older mice. There are no comparable data in man, but contrary to popular belief, the human thymus does not disappear after puberty. Aging is accompanied by fatty infiltration and loss of cortical mass, so that, in older humans, the corticomedullary ratio is diminished, but thymocytes are still present and active in the aged thymus.

Immunocompetence of Thymic Cells. The thymus might be considered as the "training camp" for the big leagues in the lymphoid periphery, so it is not surprising that thymocytes themselves are not potent in T-cell effector functions (e.g., T-cell "help," cytotoxicity, graft rejection) on a cell-for-cell basis. Suspensions of thymus cells are not immunologically inert, however, and they can carry out these functions, probably because of the population of mature thymus medullary cells in every thymocyte suspension.

Bone Marrow and Bursa of Fabricius. Precursors of B lymphocytes develop in young fowl in a lymphoid organ at the lower end of the gastrointestinal tract known as the bursa of Fabricius. Animals surgically or hormonally bursectomized very early in development lack mature B cells and are severely deficient in antibody-producing capabilities but can make normal cell-mediated immune responses. Such experiments provided some of the earliest and clearest evidence for the anatomic and functional separation of the "2 universes of immune response" (i.e., T-cell and B-cell activities).

There is no bursa of Fabricius in mammals. It is now agreed that the development of B-cell precursors occurs in the yolk sac and fetal liver in the mammalian embryo and in the bone marrow in postnatal life. Thus, the earliest development of B cell precursors takes place in the same organs that develop pre-thymic T-cell precursors. There is probably a common lymphoid stem cell that is a precursor for pre-T cells as well as for pre-B cells. A descendant of this common lymphoid stem cell once committed to one of the two pathways (e.g., to the pre-T cell lineage) cannot develop along the other (e.g., B-cell) pathway. These stem cells and their developmental pathways have not been precisely identified, and this schema is based mainly on studies of clinical immunodeficiency, rare cases of which (e.g., severe combined immunodeficiency, SCID) are best explained by absence of a stem cell precursor for both T- and B-cell development (Chapter 6).

Little is known about the organization of B-cell precursors

in the bone marrow, which is not only a *primary* hematopoietic organ for B lymphocytes after birth but also the primary hematopoietic organ for erythrocyte, granulocyte, monocyte, and megakaryocyte production. It is also a very important peripheral or *secondary* lymphoid organ containing many mature post-thymic T effector cells that can be responsible for graft-vs.-host reactions following bone marrow transplantation. Bone marrow also contains many mature B cells, which may be a major source of antibody production in mature individuals.

Secondary Lymphoid Tissue

Mature lymphocytes reside in "peripheral" lymphoid tissues in which immunologic responses follow antigenic stimulation. All peripheral tissues include both B and T lymphocytes, in different proportions.

		Approximate Percentage of Lymphocytes	
		T	*B*
Primary	Thymus	100	0
	Bone marrow	10	90
Secondary	Spleen	45	55
	Lymph nodes	60	40
	Blood	80	20
	Thoracic duct	95	5
	Other lymphoid systems	Variable	Variable

Other subdivisions of the peripheral lymphoid tissue (GALT, BALT, SALT) are organized around anatomic locations and are discussed below.

Spleen. The spleen, which is a lymphoid filter within the blood-vascular system, is important as a major site of antibody response to circulating particulate antigens such as bacteria. Individuals who have been splenectomized are therefore at increased risk for septicemia. The spleen is also a major phagocytic effector organ and is the primary site for clearance of bacteria, parasites, or autologous hematopoietic cells (RBCs, platelets, etc.) if opsonized with antibody and/or complement.

Lymph Nodes. These can be considered as lymphoid filters within the lymphatic drainage system. T cells primarily occupy the deep cortex, and B cells (with some T cells) are rich in germinal follicles in the cortex. Lymph nodes are potent sites for both T-cell functions and antibody production, responding particularly to antigens introduced into distal tissues and brought to them via afferent lymphatics. Lymph nodes throughout the body have a rich blood supply and will participate in responses to blood-borne antigenic stimulants (e.g., the generalized lymphadenopathy seen in serum sickness or secondary syphilis).

Thoracic Duct. Not usually considered as a lymphoid organ, the thoracic duct contains a large number of mature T cells (and few B cells). Thoracic duct drainage has been used as a means of depleting systemic T cells.

Other Lymphoid Systems (GALT, BALT, SALT). Recently, some regional subdivisions of the immune system have been identified and given acronyms. These are immune networks based in the gastrointestinal tract (GALT), the lungs (BALT), and the skin (SALT). These are not precise entities, but such conceptual arrangements focus attention on special aspects of the immune system, particularly in the gut, the lungs, and the skin, which are the three primary interfaces between the body and the foreign antigens "outside."

Gut-Associated Lymphoid Tissue (GALT). GALT is an acronym used to describe the lymphoid accumulations primarily in the intestines and liver. These are not only anatomically somewhat segregated, but there are also many other special features associated with GALT. The GALT B cell system is greatly devoted to IgA production and secretion. Pre-B cells arise in Peyer's patches; many enter the general circulation and "home" preferentially back to the GALT, particularly to the loose lymphoid tissue of the submucosa and, to a lesser extent, to the liver. Antigen introduction into the GI tract of an animal or man may tolerize, rather than immunize, although this whole concept is still under investigation.

Bronchus-Associated Lymphoid Tissue (BALT). This embraces lymphoid tissues of the lower respiratory tract, including hilar lymph nodes and the respiratory mucosal lymphoid cells. It, too, is a secretory system predominantly for IgA.

Skin-Associated Lymphoid Tissue (SALT). This is the newest and least studied entry into the lymphoid acronym sweepstakes. It includes the non-lymphoid Langerhans cells of the epidermis (which are Ia-positive antigen-presenting cells) and lymphoid tissue draining the skin.

Blood. The blood is a complex immunologic organ in which specific cells may be present only briefly, as they travel via the circulation from one tissue to another. The total composition of the immunologic elements of the blood is nevertheless reasonably constant. The blood also contains the lymphoid population in man that is sampled and analyzed far more frequently than any other population (e.g., lymph node). The lymphoid elements in the blood are generally assumed to be in equilibrium with, if not identical to, the tissue lymphoid elements, and therefore to be an accurate reflection of what is going on in the tissues. This assumption is understandable but remains to be proved; for example, in sarcoidosis, the T-cell subpopulations of the blood have been found to be the *inverse* of those in the affected lung. Thus, more work is needed in this area.

The impressive immunologic capabilities of blood itself are manifest in the following two examples: (a) blood-borne antigens can induce apparent immunologic tolerance in prospective kidney graft recipients, and (b) blood-borne T lymphocytes can induce fatal graft-vs.-host reactions.

Circulation of Lymphocytes

Lymphocytes comprise mobile sets of cells. T cells mature in the thymus and a small fraction of them "seed" the peripheral tissues. The bulk of peripheral T cells are long-lived, and may survive—without dividing—for years! Many of the peripheral T cells belong to the pool of "long-lived recirculating T lymphocytes." They move from the blood to the lymph nodes, spleen, and other lymphoid tissues, including the bone marrow. Blood-borne T cells leave the bloodstream to enter lymph nodes by adhering to specialized venular endothelial cells in veins within the body of the lymph node and then squeeze themselves across the venule wall to enter the lymph node. They return to the circulation by way of the efferent lymphatics and by thoracic and other similar ducts. Lymphocytes also enter lymph nodes via afferent lymphatics. Lymphocytes that enter the spleen and marrow exit via the blood. There are some special features of lymphocyte circulation. The thymus is not a significant part of the recirculation pathway of T cells, which, after leaving the thymus, do not return, with the possible exception of a few cells that may reach the thymic medulla. (As the thymus contains very few B lymphocytes, it is clearly also not in the recirculation pathway of B cells). There are specialized pathways of lymphocyte circulation in the GALT, as mentioned above. Less is known about B-cell circulation and, indeed, about B-cell lifespan. Many B lymphocytes do not live as long as T cells, although there are memory cells of the B lineage.

The fact that T cells wander throughout the body has been used by the proponents of the immunologic surveillance theory of cancer to represent T cells as "patrols" of immunocompetent cells seeking out and destroying newly arisen malignancies. In a less colorful metaphor, it is obvious that the meeting of T cells and their specific antigen in one area of the body can lead to systemic T-cell memory. In practice, one sees that individuals acquiring contact sensitivity in one area of the skin are also able to have contact sensitivity elicited at *any* skin site because of the mobility of the T effector cells involved. A consequence of the mobility of the B cells is that one of the largest reservoirs for plasma cell concentration and antibody production is in the bone marrow; the B-cell antibody producers obviously were activated elsewhere and migrated to the bone marrow.

IMMUNOGLOBULIN STRUCTURE AND FUNCTION

A review of the structure and function of immunoglobulin classes is an important prelude to understanding the biology of the immune response.

Polypeptide Units

All immunoglobulin (Ig) molecules are composed of chains of polypeptides, which are connected to each other by various bonds, and are folded upon themselves. They have attached carbohydrate moieties that do not directly contribute to antibody specificity.

Heavy and light chains are the basic building units of Ig's. IgG is composed of two identical heavy (H) and two identical light (L) chains, covalently linked, as shown in Figure 2–1. Interchain disulfide bonds are susceptible to proteolytic cleavage with papain and pepsin. The other immunoglobulins are composed of similar units, which will be described below. The Ig molecules have different functions at different ends. The N-terminals of the H and L chains are the *variable* (V) regions because they are composed of chains that vary in composition from one antibody to another. The cavity between the ends of a pair of H and L chains is the antigen-combining site whose

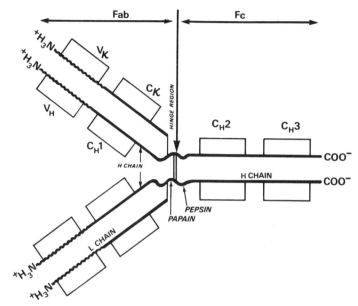

Figure 2–1. A simplified model for an IgG1(κ) human antibody molecule, showing the 4-chain basic structure and domains. V indicates variable region; C, the constant region; and the vertical arrow, the hinge region. Thick lines represent H and L chains; thin lines represent disulfide bonds. (From Goodman, J. W.: Immunoglobulins I: structure and function. *In* Stites, D. P., Stobo, J. D., Fudenberg, H. H., et al. (eds.): Basic and Clinical Immunology, 5th ed. Los Altos, CA, Lange Medical Publications, 1982, p. 30.)

unique shape is determined by the folding of the variable parts of the H and L chain. This end of the molecule is the Fab portion, and it confers immunologic specificity. As the Fab from each antibody Ig is uniquely shaped, these are called *idiotopes*.

The C-terminal end of the heavy chain of the Ig molecule is of *constant* structure for each Ig class and subclass, and confers upon the molecule various biologic functions; for example, the unique ability of IgG to pass the placenta depends on the structure of the constant end (Fc portion) of the IgG molecule.

Each H and L chain is a polypeptide sequence made from the transcription of a number of gene segments for constant and variable regions via a complex system of *gene splicing.*

Classes and Subclasses of Immunoglobulins. The constant regions of Ig's have similarities and differences. Light chains are either kappa (κ) or lambda (λ), but, in a given molecule, all the light (L) chains are identical. Heavy chains are divided into classes or *isotypes,* namely γ chains, α chains, μ chains, δ chains and ε chains for IgG, IgA, IgM, IgD, and IgE respectively. Thus, it is the constant portions of the Ig molecules that confer biologic differences on different Ig isotypes.

Immunoglobulin G (IgG)

This is the predominant Ig in the serum. IgG is a major antibacterial and antiviral Ig molecule and a potent opsonizer and toxin neutralizer. It is the only Ig molecule to cross the placenta and provides passive immunity for the newborn for the first 3 to 6 months of life. It is one of the two Ig classes that fixes complement by the classical pathway.

There are four subclasses—IgG1, IgG2, IgG3, and IgG4—which vary chemically because of small differences in the γ chains. Some differences in biologic function have been noted in these subclasses (Table 2–1). IgG2 antibodies are often opsonic and also develop in response to antitoxins and dextrans. Anti-Rh antibodies are often of the IgG1 or IgG3 subclass. There is some evidence that IgG4 antibodies can function as skin-sensitizing antibodies, akin to IgE, but the Fc portion of IgG4 has lower avidity for tissues than does Fc_{ϵ}. Undoubtedly, further research is needed to determine the biologic significance of IgG subclass types.

Immunoglobulin A (IgA)

This class of immunoglobulins has special features that are associated with the mucosal surfaces. IgA is present in the serum

Table 2–1. Human Serum Immunoglobulins

	Mean Serum Concentration (mg/dl)	Complement Fixation	Placental Transfer	Sedimentation Constant	Half-life (days)
IgG_1	900	+ +	+	7s	21
IgG_2	300	+	+	7s	20
IgG_3	100	+ + +	+	7s	7
IgG_4	50	0	+	7s	21
IgM	150	+ + +	0	19s	10
IgA	300	0	0	7s	6
sIgA	5	0	0	11s	
IgD	3	0	0	7s	3
IgE	0.005	0	0	8s	2

as a monomer of two α chains and two light chains. Some serum IgA is polymerized. IgA is the primary Ig of the secretory immunoglobulin system of the GI tract, upper and lower respiratory tracts and genitourinary tract. As such, the immunoglobulin is secreted locally by plasma cells in the lamina propria of the mucosa of these systems. In the gastrointestinal tract and other mucosal surfaces, two IgA molecules are complexed to a special polypeptide chain called secretory piece; the complex is able to resist digestion by proteolytic enzymes. IgA antibodies are believed to be particularly effective in providing antimicrobial protection at mucosal surfaces. In the gut, they are believed by some to prevent absorption of intact proteins, e.g., "immune exclusion."

Immunoglobulin M (IgM)

Serum IgM is a polymer of five units, each composed of two μ chains and two light chains. These are arranged in a pinwheel array with the Fc ends in the center, held together by special J (for joining) chains. IgM has special characteristics. It is the first Ig made in the sequence of B-cell development and is the early antibody secreted into the serum during primary antibody responses. Such antibodies may activate complement by the classic pathway, and this class also contains special antibodies such as cold agglutinins, heterophil antibodies, and isohemagglutinins.

Immunoglobulin D (IgD)

This isotype is composed of two δ chains and two light chains. It is present on immature B cells and is found in serum in low concentrations. As yet, we do not understand the full biologic significance of this particular Ig class.

Immunoglobulin E (IgE)

The classic skin-sensitizing, anaphylactic, or reaginic antibodies belong to this class. IgE molecules have two ε chains and two light chains. The Fc portion of the ε chain can bind to special Fc_ϵ receptors on mast cells and basophils. When such cells, passively sensitized with IgE of a certain antigenic specificity, are cross-linked by their appropriate antigen, the cells degranulate, releasing the pharmacologic mediators of anaphylaxis (see Chapters 11 and 13). IgE is present in the serum and tissues in very small quantities, but, because of its affinity for basophils and mast cells, it is an antibody class with very potent biologic capabilities.

Table 2–1 gives a summary of the immunoglobulins.

T-CELL BIOLOGY

Thymus-derived lymphocytes, or T cells, are pivotal elements of the immune system. They are immunologically specific, can carry immunologic memory, and can function in a variety of *regulatory* and *effector* ways.

Dual Specificity of T Cells

T cells are clonally restricted; that is, each T cell can recognize and respond to only one antigen (or to a closely related—i.e., cross-reactive—antigen). This specificity is deter- mined by the T-cell receptor. This receptor, however, has *dual* specificity. This is a crucial concept first demonstrated by Doherty and Zinkernagel and illustrated in Figure 2–2. Animals immu- nized with virus antigens were known to develop virus-specific cytotoxic T lymphocytes, capable of killing target cells infected with the same virus. The critical experiment showed that cyto-

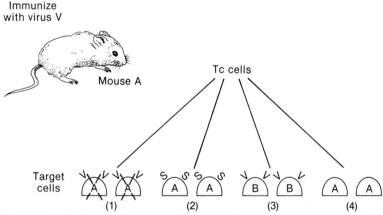

Figure 2–2. The Doherty-Zinkernagel Experiment showing that cytotoxic T cells (Tc) have specificity for antigen *and* self. Tc cells from strain A mouse immunized with virus V are cytotoxic only for target cells that have A genotype and are infected with virus V (1). Such Tc cells will not kill A targets with virus S (2), B targets with virus V (3), or uninfected A targets (4). Thus, the Tc cell recognizes both virus and self-MHC.

toxic T cells (Tc) could recognize and kill virus-infected targets only if those targets shared MHC antigens with the Tc itself. Thus, Tc cells recognize both virus and target MHC—a dual specificity. To put it another way, Tc cells recognize antigen "in the context of self-MHC products." A corollary of this concept is that T cells are triggered by antigens presented on self-membranes (containing MHC), such as a macrophage (see below). A clinical corollary of this concept is that it might be useless to "equip" a T cell–deficient person, A, with T cells from person B (assuming GVH reactions are avoided), as T cells from person B would not be effective in the milieu of person A, who is MHC-nonidentical (see below). This concept also means that T cells will not collaborate with MHC-incompatible B cells.

T-Cell Functions

T cells, which are a functionally heterogeneous collection of cells, are required for, or are involved in, a wide variety of immunologic functions. T-cell sets may interact with each other, one set promoting or inhibiting the function of another set. These networks are complex and incompletely understood; some simplification is attempted by categorizing T cells as either *effector* or *regulator*.

Effector T Cells

Cytotoxic T Cells (Tc). These cells, the most studied and best understood subset of T effector cells, recognize antigens, such as viral products, in the context of self-MHC. They are probably important in allograft destruction (although, in this case, it is difficult to see how the foreign MHC alloantigen can be seen as "self" antigen-presenting cells unless the foreign antigen is first "processed"). Such Tc cells are considered to be important in eliminating the cellular phase of viral infections (as shown experimentally in the Doherty-Zinkernagel experiment), although it appears that the price paid for viral clearance is the death of the virus-infected cell itself. Thus, much of the hepatic necrosis seen in acute hepatitis B infection is probably a result of destruction of hepatocytes bearing viral antigens—destruction that is mediated, at least in part, by Tc cells. Tc cells are cells carrying certain antigenic markers—Lyt-2 in the mouse and OKT8 and Leu2a in man. These are the same markers carried by suppressor T cells (Ts). Cytotoxic cells interact with targets bearing the appropriate antigen in the context of certain parts of the MHC (K or D regions in the mouse and HLA-A in man).

Delayed-type Hypersensitivity T Cells (Tdh). These effector cells are responsible for initiating delayed-type hypersensitivity reactions (Type IV; see Chapter 10) via secretion of lymphokines (see below). They appear to be of the Lyt-1 phenotype in the mouse and to be OKT4- and Leu3a-positive in man. Tdh recognize and respond to antigen in the context of the I region of the MHC (I region in the mouse and DR region in man).

Regulator T Cells

These lymphocytes appear to control the development of effector T or B lymphocytes. Thus, they are active in T-T and T-B collaborative systems.

T Helper Cells (Th). These were the first regulatory cells recognized and were defined by their ability to "help" B cells in typical T-B collaborative situations (see below). They carry the Lyt-1 phenotype in the mouse and the OKT4 and Leu3a antigens in man. Many in vitro proliferative responses to foreign antigens are primarily responses of Th cells. Many Th cells are important in the full development of T-cell effector functions, such as Tc activity; this would be an example of T-T interaction.

T Suppressor Cells (Ts). Ts cells are involved in negatively regulating responses. Ts are Lyt-2 cells in the mouse and OKT8- and Leu2a-positive cells in man. Ts cells are considered responsible for some forms of acquired immune tolerance; that is, the introduction of specific tolerogens activates Ts circuits to down-regulate positive immune reactions. Some investigators believe that tolerance to self-antigens is not necessarily due to the *absence* of self-reactive T-cell clones (i.e., Th) but rather to the *presence* of Ts cells, which keep autoreactive Th cells in check. According to this view (not held by all), autoimmunity could be seen as a defect in Ts function.

Other Regulator T Cells. Still other examples of regulator T cells can be found, including inducers, amplifiers, and contrasuppressors (all in the mouse). We await further clarification of this most complex system in man.

T-Cell Activation

T cells, ordinarily in unactivated or resting phases (G_0 or G_1), are activated upon receiving the proper signals. Activation may involve any or all of the following; proliferation, differentiation, secretion of lymphokines, and development of effector function. Activation of T-cell clones can occur *specifically* (i.e., by the antigen corresponding to the clonally selected T-cell receptor) or *nonspecifically* (i.e., by a mitogen that activates T cells irrespective of their particular antigen reactivity). Nonspecific activation is, therefore, polyclonal.

Activating Signals for T Cells. Both specific antigen and nonspecific mitogen must be "presented" to T cells in certain ways.

Specific T-Cell Activation. A specific antigen, e.g., tetanus toxoid, is taken up by macrophages (any macrophage will probably be sufficient) and the T-cell receptors on the clone of T cells able to respond to tetanus toxoid "see" that antigen on the macrophage surface, together with products of the MHC, namely Ia or DR antigens. It is not entirely clear whether antigens must be digested or "processed" by macrophages before they are displayed in the proper fashion; it is likely that some antigens, particularly complex ones, are degraded, whereas simple ones, such as haptens, are not. (The presentation mode of allohistocompatibility—i.e., transplantation antigens—is obscure.)

Current paradigms indicate that T cells require at least two signals for activation (Fig. 2–3). In the case described here, the specific signal (signal #1) is tetanus toxoid antigen with MHC products. Another nonspecific signal (signal #2) is provided by the macrophage antigen-presenting cell in the form of interleukin-1 (IL-1), a nonspecific short-range lymphokine (see under Lymphokines and Interleukins, below). T cells may bind antigen in response to signal #1 but require both signals for activation.

Specific T-cell memory is often tested in systems using these concepts. For instance, the T cells of the peripheral blood of a non-immune subject that contains the relevant machinery (antigen-presenting monocytes and responding T cells, among other elements) will not proliferate in culture in response to the addition of tetanus toxoid antigen (because the clone size of the relevant T cells is too small to be "seen " in such an assay). On the contrary, culture of peripheral blood cells from a recently immunized subject, together with tetanus toxoid, will result—after 5 to 7 days—in T-cell proliferation. The latter is usually measured by incorporation of ^{3}H-thymidine, as an index of cell proliferation.

Nonspecific T-Cell Activation. A number of substances, called mitogens, are capable of activating large groups of T cells to proliferate (and sometimes to develop effector cell function). In

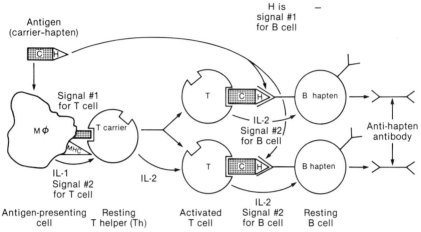

Figure 2–3. For efficient B-cell triggering, 3 cells are needed—an antigen-presenting macrophage to "present" (and usually to process) the complete antigen (C-H), a T helper cell able specifically to recognize the carrier C as foreign and to respond to it, and a B cell specific for hapten H. When all cells and antigen (C-H) are present, the following seems to happen. The macrophage "presents" the C part of the antigen in the context of its own MHC to the Th cell, (signal #1 for the T cell) and also makes IL-1 (signal #2 for the T cell). The cell clone expands, making IL-2. The T cells also provide "T-cell help" to the B cell, probably via lymphokines (such as IL-2 itself and B cell growth and differentiation factors) (signal #2 for the B cell). The B cell also recognizes the hapten, H, via its sIgM receptors for H, (signal #1 for the B cell) and is subsequently triggered to differentiate and mature into B cells and plasma cells secreting anti-H.

this case, the mitogen must also be presented to responding T cells on antigen-presenting cells of the reticuloendothelial system, e.g., monocytes and macrophages. It is not clear whether IL-1 secretion is also necessary for such T-cell activation; it is possible that T-cell mitogens can deliver all the signals needed for T-cell activation. In any event, this type of T-cell stimulation is different in that T-cell mitogens, including phytohemagglutinin (PHA) or concanavalin A (Con A), do not involve triggering of T cells via clonally selected specific T-cell receptors. Instead, these mitogens, which are lectins of plant origin, bind to glycoprotein receptors present on most T cells, regardless of the antigen specificity of those T cells.

In the example given above, the peripheral blood T cells of both tetanus-immunized and tetanus-naive individuals will proliferate well after stimulation with PHA or Con A. Such mitogen responsiveness is frequently used in clinical immunologic assessments to determine *overall* T-cell competence.

The Mixed Leukocyte Reaction (MLR). The MLR is a special system of lymphocyte activation. In its simplest form, the peripheral blood cells of two individuals are mixed and, after 3 to 5 days' culture, are assessed for cell proliferation, again using ^{3}H-thymidine uptake as a measure of DNA synthesis and cell proliferation. If the cells come from identical twins or sibs identical at the HLA (major histocompatibility) locus, cells do not proliferate. If the individuals, e.g., M and N, are *not* HLA-identical, vigorous T-cell proliferation occurs. Of course, in this example, it is impossible to tell whether the proliferating cells are from donor M, responding to HLA antigens of donor N, or vice versa. This is a "two-way MLR" since, under ordinary circumstances, it will contain M–anti-N and N–anti-M reactions. Most often, the reaction is converted to a "one-way MLR" by pretreatment of one cell population (e.g., M), with mitomycin C or X-irradiation. These treatments allow M cells to stimulate the MLR (i.e., to "present" their MHC antigens to the N cells), but the M cells cannot proliferate in response to N-MHC antigens. Thus, in this example, M cells are the stimulators and N cells are the responders.

The vigor of such an N–anti-M reaction has been used to predict allograft rejection and GVH responses.

Why Are MLRs So Potent? There is a paradox inherent in the comparison between the T-cell proliferation induced by tetanus toxoid (as an example of a foreign antigen) and the T-cell proliferation induced by an allohistocompatibility antigen, as in N–anti-M MLR. The T cells of individuals not immunized to tetanus toxoid do not proliferate in response to that antigen but the T cells of a given individual will respond to alloantigens of all MHC-incompatible genotypes! In cellular terms, there seems to be a very high frequency of alloreactive T cells normally present, the reason for which has recently become clearer. The high frequency of alloreactive T cells (or the larger size of alloreactive T-cell clones) does not appear to be due to "natural" immunization with MHC antigens in the environment, as occurs with the development of anti-A and anti-B isohemagglutinins in persons with type O erythrocytes. Instead, alloreactivity appears to be some kind of cross-reaction to antigens that resemble self-MHC. Individuals have T cells that recognize self-MHC on antigen-presenting cells in the normal course of T-cell activation. That is, the T cells respond to self + X, where "self" is self-

MHC, and "X" is the nominal foreign antigen, e.g., tetanus toxoid. In alloreactivity, there may be T cells that see a foreign MHC as altered-self (resembling self + X) without the nominal antigen, and thus respond to allo-MHC.

Lymphokines and Interleukins

Lymphokines. Although activated T cells do not synthesize and secrete conventional antibodies, it has been known for a long time that they do make a variety of soluble substances. Collectively, these have been called *lymphokines* as a family name for products of lymphocytes that may be responsible for many of the functions of lymphocytes. As the name implies, lymphokines would be a subset of *cytokines*, which include products of other types of cells, e.g., monokines from monocytes.

There has been much confusion in the immunology literature concerning lymphokines. While it is agreed that lymphokines are small molecules that act at short range, are unrelated to immunoglobulins, and are not immunologically specific in their actions, there is disagreement about many other of their features. This disagreement stems from the fact that, until recently, lymphokines had not been purified to homogeneity and so had to be identified via bioassays.

The best known lymphokine is MIF (migration inhibition factor). This is a product of activated T cells (probably Tdh cells) that can inhibit the migration of, and activate, tissue macrophages. Conceptually, it is easy to see that the activation of a few immunologically specific T cells at the site of a DH reaction (e.g., a positive tuberculin test) could amplify that reaction greatly by releasing MIF, which would cause the accumulation and activation of the large numbers of nonspecific macrophages that are seen in such reactions. Indeed, since activated macrophages are far more potent than resting macrophages in phagocytosis and intracellular killing, such a recruitment and activation mechanism would be highly beneficial as an amplification system for immunity to many microbes.

In addition to MIF, there is a bewildering variety of other lymphokines, including MAF (macrophage aggregation factor), BF (blastogenic factor), and others.

Interleukins. The situation has become somewhat simpler in recent years. The term *interleukin* has been given to substances that act on leukocytes. Interleukins have all the characteristics of lymphokines mentioned above, i.e., they are small, immunologically nonspecific, and act at short range. An interleukin, however, need not be a lymphocyte product.

Interleukin-1 (IL-1). This substance, formerly called lymphocyte activating factor (LAF), is a product of antigen-presenting monocyte-macrophages and a related substance (epidermally derived thymocyte activating factor, ETAF), which is made by stimulated epidermal cells. IL-1 is weakly mitogenic by itself, but is a potent T-cell co-mitogen when present with PHA or Con A. It appears that the latter two substances induce IL-1 production from macrophages. The secreted IL-1, together with the mitogen, greatly enhances the resultant polyclonal T-cell activation. Human IL-1 has a molecular weight of about 12,000.

Interleukin-2 (IL-2). Interleukin-2 (IL-2) is a true T-cell lymphokine. It is released by T cells under the influence of IL-1. T cells stimulated by mitogen and IL-1 not only synthesize and secrete IL-2, which is a potent stimulator of blastogenesis, but also synthesize more IL-2 receptors, making them even more receptive to IL-2. Cells with significant numbers of IL-2 receptors can be kept in continuous culture if IL-2 is supplied. It is this function that gives the name "T-Cell Growth Factor" (TCGF) to supernatants of activated T cells that contain IL-2. It is likely that TCGF, and probably also IL-2, are mixtures of substances. A purified IL-2 preparation has a molecular weight of about 15,000.

In Vivo Effects of Interleukins. Recent work that has looked at the in vivo effects of interleukins indicates that IL-1 is identical with endogenous pyrogen (derived from PMNs) and can also stimulate fibroblast growth. IL-2 allows T-cell–deprived (nude) mice to mount certain T-cell effector functions and appears to be a very effective "signal #2" for T cells.

Interferons (IFN). These substances are also cytokines. While α and β interferons have been shown to have effects on the immune system, it is IFN-γ (immune interferon) that has provoked the most interest in immunology. IFN-γ can be produced by both T and B lymphocytes after appropriate inductive signals. IFN-γ has been shown to modulate a variety of T- and B-cell functions. The results include both augmentation and diminution of immune responses, depending upon the variables in the particular system used. Clearly, investigations into the immunomodulatory effects of IFN are still in the early phases.

B-CELL BIOLOGY

B-Cell Development

More is known about B-cell development than about most other cell lines, because we have better markers for different stages of B-cell differentiation. The development of mature B cells from precursors proceeds in fetal life and also in mature postnatal life. The most primitive B cell precursors have cytoplasmic μ chains only and no detectable surface immunoglobulin (sIg). These cells differentiate into pre-B cells that have cytoplasmic IgM (μ chains plus light chains) but still no sIg. The next stage is the development of immature B cells that have cytoplasmic IgM and also sIgM. Mature B cells lose cytoplasmic IgM and add sIgD to the sIgM. This developmental progression, which appears to proceed in the absence of antigen, involves some gene rearrangement. This knowledge of B-cell development has been useful in understanding certain leukemias, the cells of which appear, in various patients, to be "fixed" at different stages of their development. A recent field of study is concerned with the recognition of various soluble factors that promote the development and differentiation of B cells.

Mature B Cells and Their Markers

The mature resting B cell is one with sIgM ($\pm$ sIgD), and the sIgM is the receptor for its appropriate antigen. B cells also express products of the MHC—not only HLA-A, B, and C antigens but also the DR (or in the mouse, Ia) antigens. B cells also have receptors for the Fc part of some Ig classes and may also have receptors for C3b.

The sIgM is a classic example of a cell membrane protein "floating in a sea of lipid." This is most dramatically seen in "capping" experiments in which the pattern of sIgM is followed sequentially. In the resting B cell, sIgM is diffusely spread over the cell surface. When an antibody to IgM (e.g., of rabbit origin) is added, the sIgM is aggregated into "patches" that, with time, gather together at one pole of the cell in a "cap" that is later either endocytosed or shed (or both). This leaves a B cell temporarily without sIgM, but the cell resynthesizes sIgM and reexpresses it on the cell surface. This sequence of patching and capping with anti-IgM can also be mimicked, in some circumstances, by adding the appropriate antigen, which can cross-link sIgM specific for that antigen. Nevertheless, the relation between capping and B-cell triggering and antibody production is not settled.

B-Cell Activation

B cells, like T cells, can be stimulated to divide, mature, and secrete their particular products (in the case of B cells, antibody) when triggered by the appropriate signals. Again, as with T cells, the triggering can be specific—activating a particular clone of B cells—or nonspecific and polyclonal. Specific activation is antigen-specific, and nonspecific activation occurs via B cell mitogens.

T-Dependent Antigen Triggering. Most antigens are complex molecules, usually with more than one kind of antigenic determinant (epitope) on each molecule. B cells specific for a given epitope on the molecule, e.g., W, cannot develop into plasma cells secreting anti-W, without the collaboration of T helper cells (Th). In other words, binding of epitope W to the B cell (signal #1) may be necessary, but it is not sufficient for B-cell activation.

The simplest model is to consider a protein molecule, e.g., a "carrier" (C), to which has been added a hapten (H) as an identifiable epitope. For efficient B-cell triggering, three cells are needed: an antigen-presenting macrophage to "present" (and usually to process) the complete antigen (C-H), a T helper cell able specifically to recognize the carrier C as foreign and to respond to it, and a B cell specific for hapten H. When all cells and antigen (C-H) are present, the following seems to happen. The macrophage "presents" the C part of the antigen in the context of its own MHC to the Th cell (signal #1 for the T cell) and also makes IL-1 (signal #2 for the T cell). The T-cell clone expands, making IL-2. The T cells provide "T-cell help" to the B cell, probably via lymphokines such as IL-2 itself and B-cell growth and differentiation factors (signal #2 for the B cell). The B cell also recognizes the hapten, H, via its sIgM receptors for H (signal #1 for the B cell) and is subsequently triggered to differentiate and mature into B cells and plasma cells secreting anti-H. This sequence is diagrammed in Figure 2–3.

The Primary Antibody Response. The primary antibody response, after a T-dependent immunogen is seen by the immune system, consists of the following sequence: a lag period of several days before antibody is seen, a rise in serum antibody (which is mostly IgM at first, and then a mixture of IgM and IgG), and usually a fall in antibody titer after several weeks. The affinity of the antibodies for the antigen's determinants is low to moderate.

Immunologic Memory. In terms of the possible efficiency of this antibody (consider if it were diphtheria antitoxin), this primary response might be considered a weak response. Nevertheless, the immune system is now *primed* by the first exposure to antigen, and the system shows *specific immunologic memory,* i.e., after the primary antibody response has faded, the immune system still has expanded clones of B (and particularly T) "memory cells" able to mount a heightened or *anamnestic* response to a further injection of the same antigen. This state of memory, which lasts for years because of the long lifespan of T cells, accounts for the fact that, following a primary series of tetanus toxoid injections, the body can probably mount an anamnestic response to a "booster" tetanus toxoid injection at *any* time after the priming series.

The Secondary Antibody Response. The response of a primed individual to a booster antigenic challenge includes the following: a shorter lag period, a more rapid rise of antibody, a higher peak titer of antibody, a predominance of the IgG isotypes, and higher affinity of the antibody. The higher affinity is a result of cell selection during the primary and secondary responses. T-dependent antigens such as C-H will trigger a number of B-cell clones, some of which have high affinity sIg for H, and some low affinity. (These activated B cells will, in turn, secrete Ig with high or low affinity for H, respectively.) When the antigenic supply is plentiful, there will be no selective advantage to high- or low-affinity B cells. When the antigenic supply wanes, toward the end of the primary response (due to catabolism and/or binding to the newly formed anti-H), those cells with higher affinity for H will have an advantage in binding H and being triggered by it. Thus, the *average* affinity of the anti-H antibody rises during the primary and secondary responses. In the case of tetanus toxoid, it is of great advantage to have not only increased titers of antibody but also that antibody of the highest affinity for binding its antigen, tetanus toxin.

T-Independent Antigen Triggering. Not all antibody responses require T-cell "help." There are antigens that will trigger B cells into immunoglobulin production without T-cell cooperation (but the requirements for antigen-presenting cells are not yet certain). These antigens, called "T-independent," and the antibody responses they elicit have certain properties. The antigens are polymeric, often polysaccharides, such as dextran or levan, or pneumococcal capsular polysaccharides. They provoke almost exclusively IgM antibody; there is little switching to IgG production. The antibody produced is generally of low avidity, and it is difficult to demonstrate specific immunologic memory to these antigens (i.e., there is no anamnestic boost following a second antigenic exposure). Not only are these substances relatively weak immunogens, they easily tolerize the immune system if enough is given (Chapter 7). As with all immune responses, however, the *form* of the antigen is important in determining the response. Pneumococcal polysaccharides may behave as T-independent antigens in their pure, soluble form, but behave as T-dependent antigens on the intact bacillus. Perhaps the bacterium acts as a carrier, provoking T-cell "help."

The mechanism for activation of T-independent antigens probably depends on their polymeric structure. They are large molecules presenting a matrix array of identical epitopes to a B cell specific for that determinant. The multivalent nature of the ligand-cell–receptor (IgM) interaction is such that cell activation occurs and IgM is secreted. There is no T-cell "help" required, but, on the other hand, the absence of T-cell help does not allow the cell to switch over to high-affinity IgG production.

B-Cell Mitogens

There are substances that nonspecifically and polyclonally trigger large groups of B cells into cell activation and mitosis, resulting in the production of small amounts of the B-cell product, e.g., IgM. This is not, however, a replica of a potent B-cell reaction to either a T-dependent or a T-independent specific antigen.

Bacterial endotoxins (lipopolysaccharides [LPS]) are potent B-cell mitogens in mice. They need little, if any, T-cell "help" and so can function as indicators of B-cell integrity. Unfortunately, LPS is not a good B-cell mitogen in man and cannot be used clinically in assessment of immunocompetence. Pokeweed mitogen (PWM) is the most frequently used B-cell mitogen for human cells, but it has been recently found to be T-dependent itself.

The B-cell mitogenic response, like the T-cell response, is measured by culturing cells with the mitogen for several days and assaying cell division by uptake of ^{3}H-thymidine. A more sophisticated assay measures the amounts of IgG, IgA, and IgM (and occasionally IgE) secreted into the culture medium by mitogen-activated lymphocytes.

B-Cell "Switching" Mechanisms

B cells, early in life and early in the immune response, carry mainly sIgM. As the immune response proceeds, more IgG is produced because more of the stimulated cells bear sIgG. This conversion from IgM to IgG production has been called "isotype switching." It is an antigen-driven step in which the heavy chain of the predominant Ig molecule is now γ instead of μ. It is essential to understand that the antibody is of the same specificity—i.e., the idiotype does not change. This process involves a change in the readout of the cellular DNA so that the genes for γ chains (which lie next to those for μ chains) are now transcribed. This process is somehow controlled by Th cells, as it is impaired or absent in T-deprived subjects.

The production of IgA also involves "switching" from IgM, probably without the intermediary IgG state. This mechanism occurs mainly in the secretory immune systems and may require a separate subset of IgA-specific Th cells that are involved in the switch process. IgE production probably is controlled by a similar mechanism.

Hybridomas and Monoclonal Antibodies

Prior to the development of these remarkable materials, research had been hampered by the unavoidable diversity of the immune response. The injection of even the most purified hapten-carrier was followed by production of an array of anti-hapten antibodies (making up what was called an *antiserum*) differing in their avidity for the hapten, and, therefore, constituting a mixture of idiotypes. Immunochemical analysis of this mixture was not possible at the first level of resolution. An "experiment of nature" that first allowed the fine definition of immunoglobulin structure was plasma cell myeloma, in which large quantities of homogeneous immunoglobulins were noted to be produced by various malignant B-cell clones, differing in each patient. Hybridoma technology permits the controlled formation of homogeneous clones of B cells, each clone producing a single monoclonal antibody.

In practice, an animal is immunized with an antigen, even a complex one. During the antibody response, individual B cells are fused with nonsecreting mouse myeloma cells. The surviving secreting hybrids are selected and grown up from single cells, yielding a series of B-cell clones or hybridomas. Each clone produces an antibody of a single idiotype, hence a monoclonal antibody. The B cells of the immunized animal provide the hybridized clone with the information for the particular antibody being produced, while the myeloma partner confers "immortality." Monoclonal antibodies have almost no limits to their usefulness as laboratory reagents or even as therapeutic reagents, e.g., in recognizing tumor-specific antigens without reacting with normal cell constituents.

A T-cell hybridoma may be similarly produced by fusing an individual antigen-reactive T cell with a "malignant" but apparently antigen-nonspecific T cell. The progeny of such a fusion can be developed, in the presence of T-cell growth factor, into an expanded clone of identical T cells able to react only to a single antigenic determinant on an antigen-presenting cell. Such hybridomas have been essential in defining the fine structure of the T-cell receptor for antigen.

REGULATION OF THE IMMUNE RESPONSE

A current area of great interest is the regulation of immune responsiveness. As mentioned earlier, the immune system has units (lymphocytes) that can multiply during the course of the immune response and can increase their cellular machinery *per cell* at the same time. What keeps immune responses at reasonable levels? Although the secondary antibody response is larger and more efficient than the primary, why are the tertiary and quarternary responses to that antigen usually little different from the secondary? What maintains tolerance to self, and why doesn't this break down more often, leading to autoimmunity?

It is now clear that virtually all aspects of immune responses are under quantitative and qualitative control. The result—what is measured—is the net outcome of a variety of factors involved in that control. The subject is extremely complex, its details are not well understood, and there are many types of control. As an example, a diminished serum immunoglobulin level could result either from an insufficient number of T helpers or B effector cells or from an excess of T suppressors.

Normal Immune Regulation and the Network Hypothesis

Induction of immune responses normally involves both positive and negative regulatory elements. For instance, in experimental delayed hypersensitivity (DH) the degree of hypersensitivity results from the balance of induction of Tdh and the development of Ts. It is almost certain that both antigen-specific Tdh and Ts are activated in each reaction. The amount of DH provoked by a given dose of antigen can be increased merely by adding small doses of cyclophosphamide to the regimen. The drug selectively inhibits Ts and so increases the net effectiveness of the induced Tdh. Conversely, raising the antigen dose above the optimum can decrease the observed DH by activating more Ts and tipping the scales more toward the negative regulatory side.

The Network Hypothesis (Jerne). One attempt to explain immunoregulation is the idiotype network hypothesis proposed by Jerne. He stated that for every antigen receptor (idiotype) on a T or B cell, there existed another anti-idiotypic receptor on another set of T or B cells. Normally, these idiotypes and anti-idiotypes are in a kind of equilibrium. Perturbation of the network equilibrium by antigenic stimulation increases the clone of cells bearing idiotypes (T cells) and (for B cells) secreting idiotypic molecules. This increase is sensed by the system, which, after a lag, increases anti-idiotype production, which in turn, negatively feeds back onto and down-regulates the idiotype system. This is a form of servo-mechanism. There is evidence at both the T-cell and B-cell levels that such network regulatory mechanisms exist. As an example, the induction of anti-hapten antibody is soon followed by the appearance of anti-anti-hapten antibody, which down-regulates the production of anti-hapten antibody.

Genetic Aspects of Immunoregulation

The individual's genetic constitution also controls immune responses to some extent. This is most easily observed in laboratory animals whose genetic constitutions are more easily analyzed. Mice of certain inbred strains fail to mount immune responses to certain specific antigens that are, however, good immunogens in other strains. In virtually every case, the genetic defect is associated with components of the MHC. In some instances, the animal may have "a genetic hole in the repertory"—perhaps an inability to make the B- or T-cell receptor for that antigen. In other cases the particular antigen induces tolerance and stimulates Ts, rather than inducing Th and B cells.

Genetic aspects of immunoregulation are seen in man as well. This is manifested by the tendency of certain diseases to occur more frequently than expected in people of certain HLA haplotypes. The best studied example is that of ankylosing spondylitis, in which 95 percent of those with the disease have the HLA-B27 genotype, while only about 10 percent of the population is HLA-B27–positive. The nature of the abnormality involved, and its linkage to B27, is not known, however. There are other HLA-linked diseases, such as Type I diabetes mellitus, although the association with a particular genotype is not nearly as close as in ankylosing spondylitis.

Other genetic abnormalities of immunoregulation are of still another type, which might be called "immunoglobulin isotype–specific" immunoregulation. This is the inherited tendency of some individuals to make more IgE than normal. This "atopic" constitution is not linked to any particular HLA haplotype, and its ultimate genetic basis is still not understood.

Immunoregulation and Immunodeficiency

Immunodeficiency is discussed in Chapter 6. Some immunodeficiency syndromes are clearly failures of development (e.g., the DiGeorge syndrome), but others appear to be the result of imbalances in immune regulation; two examples may be instructive. A subgroup of patients with acquired common variable hypogammaglobulinemia have a defect in immunoglobulin production that is not a deficit in B-cell number or capability but an excess of Ts activity. The hypogammaglobulinemia that occasionally follows acute infectious mononucleosis due to Epstein-Barr infection is believed to be caused by down-regulation of Th by excessive activity of Ts. The diminished Th activity is associated with B-cell hypofunction.

Autoimmunity and Immunoregulation

Some autoimmune reactions can also be considered as failures of normal immunoregulatory processes. The emergence of autoimmunity and the loss of tolerance to self may occur through modulation of immunoregulatory circuits. This subject is still not entirely understood, but it is clear that there are some autoreactive cells that are normally present but ordinarily not activated. For example, B cells capable of making anti-thyroglobulin can be detected in subjects who are not making anti-thyroglobulin. Some investigators believe that constant Ts activity is normally present, keeping these "autoimmune" B cells in check. In this context, the emergence of functional clones of B cells making anti-thyroglobulin would represent a failure of normal Ts regulation. Perhaps the more frequent occurrence of rheumatoid factor in elderly people also represents a loss of Ts control of normal B cells able to make anti-IgG.

Bibliography

Crystal, R. G., Roberts, W. C., Hunninghake, G. W., et al.: Pulmonary sarcoidosis: a disease characterized and perpetuated by activated lung T-lymphocytes. Ann. Intern. Med. 94:73, 1981.

Eichner, E. R.: Splenic function: normal, too much and too little. Am. J. Med. 66:311, 1979.

Farrar, J. J., Benjamin, W. R., Hilfiker, M. L., et al.: The biochemistry, biology, and role of interleukin 2 in the induction of cytotoxic T cells and antibody-forming B cell responses. Immunol. Rev. 63:129, 1982.

Germain, R. N., and Benacerraf, B.: Helper and suppressor T cell factors. Springer Semin. Immunopathol. 3:93, 1980.

Katz, D. H.: Genetic control of cell-cell interactions. Pharmacol. Rev. 34:51, 1982.

Shorter, R. G., and Tomasi, T. B.: Gut immune mechanisms. Adv. Intern. Med. 27:247, 1982.

Streilein, J. W.: Skin associated lymphoid tissues. Exp. Clin. Immunol. 1:151, 1983.

Wall, R., and Kuehl, M.: Biosynthesis and regulation of immunoglobulins. Ann. Rev. Immunol. 1:393, 1983.

3

The Complement System

MICHAEL M. FRANK, M.D.

Introduction	Genetic Defects in the
The Classical Pathway	Complement Cascade
The Alternative Pathway	Synthesis and Control
	Overview of Complement
	Function

INTRODUCTION

The complement system is composed of a group of circulating plasma proteins that play a major role in the host defense response. Although best known for their ability to lyse antibody-coated erythrocytes and bacteria, the complement proteins also have important activities as mediators of inflammation, as attractants for phagocytic cells, and as opsonins, substances that coat particles to make them more easily phagocytosed. One of the interesting biologic features of the complement cascade is that it provides an amplification of the effect of antibody. Complement activation leads to the generation of active enzymes that cleave, and thereby activate, later components in the complement cascade. Activation of a limited number of components early in the cascade can lead to the generation of large numbers of inflammatory and cell-damaging factors at later steps. Hence a few specific antibody molecules can have a major influence on cell survival, induction of inflammation, and so on. For these reasons an understanding of the mechanisms of activation, biologic effects, and homeostatic controls of the complement system has become important in modern clinical immunologic and allergic practice.

As originally described, complement referred to the heat-labile components of serum that were required for lysis of bacteria or erythrocytes that had reacted with heat-stable specific antibody. Analysis of these requirements for lysis has uncovered a large group of proteins that act in a precise biochemical sequence and are responsible for the lytic reactions. The proteins become activated in a precise order and bind to the surface of bacteria or other targets coated with antibody. These targets, coated with antibody and complement components, often are recognized as abnormal by phagocytic cells via the interaction of specific receptors on the phagocytic cells, with specific fragments of complement proteins deposited on the particle targeted for destruction. Completion of the sequence of complement protein interactions leads to the lysis of the target.

Many of the complement proteins circulate as inactive precursors (zymogens) that are activated by specific cleavage reactions that generate a small and a large fragment of the complement protein. The larger fragment often attaches to the particle to be phagocytosed or lysed, and the small fragment is released into the fluid surrounding the cell. In many cases the small fragment has biologic activity and is capable of mediating one or another feature of the inflammatory response.

It is now known that there are two separate pathways of complement activation (Fig. 3–1). The first, termed the classical pathway because it was the first pathway recognized and studied, is initiated by the interaction of antibody-coated targets or antigens with C1, the first component of the complement cascade. It proceeds through a series of numbered components, of which all but one are in numerical order, to the activation of C9, the last component in the sequence, and to lysis of the target. In addition, non–antibody-coated particles of certain types, particularly those with repeating polysaccharide subunits (like the surface of bacteria or fungi), are capable of interacting directly with components of complement, leading to the opsonization and destruction of the uncoated particles. This phenomenon is now recognized as being due to a second pathway of complement activation that may be very important in the lysis of bacteria exposed to body fluids before there is time for an antibody response; this is termed the alternative pathway. The compo-

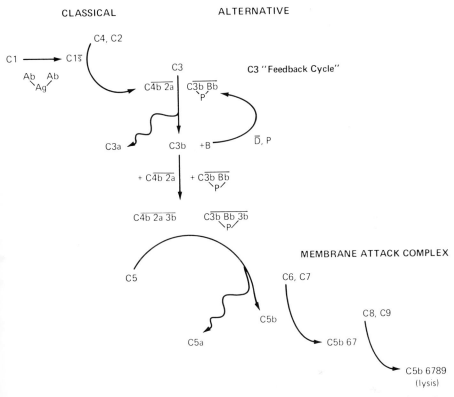

Figure 3–1. The classical and alternative complement pathways, showing interaction of proteins and generation of major cleavage fragments. Components acting as active enzymes are designated by placement of a bar above the appropriate component (e.g., C1s̄). The C3 "Feedback Cycle" is often designated as the C3b-dependent Amplification Pathway.

nents of the classical pathway through C9 are numbered, while the components of the alternative pathway are given letter designations (Table 3–1). A number of control steps occur in the complement cascade, and the several proteins that function to turn off activated components are also designated by letters. Exceptions will be discussed below.

THE CLASSICAL PATHWAY

The classical pathway is initiated by the interaction of antibody with a target cell, be it an erythrocyte, a nucleated cell, or a bacterium (Fig. 3–1). IgG subclasses 1, 2, and 3, and IgM are the only immunoglobulins capable of activating the classical

Table 3–1. Proteins of the Complement Cascade

Protein	Concentration in Serum (mg/ml)	Biologic Function
C1 q	80	Binds to Ag-Ab complexes
r	34	Subunit of C1
s	30	Enzymatic activity cleaves C4 and C2
C4	350	C4a anaphylatoxin
		C4b viral neutralization
C2	15	
C3	1200	C3a anaphylatoxin, immunoregulatory
		C3b key component of alternative path-
		way; major opsonin in serum
		C3e fragment induces leukocytosis
C5	75	C5a anaphylatoxin; principal chemotac-
		tic factor in serum; induces neutrophil
		attachment to endothelium
		C5b initiates membrane attack
C6	70	Participates with C5b in formation of
C7	60	membrane attack complex (MAC)
C8	80	that lyses cells
C9	60	
Factor B	225	Bb causes macrophage spreading on
		surfaces
Factor D	1	
Properdin	25	Stabilizes alternative pathway conver-
		tase

pathway. Activation is initiated by the binding of C1 to the Fc fragment of the activating antibody. C1 is composed of three subunits, termed C1q, C1r, and C1s, that remain bound together in the presence of Ca^{++}. C1q, which binds to the antigen antibody complex, is a molecule that, as visualized under the electron microscope, has a core-like structure and six radiating arms, each of which ends in a pod. The pods are capable of attaching to the Fc portion of the antibody molecule, an attachment presumably stabilized by the conformational change occurring within the Fc fragment when antibody binds to the antigen. One molecule of C1q is capable of binding to one molecule of IgM attached to an antigenic surface through several of its combining sites. An IgG doublet (two molecules of IgG side-by-side) is required to perform the same function, because multiple Fc fragments are required to give sufficient stability to the C1q to form a firm bond. For this reason, not only is the class and type of antibody important in determining whether complement will be activated but so also is the nature of the antigenic surface. For example, if the surface has antigenic groupings that are too far apart to permit the formation of IgG doublets, IgG will not activate complement and induce complement-mediated damage. It is believed that IgG anti-Rh antibody is a poor complement activator because it is unable to form such doublets efficiently on an erythrocyte surface.

Information that the C1q portion of the C1 molecule has bound to the antigen antibody complex is transmitted to the r and s portions of the molecule. The chains of C1r and C1s are cleaved, and new enzymatic activities appear that were not associated with unactivated C1. Acting as an esterase, C1 cleaves the next two components in the complement cascade, C4 and C2, each into a large fragment and a small fragment. The large fragment of C4 attaches covalently to the surface of the particle to be destroyed. The small fragment has anaphylatoxic activity as described in Table 3–1. The bound C4, in the presence of Mg^{++} ion, associates with and binds the next component in the complement cascade, C2. The C2 bound to the C4 is cleaved by activated C1 esterase. A large fragment of this cleavage is left behind—still bound to the C4—and a small fragment enters the fluid surrounding the target. Activated C1 cleaves many molecules of C4 before it is inactivated. C4 binds to the target and, in turn, can bind many molecules of C2 that can be cleaved. The C1 enzyme continues to form C4,2 complexes bound to the target, unless its activity is destroyed by a protein termed the C1 esterase inactivator or inhibitor. This protein destroys the enzymatic activity of C1r and C1s by directly binding to the active binding site on each of these subunits of the C1 molecule. Thus, unlike an enzyme, the protein is utilized during the inactivation reaction.

An inherited autosomal dominant disease, hereditary angioedema (HAE), is characterized biochemically by the failure to synthesize adequate quantities of the C$\overline{1}$ esterase inhibitor (C$\overline{1}$ INH) and, clinically, by episodic attacks of deep subcutaneous or subepithelial edema (angioedema). These patients can have angioedema attacks of any part of the body, but attacks primarily involve the extremities and gastrointestinal mucosa. Attacks involving the oral pharynx may lead to death from swelling and asphyxiation. Patients with this disorder have unregulated activation of C1, which continues to cleave C4 and C2, thus markedly reducing the levels of these two components of the complement cascade. It is believed that biologically active fragments of C4 and C2, following further enzymatic cleavage, are responsible for the swelling in hereditary angioedema. However, the C$\overline{1}$ esterase inhibitor not only inactivates C$\overline{1}$ esterase but also inactives enzyme systems activated by Hageman factor and its fragments. Thus, this protein inactivates activated Hageman factor and its fragments as well as components of the fibrinolytic, clotting, and kinin cascades. Any or all of these may contribute to the edema in this patient group.

The complex of C4 and C2 in the presence of magnesium ion is associated with the development of a new enzyme composed of the large fragments of C4 and C2. This enzyme interacts with C3 and cleaves it in turn into a larger fragment, C3b, and a smaller fragment, C3a. Again, the small fragment is released and the large fragment may bind to the surface of the target particle to continue the cascade. C3 is a critical component in the complement cascade. C3, present in high concentrations in plasma, functions in both classical and alternative pathways, since the pathways join at the level of this important protein and thereafter proceed together. Moreover, the binding of C3b to the surface of a target particle is an important opsonic event, since receptors for C3b are present on all phagocytic cells. Target particles coated with C3b, by binding to this receptor, become fixed to the membrane of phagocytic cells, facilitating ingestion of the target. Particle-bound C3b undergoes a complex set of decay reactions (see below). Specific receptors for certain of these decay products are also present on phagocytic and lymphoid cells. These receptors may also aid phagocytosis or play an immunoregulatory role in the immune response, but their precise role has not been determined. The binding of C3b to a target particle is of extreme importance in regulating activation of the alternative pathway as well.

C3a—the small fragment of C3 that is released upon cleavage of the C3 molecule by the C4,2 enzyme—also has important biologic activity. C3a acts as an anaphylatoxin, causing mast cells to degranulate and release their mediator contents. It is elevated in such diseases as the adult respiratory distress syndrome and in other situations in which complement is activated, suggesting that this fragment induces mast cell degranulation, release of mediators, and other immunopathologic effects. C3b bound to the cell surface is capable of binding C5, the next component in the sequence. C5 bound to surface C3b can be cleaved by the C3 cleaving enzyme (C4,2) into a small fragment, C5a, and a large fragment, C5b, each of which has important biologic and biochemical functions.

C5a, released from the C5 molecule, functions in a number of important biologic systems. Like C3a, C5a is an anaphylatoxin, causing mast cells to degranulate and release their mediators. C5a also acts as a potent chemotactic factor. Neutrophils, monocytes, and macrophages have on their surface a C5a receptor, the triggering of which by C5a induces movement of the cell. If these receptors are triggered selectively on one side of the cell, the cell will move in that direction. Thus a phagocyte will move up a C5a gradient toward the site of C5a generation. C5a has other potent effects on neutrophils, causing them to aggregate and stick to endothelium, which also has important biologic consequences. The generation of C5a in the circulation tends to aggregate neutrophils, and these aggregates may embolize to the lung, where they may cause marked respiratory distress. Patients on renal dialysis and on heart-lung machines may generate C5a in their circulation as a result of activation of the alternative complement pathway by the dialysis membranes. This may be followed by embolization of aggregated neutrophils with attendant marked respiratory distress. This may also occur in the adult respiratory distress syndrome, in which the complement activation results from marked tissue trauma or the presence of bacteria in the circulation.

C5b, the major fragment of C5, functions differently from the earlier large fragments. C5b binds to the cell but does not link itself to the cell surface; the molecule, which is quite hydrophobic, is stabilized by the next component in the sequence, C6. The C5b6 complex, in the presence of the following component C7, is capable of inserting into the lipid bilayer of the cell surface via its hydrophobic domain. This insertion into the lipid bilayer begins the lytic sequence. In the presence of the next component, C8, and markedly augmented by the final component, C9, these proteins associate into a cylinder-like structure with a hydrophilic center and a hydrophobic outer ring. The hydrophobic exterior holds the cylinder in the cell membrane. This structure in the lipid bilayer allows water and small ions to enter and leave the cell freely through the hydrophilic center, causing the cell to lose its capacity to retain osmotic equilibrium. Water enters the cell and it swells and lyses. Thus the presence of the complement proteins, operating in a precise functional sequence, leads first to membrane alteration or opsonization of the target cell and, later in the sequence, to actual direct cellular cytotoxicity.

THE ALTERNATIVE PATHWAY

Complement may also be activated by mechanisms that do not require antibody. Certain chemical structures, such as the repeating polysaccharide units or the lipopolysaccharide found on the surface of some microoganisms, may activate complement directly via a series of proteins that constitute the alternative pathway (Fig. 3–1). The key to an understanding of the proteins of the alternative pathway is knowledge of the structure and chemistry of C3. C3 is a two-chain molecule, the larger of which, termed the α chain, has within it a tight thiol-ester loop linking a glutamic acid and cysteine of the protein backbone. This is a highly reactive group and is usually buried within the interior of the protein. Upon the cleavage of C3a, this group is exposed and will be attacked either by water, leading to hydrolysis, or by the surface of an organism or foreign substance to which it may bind by an amide or ester linkage. Water can slowly penetrate to the thiol-ester loop in intact C3 as well. After cleavage of the thiol-ester loop in the intact C3 molecule or in C3b, the protein is capable of interacting with another protein of the alternative pathway, termed factor B. In the presence of a third protein, factor D, the B bound to C3 is cleaved into a large fragment, Bb, that remains bound to the C3, and a small fragment, Ba.

In essence, the function of the proteins of the alternative pathway is exactly analogous to that of the proteins of the classical pathway. One can think of C1 and D as serving equivalent functions. Both are serine proteases that cleave other proteins in the cascade. B itself is analogous to C2 and appears to represent a gene duplication of C2. In the presence of magnesium ion it is cleaved into a small fragment and a large fragment. The large fragment forms an enzyme complex with a cell-bound protein that has C3 cleaving activity. In this formulation, C3, with its open thiol-ester loop, is exactly analogous to C4b in its function, in that it acts as an acceptor for a protein fragment to form a complex enzyme capable of cleaving additional C3. Thus, there are two molecular forms of C3 capable of activating the alternative pathway. The first is simply intact C3 with the thiol-ester cleaved. Presumably, this cleavage of the internal loop occurs slowly and spontaneously in the circulation at all times. The second is C3 with the C3a fragment removed, or C3b. The C4,2 complex of the classical pathway described earlier, and the C3b complex described in this section are both physiologically unstable. C3bBb, the C3 convertase of the alternative pathway, is so unstable that it decays rapidly in the absence of stabilizing factors. A natural circulating protein termed properdin (P) is capable of stabilizing C3bBb, thereby permitting the alternative pathway to proceed.

There are a number of proteins in blood that regulate and

mediate the rapid cleavage of C3b, which, after cleavage, can no longer activate the alternative pathway. A major problem associated with normal complement function in vivo is that the proteins may be activated and bind to normal host structures. This could lead to inflammatory responses and direct cytotoxicity of cells within the host structure, such as the kidney. Presumably, the C3b regulatory proteins act to destroy C3b if associated with host tissues. Two plasma proteins, termed factors H and I, are responsible for mediating the rapid decay of C3b. The α chain of C3b undergoes proteolytic cleavage in the presence of these two factors, forming a product termed iC3b, or inactive C3b. This further cleavage product can no longer activate the proteins of the alternative pathway. The ability of factors H and I to cleave C3b is influenced by the site to which the C3b is bound. If the C3b is bound to a bacterial surface, factors H and I interact with it rather inefficiently, leading to the persistence of C3b on the bacterial surface, activation of the alternative pathway, and destruction of the bacterium. If the C3b is bound to a normal host structure, factors H and I interact with it efficiently, leading to its cleavage. The control of tissue-bound C3b is yet more complex. One of the receptors for C3b, termed C3b complement receptor or CR1, can bind to C3b. In this situation it replaces the need for factor H. Factor I, an enzyme, is capable of cleaving receptor-bound C3b, and the cleavage is very much more extensive than that produced by factors H and I. The product of such cleavage, C3dg, is a 41,000 molecular weight complement fragment that is capable of interacting with cells with specific receptors for this small fragment. In summary, C3 undergoes a complex set of degradation reactions. There appear to be a series of specific cellular receptors for products formed in the different stages of C3 degradation, suggesting that these degradation products interact with cells in a highly specific manner to determine how they will react. Presumably, in some cases the formation of such fragments will in some way regulate the production of antibody, while in other cases, the fragments will mediate the phagocytic response by neutrophils and macrophages.

    In summary, the two pathways of activation of the complement cascade converge at the C3 utilization step. The classical pathway proceeds through the attachment of antibody to the antigenic surface, leading to activation and binding of C1, C4, and C2. This, in turn, leads to activation of binding of C3 and the later components of the cascade. Ultimately the lytic event may ensue. Alternative pathway factors, even in the absence of antibody, can be activated and protein fragments generated that are capable of binding to acceptor surfaces. The proteins of the alternative pathway are similar to those of the classical pathway and produce similar enzymes. C3 activated by either pathway can bind to acceptor surfaces. If these acceptor surfaces are chemically suitable, the alternative pathway will proceed. If these acceptor surfaces are not suitable, as is presumably the case with those that exist on host tissues, alternative pathway factors will be destroyed by regulatory proteins present in the circulation, such as factors H and I, and on cells, such as the C3b receptor.

GENETIC DEFECTS IN THE COMPLEMENT CASCADE

A small number of patients with deficiencies of each of the numbered components in the classical system have been described, and a very limited number of patients with alternative pathway deficiencies have been noted. Patients with deficiencies in the early components of the classical pathway, C1, C4, and C2, can mount a normal response to small numbers of invading bacteria via the alternative pathway and late component activation. In fact, patients with C4 and C2 deficiency do well with infection except when under extreme stress. Patients with C1q deficiency seem to have a greater problem with infection, for undetermined reasons. Patients with C3 deficiency have a major problem with infection, particularly early in life, before large quantities of protective antibody have been formed. Patients with deficiencies of proteins later than C3 in the lytic sequence tend to do well with infection, because they are capable of opsonizing bacteria via the C3 mechanism. The major exception to this general rule is infection with neisserial organisms. Patients with late component deficiencies, from C5 to C8, have a much higher than normal incidence of disseminated meningococcal and gonococcal infections. The presence of the lytic mechanism apparently is required for complete host defense against this class of organisms. As might be expected, patients with defects in the early components of the alternative pathway have a great deal of difficulty with bacterial infection because this pathway appears important in host defense, before antibody production has had a chance to commence.

Patients with many defects of complement proteins appear to be at high risk for the development of a wide variety of autoimmune diseases ranging from systemic lupus erythematosus to glomerulonephritis.

SYNTHESIS AND CONTROL

The genes for C2, B, and C4 are located within the MHC (major histocompatibility complex), and these three proteins are considered the Class III antigens of the major histocompatibility locus. Several of the complement proteins appear to be synthesized by multiple cells, at least in vitro. For example, B, C2, C3, and C4 can be synthesized by macrophages, particularly when those macrophages are stimulated by the phagocytic process. Components such as C3 appear also to be synthesized by hepatocytes, and the normal plasma level of C3 appears to result from hepatocyte synthesis. Presumably the liver is primarily responsible for the production of most components. Complement component synthesis may also occur at the site of local inflammation, facilitating host defense. C1 appears to be synthesized in vitro by many types of epithelial cells, including gastrointestinal and bladder mucosal epithelium.

OVERVIEW OF COMPLEMENT FUNCTION

This analysis of complement component function allows consideration of the function of complement as an integrated system during host defense. Bacteria arriving at a local tissue site will interact with components of the alternative pathway, resulting in the generation of biologically active fragments, opsonization of the bacteria, and initiation of the lytic sequence. If the bacteria persist or are invading the host a second time, the antibody response will also play an important role leading to activation of the classical pathway, which is much more rapid and efficient in mediating opsonization and complement fragment generation. The generation of complement fragments leads to a number of important inflammatory effects. Mast cells release their contents, and the blood supply to the area increases markedly as vessels dilate. Although complement fragments, acting as anaphylatoxins, produce many of the same effects as IgE, there is no certain evidence that they mediate any of the common allergic diseases. Complement fragments have important effects on the release of neutrophils from the bone marrow, apparently mediated by C3e, a fragment of C3 that is still being characterized. Neutrophils in the circulation arrive at the site of hyperemia, where, in the presence of C5a, they attach to endothelium and leave the blood vessels. C5a causes a directed migration of these cells, which tend to enter the area where the complement is being activated. Local synthesis by macrophages leads to the formation of even more complement components, which may interact with the bacteria. All of these effects promote the ingestion and ultimate destruction of the bacteria by neutrophils and macrophages.

Thus, complement is capable of mediating the host defense process under normal circumstances. In some cases an immunoregulatory defect leads to the formation of autoantibody (antibody against one's own tissues). Complement, acting in its normal capacity, may be activated by such antibody, causing damage of local tissues. Regulatory factors help to contain this damage by destroying some of the important complement protein fragments when they are attached to host tissues (see Chapter 19 in *Principles of Immunology and Allergy*).

Complement activation may cause disease even in the absence of specific antibody. For example, paroxysmal nocturnal hemoglobinuria (PNH) is associated with defective formation of a complement regulatory protein that is cell-surface bound. This protein, found on erythrocytes, neutrophils, and platelets, promotes the decay of active complement fragments after they have bound to the cell surfaces. Deficiency of this protein in patients with PNH permits increased complement activation at the surface of these cells and their ultimate destruction.

Bibliography

Atkinson, J. P., and Frank, M. M.: Complement. *In* Parker, C. W. (ed.): Clinical Immunology. Philadelphia, W. B. Saunders Co., 1980, p. 219.

Brown, E. J., Joiner, K. A., and Frank, M. M.: Complement. *In* Paul, W. E. (ed.): Fundamental Immunology. New York, Raven Press, 1984, p. 645.

Cooper, N. R.: The complement system. *In* Stites, D. P., et al.: Basic and Clinical Immunology, 5th ed. Los Altos, CA, Lange Medical Publications, 1984, p. 119.

4

Phagocytosis

PETER DENSEN, M.D.,
and GERALD L. MANDELL, M.D.

INTRODUCTION

Phagocytosis is the active ingestion by cells of particulate matter, such as microorganisms. Eosinophils, basophils, monocytes, and polymorphonuclear neutrophils have this capability. The role of the eosinophil and the basophil in the immunologic responses of the host is dealt with in Chapters 11 and 14 respectively. These two cell types are capable of phagocytosis, as evidenced by their numbers, motility, appearance at sites of inflammation, and by the presence of ingested microorganisms in exudates from acute and chronic infections. Circulating monocytes enter the tissues, where they give rise to resident, mobile tissue macrophages and the fixed macrophages of the reticuloendothelial system. Ingestion of organisms, cellular debris, and other foreign antigens, as well as exposure to humoral mediators, activates these cells, enabling them to kill ingested pathogens and to play an important role in antigen processing, functions that are discussed in Chapter 2. The neutrophil, which is the preeminent phagocytic cell, patrols the circulation until some infectious or inflammatory stimulus causes it to enter the tissues on a suicidal mission. The remainder of this chapter will examine the biologic basis of neutrophil function as it relates to both normal and abnormal host defense and to immune-mediated mechanisms of tissue injury.

BIOLOGY OF NEUTROPHILS AND PHAGOCYTOSIS

Neutrophils

Morphology and Development

Neutrophils (Fig. 4–1), derived from pluripotential stem cells located in the bone marrow, mature in two phases, a mitotic and a nonmitotic phase, each lasting approximately 1 week. The mature neutrophil contains two populations of cytoplasmic granules: the primary or azurophil granules and the specific or secondary granules. Specific granules outnumber primary granules by a ratio of 2–3:1, because the latter undergo numerical reduction during cell division whereas the former arise during the nonmitotic phase of development and therefore are not reduced in number. Primary granules contain acid hydrolases, neutral proteases, cationic proteins, lysozyme, acid mucopolysaccharide, and, most important, myeloperoxidase. Specific granules contain lactoferrin, lysozyme, vitamin B_{12} binding proteins, and cytochrome b.

During maturation, a thin, clear area of cytoplasm becomes apparent around the periphery of the cell. As the cell acquires the capability for directional motility, this veil, which is composed of a meshwork of microfilaments, extends to form a broader, clear area at the advancing edge of the cell. Microfilaments are

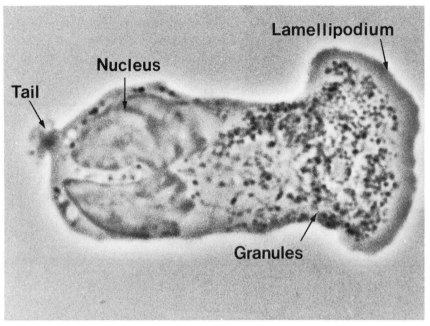

Figure 4–1. Polymorphonuclear neutrophil—phase contrast microscopy.

polymers of actin, a contractile protein. Actin and a number of interacting proteins constitute the contractile machinery of the cell that provides for locomotion. Regulation of the length of the filaments and their degree of cross-linking permits the physico-chemical fluctuation of actin between the gel and the sol state. Changes in calcium concentration during membrane stimulation help to provide for a flow of actin from regions of high to low calcium concentrations, thereby generating cell motility. Micro-tubules—other intracytoplasmic structures—are involved in de-granulation and in the regulation of cell-surface microviscosity during phagocytosis.

As the cells become metamyelocytes, they acquire the ability to reduce nitroblue tetrazolium dye (an indicator of stimulated oxidative metabolism). These changes are further accompanied by the appearance of specific cell-surface antigens and receptors. These receptors are distributed homogeneously over the surface of the resting cell but may become asymmetrically distributed during cell stimulation. Receptors for IgG, C3b, and C5a appear to be most important from the standpoint of cell function. IgG and C3b, a fragment of the third component of complement, play an important role in promoting ingestion of bacteria by neutrophils. C5a, a fragment of the fifth component of complement, is an important stimulus of neutrophil motility (see Chapter 3).

Neutrophil Kinetics

Approximately one hundred billion mature polymorphonuclear neutrophils are released from the bone marrow daily. Moreover, the mature granulocyte reserve in the bone marrow contains up to 10 times the normal daily neutrophil requirements. In the face of a continuing demand for neutrophils, as occurs during infection, this reserve may be depleted. As a consequence of this depletion, immature neutrophil precursors appear in the peripheral circulation, a phenomenon that is referred to as "a shift to the left." About 10 percent of the body's mature neutrophils are present within the intravascular space, half in a circulating pool and half in a marginating pool. The marginating pool is located along the vascular endothelium, primarily in the venous circulation. The intravascular half-life of mature neutrophils is about 6 to 8 hours. They may survive in the tissues for up to 4 days once the cells leave the circulation.

Granulocytosis can be produced by a number of physiologic and pharmacologic stimuli in addition to infection. Most often these stimuli cause granulocytosis by altering the distribution of neutrophils in the various bone marrow and vascular compartments rather than by an absolute increase in cell production. For example, the acute administration of glucocorticosteroids produces granulocytosis by stimulating the release of cells from the marrow granulocyte reserve. Exercise, stress, epinephrine, alcohol, and hypoxia all produce granulocytosis by mobilizing the pool of marginated granulocytes. Chronic glucocorticosteroid administration produces granulocytosis by inhibiting the egress of neutrophils from the circulation.

Delivery to the Inflammatory Site

Humoral mediators diffusing from the site of inflammation alter the surface properties of vascular endothelium and circulating neutrophils. In the latter case, these changes result in a decrease in surface charge, an increase in receptor number, and an increase in adhesiveness as a consequence of limited degranulation by the cell. These changes facilitate neutrophil adherence to vascular endothelium and subsequent entry into tissues.

Neutrophils arrive at the inflammatory site by following a concentration gradient of inflammatory mediators in a directional manner (chemotaxis). A number of factors have been characterized that promote chemotaxis at extremely low concentrations (10^{-11} M). Among these factors are C5a (a complement chemotactic factor generated during the interaction of microorganisms with the complement system), products of arachidonic acid metabolism (the hydroxy-eicosatetraenoic acids and leucotrienes), and microbe-derived formyl peptides. In addition, during degranulation, granule constituents are released that exert a chemotactic effect on neutrophils and other granulocytes. Modulation of chemotactic responsiveness occurs when inflammatory mediators stimulate limited degranulation with the addition of fresh membrane to the cell surface. There is a concomitant increase in the number of receptors for chemotactic factors (upregulation). These receptors are occupied and rapidly internalized as the cell moves in an increasing chemotactic gradient. The resultant decrease in receptor numbers (down-regulation) serves to control chemotactic responsiveness. In addition, the release of toxic metabolites of oxygen and of granule proteases during stimulation of the cell can inactivate a number of soluble, chemotactic factors. This multitude of effects serves in concert to attract and retain the neutrophil at the site of microbial invasion.

Phagocytosis

Phagocytosis is a two-step process involving attachment and then ingestion of the phagocytic particle. The major opsonic factors (humoral substances that promote ingestion) are the C3b fragment of complement and specific immunoglobulin of the IgG class. Opsonization occurs when IgG binds to specific antigenic determinants on the surface of the organism. This interaction leads to the activation of complement and the deposition of C3b (see Chapter 3). The surface of many bacteria contains antiphagocytic structures, for example, the pneumococcal capsule. Antibody and complement bound to the bacterial surface promote phagocytosis by neutralizing the antiphagocytic properties of the organism and by acting as ligands between the organism and specific receptors in the phagocytic cell membrane. The progressive, sequential engagement of these receptors initiates microfilament polymerization in the underlying cytoplasm and results in the circumferential flow of the phagocytic membrane around the organism, enclosing it in a phagocytic vacuole.

The Respiratory Burst

The metabolic or respiratory burst is a series of enzymatic reactions that occurs when phagocytic cells are stimulated by the attachment of opsonized particles to the cell membrane or by perturbation of the cell membrane by some inflammatory mediators such as C5a. These reactions serve to convert oxygen to a variety of toxic metabolites important in the bactericidal reactions of the cell and to regenerate the substrate for this reaction. Initiation of the respiratory burst is due to the activation of an intramembrane nicotinamide-adenine dinucleotide phosphate (NADPH)–reduced oxidase. The oxidase activity is not the result of a single enzyme but rather is due to a transmembrane electron transport system involving a b-type cytochrome. Since the cytochrome is present in the specific granules of resting cells, its translocation to the cell membrane may be important in the assembly and activation of the membrane NADPH oxidase system. The NADPH binding site is believed to be located on the cytoplasmic face of this system, and the oxygen binding site on the external surface of the cell. Thus, the system shuttles electrons across the membrane from NADPH to oxygen. The toxic metabolites formed during the reduction of oxygen are released from the external cell surface as it invaginates to become the inner lining of the phagocytic vacuole encompassing the ingested microbe.

The chief consequences of the respiratory burst are oxygen consumption, superoxide and hydrogen peroxide production, and stimulation of the hexose monophosphate shunt. The transfer of an electron from NADPH to oxygen results in the reduction (consumption) of oxygen to form superoxide (O_2^-), as shown in the following reaction:

$$2\ O_2 + NADPH \rightarrow 2\ O_2^- + H^+ + NADP^+$$

At the acidic pH present in the phagocytic vacuole, hydrogen peroxide is rapidly generated by the spontaneous dismutation of superoxide:

$$2\ O_2^- + 2\ H^+ \rightarrow H_2O_2 + O_2$$

Superoxide dismutase and the glutathione synthetase/reductase system present in the cytoplasm of neutrophils protect the cell from the toxic effect of these substances as they diffuse into the cell. The latter reaction system uses NADPH to regenerate reduced glutathione. Thus, NADPH plays a critical role both in the primary reduction of oxygen and in the protection of the cell from toxic metabolites of oxygen. The hexose monophosphate shunt, a series of reactions oxidizing glucose to a 5 carbon sugar and carbon dioxide, serves to regenerate NADPH.

Degranulation

Degranulation is the process by which the cytoplasmic granules fuse with the neutrophil membrane and empty their contents into the phagosome or the extracellular milieu. It is stimulated by ingestion and by inflammatory mediators as a result of the binding of these substances to their specific receptors in the cell membrane. Degranulation is initiated before ingestion is complete, allowing active enzymes to leak out of the nascent phagocytic vacuole into the environment. Since soluble mediators do not promote phagosome formation, these substances can stimulate direct external degranulation.

Microbicidal Mechanisms

Degranulation and the respiratory burst are closely linked events that serve to deliver highly toxic substances into the phagocytic vacuole. The phagosome is important because it concentrates these toxic substances around the ingested particle and minimizes their noxious effect on the phagocyte and surrounding cells. Another important aspect of neutrophil microbicidal activity is redundancy. Redundancy allows for several general mechanisms by which most microorganisms can be damaged. Neutrophils can ingest and kill organisms under both aerobic and anaerobic conditions; thus, killing mechanisms are generally divided into oxygen-dependent and oxygen-independent subsets. Factors and substances that exert a bactericidal or bacteriostatic effect, in the absence of oxygen, include the acid environment present in the phagocytic vacuole; lactoferrin, a protein that binds iron necessary for bacterial growth; lysozyme, an enzyme that plays an important role in the hydrolysis of the peptidoglycan backbone of bacterial cell walls; and cationic proteins that interact with the bacterial cell surface to alter permeability and inhibit growth.

Oxygen-dependent killing is divided into myeloperoxidase-independent, and myeloperoxidase-dependent mechanisms. Hydrogen peroxide, superoxide, singlet oxygen, and the hydroxyl radical are toxic substances produced during the reduction of oxygen that exert a direct bactericidal effect. Although hydrogen peroxide by itself has important bactericidal properties, when it is combined with myeloperoxidase released from the primary granule and with a halide ion such as chloride (present in the environment), a bactericidal system is formed that has 50 times the activity of hydrogen peroxide alone. The microbicidal activity of this system probably results from halogenation or oxidation of critical microbial structures.

Toxic products released by neutrophils are largely confined to the phagocytic vacuole. Nevertheless, ample opportunity exists for these substances to escape into the extracellular milieu. Neutrophils respond in a stereotypic fashion with a respiratory burst and degranulation, regardless of the nature of the stimulus (e.g., invasive bacteria vs. synovium to which antibody and complement have been bound). Therefore, it is not surprising that these beneficial microbicidal systems have been implicated in the pathogenesis of both immune and non-immune mediated arthropathies and nephropathies. Evidence also suggests that neutrophils play an important role in the development of the adult respiratory distress syndrome and pulmonary emphysema.

DEFECTS IN NEUTROPHIL FUNCTION

Infections resulting from defects in granulocyte function tend to be prolonged, to respond slowly to antibiotics, and to recur. Staphylococci, gram-negative organisms, and fungi are the major pathogens responsible for these infections. Chemotactic defects frequently are manifested as persistent cutaneous infections with associated adenitis. Bacteremia and metastatic spread of infection is unusual in patients with pure chemotactic defects, probably because phagocytosis frequently proceeds normally once neutrophils arrive at the site of infection.

Quantitative Defects of Neutrophil Function

The most common defect in granulocyte function results from an absolute reduction in the number of circulating neutrophils. The risk of infection increases progressively with both the duration and the magnitude of neutropenia below 1500 cells/mm^3, with a dramatic increase as levels fall below 500 neutrophils/mm^3. Neutropenias most often occur as a predictable result of chemotherapy for underlying malignancy, or as an idiosyncratic reaction to a pharmacologic agent. Less commonly, neutropenia may be inherited or result from hypersplenism or splenic sequestration of antibody-coated neutrophils.

Chemotactic Defects—Extrinsic Abnormalities

Decreased neutrophil chemotaxis is a feature of some diseases affecting the complement cascade, e.g., C3 and C5 deficiency. Chemotactic inhibitors have been described in patients with cirrhosis and increased levels of circulating IgA, and in diseases characterized by the presence of circulating immune complexes, such as rheumatoid arthritis and systemic lupus erythematosus. An inhibitor of chemotaxis has also been described in some patients with juvenile periodontitis, a familial disorder characterized by periodontitis in the absence of severe dental disease. Of particular note is the report of an acquired neutrophil chemotactic defect in two adults with gingival infection due to capnocytophaga. Sonicates of the organism inhibited the chemotactic response of neutrophils, and the patients' neutrophil function returned to normal with the eradication of the infection. These findings suggest that the chemotactic defect associated with some forms of periodontal disease may be due to the presence of bacterial products in the circulation.

Chemotactic Defects—Intrinsic Abnormalities

The Chédiak-Higashi syndrome is a rare autosomal recessive syndrome characterized by partial oculocutaneous albinism, rotatory nystagmus, peripheral neuropathy, abnormal NK cell function, and recurrent infection. There is a generalized dysfunction of granule-containing cells, and giant granules may appear in all types of leukocytes, melanocytes, Schwann cells, renal tubular cells, and thyroid cells. A primary neutrophil chemotactic defect is present, and cutaneous infection in these patients is common (see Chapter 6). Phagocytosis and the metabolic burst occur normally; however, bacterial killing rates are delayed because of abnormal degranulation and delayed delivery of granule enzymes to the phagosome. The biochemical abnormality underlying the neutrophil dysfunction in the Chédiak-Higashi syndrome is unknown, but amelioration of the chemotactic defect has been reported in some patients who have been treated with pharmacologic agents that affect microtubule assembly.

The hyperimmunoglobulinemia E (Job's) syndrome is characterized by eczema, recurrent cold staphylococcal skin abscesses, sinusitis, otitis media, recurrent pneumonia, and mucocutaneous candidiasis (see Chapter 6). The variable defect in neutrophil chemotactic activity of these patients correlates best with the severity of the eczema, but the biologic basis of this syndrome is unknown. IgE levels are markedly elevated, and the serum from these patients contains specific antistaphylococcal and anticandidal IgE antibodies. Such antibodies are not found in normal individuals, in patients with hyperimmunoglobulinemia E due to atopic disease or parasitic infection, or in patients with chronic staphylococcal infections. The mononuclear cells from patients with Job's syndrome spontaneously produce a factor that inhibits the chemotactic responses of normal neutrophils and of monocytes. Monocytes from other individuals, either with or without atopy, fail to produce this factor. These clinical and laboratory findings suggest that endogenous histamine, an inhibitor of neutrophil chemotaxis, may play an important role in the pathogenesis of this syndrome. This contention is supported by the fact that certain histamine inhibitors improve the chemotactic responsiveness of some patients' neutrophils in vitro.

Other, rarer abnormalities of neutrophil function were found in a patient with defective actin polymerization and in another patient whose cells lacked a membrane glycoprotein (GP-110).

ABNORMAL PHAGOCYTOSIS

Impaired Opsonization

The serum from patients with inherited or acquired hypo- gammaglobulinemia or deficiencies of the early complement components, especially C3, is unable to support normal opsonization. Consequently, these patients suffer from recurrent infections due to encapsulated bacteria such as pneumococci, *Haemophilus influenzae,* and *Neisseria meningitidis.*

Impaired Internalization

An individual has been described whose neutrophils exhibited normal chemotaxis but abnormal phagocytosis. Opsonization was unimpaired, and the number of C3 and IgG receptors on the neutrophils' cell membrane was normal. However, neutrophil functions coupled to these receptors (ingestion, degranulation, metabolic burst) were impaired. Most important, these same responses were normal when certain soluble stimuli were used to bypass these receptors. A glycoprotein, GP-150, was missing from the cell membrane of the neutrophils. The demonstration of the underlying cause of this patient's defect is important because it serves to underscore the specificity of structure function relationships at the level of the neutrophil cell surface.

Abnormal Intracellular Killing—Defective Membrane Oxidase System

Decreased Respiratory Burst

Chronic Granulomatous Disease (CGD). Although autosomal forms have been described, CGD is most commonly inherited in an X-linked manner. Seventy-eight percent of affected individuals present with recurrent and prolonged infection during the first year of life. Infections include pyogenic dermatitis, suppurative adenitis, recurrent pneumonia with abscess formation, stomatitis, enteritis, and colitis. One third of the patients may have abscesses in the liver or perihepatic region. Osteomyelitis is common and is noteworthy for its relatively frequent causation by *Serratia marcescens,* and involvement of the metacarpal and metatarsal bones. Although *Staphylococcus aureus* is the pathogen isolated from infected areas in slightly over half the cases, gram-negative bacteria account for 75 percent of all septic episodes and 80 percent of fatal septicemias. Infections caused by catalase-negative organisms, e.g., streptococci, are uncommon because hydrogen peroxide produced by these bacteria effectively circumvents the biochemical lesion in the neutrophil. Physical findings commonly include failure to thrive, dermatitis, adenopathy, and hepatosplenomegaly, which on pathologic examination frequently demonstrates noncaseating granulomata. Leukocytosis, anemia, and hyperglobulinemia are common.

Chemotaxis, phagocytosis, and degranulation are normal. (The defect in CGD lies in the membrane oxidase system.) Various defects have been described: (1) ability to activate the oxidase system; (2) presence of an oxidase system that is functionally abnormal; and (3) absence of a nonfunctional oxidase system (see Chapter 6).

The diagnosis of CGD is established with the aid of the nitroblue tetrazolium (NBT) dye test. Reduction of this dye by neutrophils is primarily dependent on the production of superoxide; therefore it is negative in CGD. Diagnosis of CGD should be confirmed by the demonstration of normal phagocytosis and a marked reduction in the parameters of the metabolic burst. In order to detect abnormalities in the activation system, both soluble and particulate stimuli should be used in tests of oxidative function.

Glucose-6-Phosphate Dehydrogenase (G6PD) Deficiency. Neutrophil dysfunction is not observed in the common form of G6PD deficiency in blacks, which is due to the presence of an unstable enzyme. However, it does occur in rare cases of this deficiency in Caucasians who have less than 5 percent of the normal levels of G6PD. In the absence of G6PD, glucose cannot be metabolized by the hexose monophosphate shunt, and therefore NADPH, the critical substrate for the membrane oxidase system, cannot be regenerated from NADP. Neutrophils from these patients have an abnormal NBT test, but, in contrast to the classic form of CGD, additional stimulation of the cells with methylene blue fails to activate the hexose monophosphate shunt.

Enhanced Respiratory Burst

Myeloperoxidase Deficiency. Neutrophil myeloperoxidase deficiency is the most common qualitative defect in neutrophil function, with a frequency of 1 to 2 per 4000 people for whom leukocyte counts are performed. The mode of inheritance is uncertain, owing to the heterogeneous expression of the defect. The majority of these individuals are healthy, and only five have been reported who have had serious infections. Systemic candidiasis occurred in four of these patients, three of whom had diabetes mellitus. Neutrophils from these patients exhibit normal chemotaxis, phagocytosis, and degranulation, but the respiratory burst is enhanced. Although devoid of myeloperoxidase, these neutrophils are able to use an enhanced oxidative burst to kill ingested microorganisms. Nevertheless, there is a delay in intracellular killing that is more pronounced for fungi than for bacteria. These findings explain the apparent well-being of the majority of these individuals and the susceptibility of a few to fungal infections.

EVALUATING PHAGOCYTE FUNCTION

A total and differential white blood cell count and examination of the peripheral blood smear are the most important initial steps in the workup of patients with suspected abnormalities in neutrophil function. Given an appropriate clinical history and physical examination, determinations should be made of serum Ig and complement levels, and an NBT test should be performed. Further evaluation depends on the results of these screening tests.

THERAPY FOR NEUTROPHIL DEFECTS

Antimicrobial Therapy

Prophylactic antibiotics such as dicloxacillin, rifampin, and trimethoprim-sulfamethoxazole are commonly administered to patients with abnormal neutrophil function, to prevent the recurrent and severe infections to which they are susceptible. The broad antimicrobial spectrum of trimethoprim-sulfamethoxazole against both gram-positive and gram-negative bacteria, coupled with its penetration and concentration within neutrophils, probably accounts for its effectiveness in reducing infections in patients with CGD. In vitro studies have also demonstrated enhanced nonoxidative killing of certain organisms by neutrophils in the presence of sublethal concentrations of cell-wall active antibiotics, but the significance of these findings for patient management has not been determined.

Granulocyte Transfusion

Neutrophil transfusions have been successfully used in granulocytopenic patients and in a limited number of individuals with neutrophil bactericidal defects and progressive infection. Although leukocyte transfusions may be lifesaving in these patients, associated complications, such as cytomegalovirus infection, allosensitization to HLA antigens, difficulties in procurement, risks to the donor, cost of the procedure, and an increased incidence of acute pulmonary reactions when transfusions are given in conjunction with amphotericin B, have limited the use of this procedure. The latter complication is of particular concern, since one accepted indication for neutrophil transfusions is the treatment of unrelenting fungal infection in the neutropenic host. In addition, some patients with CGD are missing a Kell-related antigen on the surface of their neutrophils and red cells. Failure to recognize this antigenic abnormality can result in severe transfusion reactions. Thus, leukocyte transfusions seem best reserved for the individual patient with severe granulocytopenia or functionally defective neutrophils who has a serious bacterial or fungal infection that has not responded to appropriate antimicrobial therapy.

Bibliography

Babior, B. M.: Oxygen-dependent microbial killing by phagocytes. N. Engl. J. Med. 298:659, 1978.

Babior, B. M., and Crowley, C. A.: Chronic granulomatous disease and other disorders of killing by phagocytes. *In* Steinbury, J. B., Wyngaarden, J. B., Frederickson, D. S., et al. (eds.): The Metabolic Basis of Inherited Disease, 5th ed. New York, McGraw-Hill, 1983, p. 1969.

Clark, R. A.: Chemotactic factors trigger their own oxidative inactivation by human neutrophils. J. Immunol. 129:2725, 1982.

Fletcher, M. P., and Gallin, J. I.: Degranulating stimuli increase the availability of receptors on human neutrophils for the chemoattractant f-met-leu-phe. J. Immunol. 124:1585, 1980.

Gallin, J. I.: Abnormal phagocyte chemotaxis: pathophysiology, clinical manifestations, and management of patients. Rev. Infect. Dis. 3:1196, 1981.

Gallin, J. I., Buescher, E. S., Seligmann, B. E., et al.: Recent advances in chronic granulomatous disease. Ann. Intern. Med. 99:657, 1983.

Griffin, F. M., Griffin, J. H., Leider, J. E., et al.: Studies on the mechanism of phagocytosis. I. Requirements for circumferential attachment of particle bound ligands to specific receptors on the macrophage plasma membrane. J. Exp. Med. 142:1263, 1975.

Klebanoff, S. J., and Clark, R. A.: The Neutrophil: Function and Clinical Disorders. Amsterdam, North Holland Biomedical Press, 1978.

Mandell, G. L.: Bactericidal activity of aerobic and anaerobic polymorphonuclear neutrophils. Infect. Immun. 9:337, 1974.

Segal, A. W., Cross, A. R., Garcia, R. D., et al.: Absence of cytochrome b_{-245} in chronic granulomatous disease: a multicenter European evaluation of its incidence and relevance. N. Engl. J. Med. 308:245, 1983.

Southwick, F. S., and Stossel, T. P.: Contractile proteins in leukocyte function. Semin. Hematol., 20:243, 1983.

5

HLA: The Major Histocompatibility Complex in Man*

FRITZ H. BACH, M.D.

Introduction	T-Lymphocyte Response to
Basic Genetics	HLA-Encoded Antigens
Methods Used to Define MHC-	HLA and Transplantation
Encoded Antigens	HLA and Disease
HLA—The Major Histocompati-	Concluding Remarks
bility Complex in Humans	

INTRODUCTION

In every mammalian species studied to date, there is a genetic region referred to as the major histocompatibility complex (MHC). Genes of the MHC encode cell-surface molecules that are strong transplantation antigens; i.e., they elicit a strong immunologic response in a recipient of a transplanted organ when the donor antigens are different from those of the recipient.

*This is paper #385 from the Immunobiology Research Center, Departments of Laboratory Medicine/Pathology, University of Minnesota, Minneapolis, MN 55455. This work was supported by NIH grants A1 17687, A1 18326, A1 19007, AM 13083; National Multiple Sclerosis Society grant #RG 1505-A-1, and March of Dimes grant 1–887.

65

The MHC of the mouse is referred to as H-2; in man the term for this genetic region is HLA.

The MHC-encoded antigens play a crucial role in determining the fate of transplanted tissues, but a wide variety of biologic phenomena have also been related to the MHC. Of clinical significance is the important observation that genes of the MHC control immunologic responsiveness to foreign antigens; these MHC genes are referred to as immune response (Ir) genes. A possible explanation for the association between certain MHC genes and disease is that the same genes control immune responsiveness to antigens that may be of import in any disease with which there is an association with a given MHC gene.

There is an intimate association between antigens encoded by MHC genes and the response of the various functionally disparate subpopulations of T lymphocytes. It has been hypothesized that the regulation of immune responsiveness by MHC genes relates, in large measure, to the ability of T lymphocytes to recognize the MHC products as alloantigens (foreign antigens recognized by one member of a species on cells of another member of the same species) as well as they recognize foreign antigens such as viruses. The manner by which T lymphocytes recognize the foreign antigen is referred to as "MHC-restricted recognition," i.e., the foreign antigen is not recognized alone but rather "in the context" of the animal's own MHC antigens. The phenomenon of MHC-restricted recognition will be discussed later.

The purpose of this chapter is to review briefly the basic genetics of the major histocompatibility complex in man (also referred to as the HLA region).

BASIC GENETICS

The 46 chromosomes of man are made up of 23 pairs; 22 pairs are *autosomes* and one pair consists of the *sex chromosomes*. One member of each pair of chromosomes is inherited from the father and the other member from the mother. Two such chromosomes are called *homologous chromosomes*. The sex chromosome pair of males consists of an X chromosome inherited from the mother and a Y chromosome inherited from the father; the female pair has two X chromosomes, one inherited from each parent.

Chromosomes are homologous—that is, fit into a pair—because the genetic information on each of the two chromosomes is concerned with the same phenotypic traits (with the exception of the sex chromosomes). For instance, one pair of homologous chromosomes may contain the genetic information (genes) that encodes the hemoglobin chains. A person can inherit the gene for Hgb chain B from one chromosome of the pair, perhaps from the father, and the gene for Hgb chain S from the chromosome of the mother. The region on the chromosome associated with a given trait is called a *locus* or location on the chromosome, and is very small compared to the entire length of the chromosome. The genetic material at this locus is referred to as a *gene* or *allele*. The latter term, *allele*, refers to the alternate forms of the gene that can exist at a locus. Thus, in the above example, the individual in question has a normal Hgb B allele and a mutant Hgb S allele.

Although there can be only two alleles at a given genetic locus, there may be more than two in the population. For example, in the ABO genetic system an individual can have the A allele from one parent and the B allele from the other parent, resulting in blood type AB. Another individual can have the O allele on both homologous chromosomes and thus have blood type O. These are thus three different alleles of the ABO locus. An individual with the same gene at a given locus on the two homologous chromosomes is said to be *homozygous* at that locus; with different alleles on the homologous chromosomes, the individual is said to be *heterozygous*. *Polymorphism* refers to the presence in the population of more than one allele at a given locus.

If two loci are close together on a chromosome, each of the two homologous chromosomal segments (carrying two alleles— one from each locus) will usually segregate (be transferred from parent to offspring) as a unit. Two such loci are said to be *linked*.

During meiosis, homologous chromosomes pair prior to reduction of the number of chromosomes from 46 (the *diploid* number) to 23 (the *haploid* number). During this time *recombination* can occur, resulting in an exchange or crossing-over of homologous regions of the paired chromosomes. After the recombinational event, the haploid set of chromosomes includes a chromosome, part of which was inherited from the father and part from the mother. The frequency of recombination between two linked loci is recognized as the fraction of gametes that contain alleles for both loci that had previously been on separate homologous chromosomes, indicating that a recombinational event has taken place. This recombination frequency is proportional to the genetic distance separating the loci. Two closely linked loci are usually inherited as a unit, i.e., the two alleles linked together normally segregate to the same gamete during meiosis. (Such a set of closely linked loci, which are usually inherited together, is sometimes called a *haplotype*.) Two loci relatively far apart on the chromosome may show an essentially independent assortment, segregating to the same gamete only 50 percent of the time.

A genetic concept that is important in analyzing the MHC is that of *linkage disequilibrium*, which refers to the inheritance of alleles of two closely linked loci. Given enough time in evolution, genetic theory would predict that the frequency with which alleles of two closely linked loci will be found together on the same chromosome does not differ significantly from that determined by their two individual gene frequencies. For instance, if an allele of locus A is found with a frequency of 0.1 and an allele of closely linked locus B with a frequency of 0.1, one would predict that, given equilibrium, the two alleles would be found on the same chromosome with a frequency not significantly different from $0.1 \times 0.1 = 0.01$. If these two genes are found together with a frequency significantly exceeding 0.01, this increased frequency is referred to as linkage disequilibrium.

As a general rule, in immunogenetic systems both alleles at a given histocompatibility locus are phenotypically expressed *(codominant)*.

METHODS USED TO DEFINE MHC-ENCODED ANTIGENS

Cell-surface molecules encoded by HLA genes are commonly detected by one or more of three methods. First, there are serologic techniques employing antisera, usually obtained from multiparous females who have formed antibodies to antigens present in fetal tissue inherited from the father and foreign to the mother. These antisera are used in a variety of tests, including, most commonly, complement-dependent antibody-mediated cytotoxicity.

Second, a mixed leukocyte culture (MLC) can be performed in which the stimulating cells are putatively homozygous for the HLA antigens that one wishes to measure. Such cells are referred to as homozygous typing cells (HTCs). The MLC test mixes peripheral blood leukocytes of two individuals and measures the proliferative response to T lymphocytes of one individual, the stimulating cell donor, as they recognize HLA-encoded foreign antigens present on the cells of the second individual. Stimulating cells are treated with either mitomycin C or x-irradiation so that they can present their antigens but will not themselves incorporate radioactive thymidine, the assay of the response of the responding T lymphocytes. When the stimulating cell is homozygous for a specificity that can cause stimulation in MLC, any responder cell carrying that specificity will not respond to it; thus the presence of a specificity on the responding cell is indicated by failure to respond to the relevant HTCs.

Third, a refinement of the MLC test, which allows the preparation of cellular reagents recognizing HLA-encoded antigens, is referred to as the primed lymphocyte typing (PLT) test, or secondary MLC.

The second and third tests discussed above both rely on the response of T lymphocytes to defined antigens. The utilization of both serologic and cellular methods for HLA antigen definition is valuable because the antigenic determinants on the various HLA molecules that are recognized serologically apparently differ from those that are recognized by T lymphocytes, even though the serologically defined (SD) and T lymphocyte–defined (LD) determinants may be on the same molecule.

HLA—THE MAJOR HISTOCOMPATIBILITY COMPLEX IN HUMANS

A schematic representation of the HLA complex is presented in Figure 5–1. The HLA-A, -B, and -C loci code for antigens that are present on essentially all cells of the body. The HLA-D locus was first defined using cellular techniques, i.e., proliferation in a primary MLC. The antigens associated with HLA-D, detectable by serologic methods, are referred to as the DR (D-related) antigens and are expressed on macrophages, B cells, and activated T cells. The loci of HLA have been divided into two classes. The A, B, and C loci of HLA are referred to as Class I, and the loci DR, DQ, and DP as Class II (Fig. 5–1). Although there are several differences between Class I and Class II products, the distinction is based on their molecular nature. Class I products consist of a 44,000-dalton "heavy chain" associated, noncovalently, with a 12,000-dalton protein, β_2-microglobulin (Fig. 5–2). The Class II products consist of noncovalently associated α-β heterodimers in which the α chain varies in molecular weight from 31,000 to 34,000 daltons and the β chain from 25,000 to 29,000 daltons (Fig. 5–2). It is therefore possible to refer to the HLA-A, -B and -C genes within the MHC, since only the heavy chain is encoded in the HLA region, β_2-microglobulin being

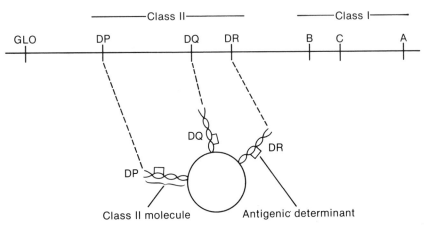

Figure 5–1. Schematic representation of the HLA complex located on the short arm of chromosome six. GLO (glyoxalase) is centromeric to the HLA complex. The DP, DQ, and DR loci encode for Class II molecules, and the A, B and C loci encode for Class I molecules.

The products of the HLA DP, DQ, and DR genes are randomly expressed on cells, e.g., macrophages, B cells, and some activated T cells. These Class II molecules express antigenic determinants that are detected by antibodies, i.e., DQ and DR, or by MLC, i.e., DP and Dw (not shown).

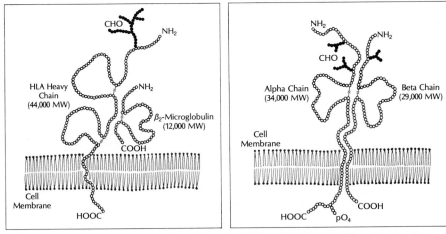

Figure 5–2. Structural diagrams of the Class I and Class II molecules. Class I molecules are expressed on all nucleated cells, whereas Class II molecules are expressed on macrophages, B cells, Langerhans cells, dendritic cells, and some activated T cells. (From Najarian, J. S.: Immunologic aspects of organ transplantation. Hosp. Pract. 17:61, 1982.)

encoded elsewhere. However, since the two separate genes (encoding the α and β chains) of each Class II product appear to be included with the HLA region, one cannot refer simply to "the DR gene," but must indicate whether the DRα or DRβ gene is meant.

Presented in Table 5–1 are the currently recognized antigens of HLA as detected by serologic methods and by both primary and secondary mixed leukocyte culture responses to HTCs. As noted, the HLA-A and -B loci are markedly polymorphic, with a finer definition of determinants that can be recognized by specific sera; the HLA-C locus is not as polymorphic as HLA-A and -B.

Table 5–1. Recognized HLA Specificities

HLA-A	HLA-B	HLA-C	HLA-D	HLA-DR	DP	DQ
HLA-A1	HLA-B5	HLA-Cw1	HLA-Dw1	HLA-DR1	DP1	DQ1
HLA-A2	HLA-B7	HLA-Cw2	HLA-Dw2	HLA-DR2	DP2	DQ2
HLA-A3	HLA-B8	HLA-Cw3	HLA-Dw3	HLA-DR3	DP3	DQ3
HLA-A9	HLA-B12	HLA-Cw4	HLA-Dw4	HLA-DR4	DP4	
HLA-A10	HLA-B13	HLA-Cw5	HLA-Dw5	HLA-DR5	DP5	
HLA-A11	HLA-B14	HLA-Cw6	HLA-Dw6	HLA-DRw6	DP6	
HLA-Aw19	HLA-B15	HLA-Cw7	HLA-Dw7	HLA-DR7		
HLA-Aw23(9)	HLA-Bw16	HLA-Cw8	HLA-Dw8	HLA-DRw8		
HLA-Aw24(9)	HLA-B17		HLA-Dw9	HLA-DRw9		
HLA-A25 (10)	HLA-B18		HLA-Dw10	HLA-DRw10		
HLA-A26 (10)	HLA-Bw21		HLA-Dw11	HLA-DRw11(5)		
HLA-A28	HLA-Bw22		HLA-Dw12	HLA-DRw12(5)		
HLA-A29	HLA-B27		HLA-Dw13	HLA-		
HLA-Aw30	HLA-Bw35		HLA-Dw14	DRw13(w6)		
HLA-Aw31	HLA-B37		HLA-Dw15	HLA-		
HLA-Aw32	HLA-Bw38(w16)		HLA-Dw16	DRw14(w6)		
HLA-Aw33	HLA-Bw39(w16)		HLA-Dw17(w7)			
HLA-Aw34	HLA-B40		HLA-Dw18(w6)			
HLA-Aw36	HLA-Bw41		HLA-Dw19(w6)			
HLA-Aw43	HLA-Bw42					
	HLA-Bw44(12)					
	HLA-Bw45(12)					
	HLA-Bw46					
	HLA-Bw47					
	HLA-Bw48					
	HLA-Bw49(w21)					
	HLA-Bw50(w21)					
	HLA-Bw51(5)					
	HLA-Bw52(5)					
	HLA-Bw53					
	HLA-Bw54(w22)					
	HLA-Bw55(w22)					
	HLA-Bw56(w22)					
	HLA-Bw57(17)					
	HLA-Bw58(17)					
	HLA-Bw59					
	HLA-Bw60(40)					
	HLA-Bw61(40)					
	HLA-Bw62(15)					
	HLA-Bw63(15)					
	HLA-Bw4[a]					
	HLA-Bw6					

The HLA-D locus is formally defined by response in a primary mixed leukocyte culture to HTCs. The HTC technique makes use of stimulating cells that are homozygous for HLA-D antigen(s). The cells of a tested individual who does not carry the antigens present on the HTC will give a strong proliferative response to the selected HTC. If an individual carries the antigen(s) present on that HTC, then there should be a relatively weak, or absent, response by the cells of that individual to the same HTC. A number of HLA-D antigens (or antigenic clusters) have been defined by this method. These are listed as HLA-Dw1 through Dw19 in Table 5–1. (The "w" designates a "workshop" number if the antigen is not yet very well defined.)

Fourteen antigens that are associated with the HLA-D region have been recognized serologically and have been referred to as HLA-DR1 through HLA-Drw14 (Table 5–1). These antigens represent a segregated series (i.e., they are apparently encoded by allelic genes). The DR antigens are expressed on Class II molecules encoded in the HLA-D region. A second series of serologically detectable antigens encoded in the HLA-D region is referred to as DQ (previously known as DS). The DQ antigens are referred to as being "supertypic" to the DR antigens, i.e., a given serologically defined determinant of the DQ series is present whenever any one of several DR specificities is present. For instance, essentially all Caucasian individuals who are DR1, DR2, or DRw6 will also be DQ1. Thus, several different DR antigens are included, at the population level, within this serologically defined DQ specificity. It is now appreciated that DQ antigens are expressed on a Class II molecule closely linked to the DR-containing Class II molecule (Fig. 5–1).

The relationship of the antigens defined with HTCs or PLT reagents to those defined serologically is uncertain. There are determinants associated both with the DR product and the DQ product that stimulate T lymphocytes. These T lymphocyte–defined (LD) determinants are, however, subtypic to the serologically defined DR specificities. As an example, individuals positive for the serologically defined specificity DR4 can carry any one of five different LD specificities defined either with HTCs or PLT reagents. Therefore, the genes coding for DR- and DQ-containing molecules are in very high linkage disequilibrium, and LD specificities defined with HTCs or PLT reagents relate largely to determinants expressed on those Class II molecules.

Other genes have been mapped to the region between the DR and DQ loci and the left-most marker of the HLA region, the locus coding for the enzyme glyoxalase (GLO). A segregated series of specificities mapping in this region and detected with PLT reagents has been referred to as the DP product (previously called SB; see Fig. 5–1).

T-LYMPHOCYTE RESPONSE TO HLA-ENCODED ANTIGENS

The HLA molecules are part of a signaling system between T lymphocytes and other immune cells, in particular antigen-presenting cells (APC) such as macrophages and dendritic cells. T-cell activation is determined by the poorly understood inter-action between Class I and Class II molecules with their specific T-cell receptors. Foreign (allogeneic) HLA molecules can act as antigen (alloantigen) by themselves in this interaction; this is characterized as allorecognition. Self (autologous) HLA mole-cules are generally not recognized by autologous T cells. When a modifying influence, such as a virus, combines with the au-tologous Class I or Class II antigen on the surface of an APC, the combination may cause activation of a T-cell receptor. This regulating function of HLA molecules is referred to as HLA-restricted recognition (Fig. 5–3). The successful activation of the T-cell receptor is a necessary step in inducing the immune

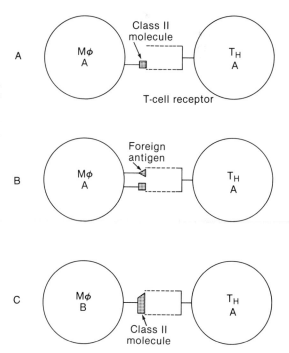

Figure 5–3. Activation of helper T cells (T$_H$) requires activation of the T-cell receptor. *A*, Class II molecules expressed on macro-phages (Mϕ) from individual A are not recognized by A's T$_H$. *B*, For-eign antigens, e.g., a virus ex-pressed on Mϕ, may combine with Class II molecules to form deter-minants that will activate T$_H$ from individual A. *C*, Class II molecules from a different individual, B, in itself may be sufficient to activate individual A's T$_H$ receptor. Activa-tion of cytotoxic T cells requires the similar recognition of Class I molecules.

response to foreign antigens (Fig. 5–4). Certain patterns have emerged from the two categories of recognition, in that there is the differential response to Class I and Class II antigens of functionally disparate subpopulations of T lymphocytes.

Cytotoxic T lymphocytes (Tc) primarily recognize Class I antigens or foreign antigens restricted by Class I antigens. Conversely, helper T lymphocytes (Th) preferentially recognize Class II antigens in both of these situations. Some exceptions have been noted to this general rule—at least for allorecognition, Class II antigens can serve as targets for Tc, and an occasional Th can respond to Class I antigens—but the general rule is applicable in most situations. Very few restricted recognition exceptions have been reported.

Suppressor T lymphocytes (Ts) also appear to be activated by HLA antigens, but less is known of this than of the Th and Tc activations. The specificity of Ts also appears to be to Class II antigens, but the exact cellular nature of the suppressive response to Class II antigens has not yet been elucidated. Ts do relate to some extent to Class II antigens as do Th, and to that extent the Class II antigens apparently "regulate" the immune response by creating the balance of help and suppression, which are the regulatory forces for immunologic responsiveness.

HLA AND TRANSPLANTATION

Clinical studies give evidence that the HLA complex is of enormous importance in determining the success of such transplanted organs as the kidney or bone marrow. Kidney graft survival, after many years of observation, is almost 100 percent when the donor is an HLA identical sibling, i.e., an individual who has inherited the same HLA chromosomes from the parents. Graft survival is significantly less if the donor differs by one HLA haplotype from the recipient, and if donor and recipient differ by both HLA haplotypes, graft survival is even worse.

Until quite recently, identity for the HLA complex was essential to achieve engraftment of a bone marrow transplant and to avoid a fatal graft-versus-host (GVH) reaction. The first successful matched bone marrow transplants were performed in 1968 after recognition that, based on murine studies, identity for the HLA might allow establishment of long-term chimerism in the recipient following bone marrow transplantation. Serious attempts to transplant without having an HLA identical sibling donor have been made only during the past few years.

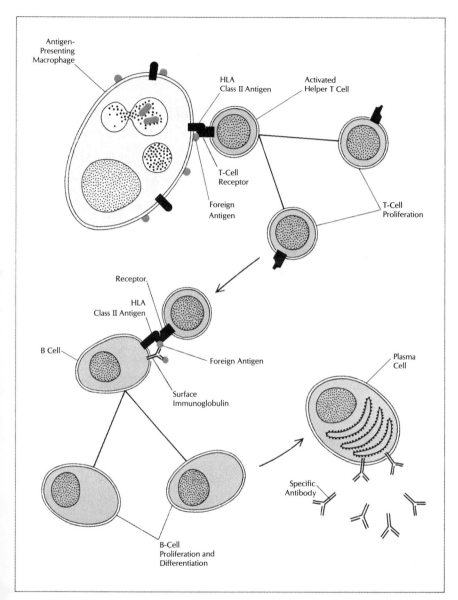

Figure 5–4. An effective antibody response to a T-cell–dependent antigen requires that class-specific HLA antigen recognition occur at three different levels. The HLA antigen must be present on the plasma membrane of the antigen-presenting macrophage; it must be recognized by the specifically activated helper T cell; and it must be present along with specific surface immunoglobulin on the B lymphocyte if that cell is to proliferate and differentiate to an antibody-secreting plasma cell. The interaction between the B cell and the helper T cell is hypothetical but in accord with experimental observation. (From McDevitt, H. O.: The HLA system and its relation to disease. Hosp. Pract. 20:61, 1985.)

The dramatic influence of HLA on kidney graft survival raised the major question of whether it is more important to match for the Class I or for the Class II antigens. The Class I antigens have for many years been considered of greater importance, but this may have been because the Class II antigens had not been very well defined. Most of the data accumulated in the last decade suggests that matching for Class II antigens is of greater importance. A large number of studies of living related donors have demonstrated that graft survival is significantly improved by utilizing a donor-recipient combination in which there is a very weak response in MLC, i.e., the donor and recipient are well-matched and do not differ for antigens that stimulate a strong proliferative response in the MLC. Typing donor and recipient serologically for the DR antigens has not yielded dramatic results equal to those obtained when MLC matching was undertaken. Many studies, however, matching for only the serologically defined DR (and in some cases DQ) antigens have revealed graft survival improvement. The complexity of LD specificities subtypic to DR, as well as the existence of the DP product, accounts for the failure of DR matching alone to yield survival results as good as those when the MLC is used as the measure of compatibility.

Whatever the relative role of Class I and Class II antigens in the matching process, the overall importance of HLA in graft survival is well-established.

HLA AND DISEASE

The demonstration by Lilly and coworkers that genes of the murine H-2 complex play a role in susceptibility to viral leukemogenesis broadened significantly the possible biologic importance of the MHC. Lilly found that certain loci of the H-2 complex affect the progression of both Gross and Friend virus–associated diseases. There are at least two genes important in the pathogenesis of both diseases; one gene segregates independently of H-2, while the other is linked to H-2. The first demonstration that genes of the MHC may be associated with certain diseases in man was provided in 1967 by Amiel, who found that there was an increased frequency in patients with Hodgkin's disease of HLA-4c (an HLA Class I antigen that has now been renamed).

Both positive and negative associations between an HLA antigen and a given disease are based on the frequency of the antigen in a normal control population as compared with the frequency of that same antigen in patients having the disease. For example, a positive association has been detected between insulin-dependent diabetes (IDD) and the antigens DR3 and DR4. The antigen DR2 is significantly decreased in those patients as compared with the normals, an example of a negative association.

Another method of defining the association with disease is to determine the relative risk of developing the disease by an individual who carries a given antigen as compared with an individual who does not carry that antigen; i.e., an individual who carries both DR3 and DR4 is approximately 50 to 60 times as likely (from our own data) to have IDD as an individual who has neither of these antigens.

A hypothesis to explain the association between HLA antigens and a given disease is to link the immune response (Ir) genes to the pathogenetic mechanisms underlying that disease. The association between the HLA antigens and a given disease would then be attributed either to that antigen itself playing a role in controlling immune responsiveness or to linkage disequilibrium between the genes coding for the antigens and the Ir genes. This seems highly likely for a number of different entities, especially those in which immune phenomena are strongly implicated.

A large number of diseases have been shown to have significant associations with various HLA antigens. One of the earliest and most dramatic of these associations is between the antigen HLA-B27 and a number of diseases, including ankylosing spondylitis and Reiter's disease. Associations for ankylosing spondylitis are very strong. HLA-B27 is present in 6 to 8 percent of the normal Caucasian population and yet is found in 85 percent or more of patients with ankylosing spondylitis. The relative risk of an individual who is HLA-B27–positive for developing ankylosing spondylitis is, in different studies, anywhere from 75-fold to 150-fold greater than for an individual negative for HLA-B27. This very strong role probably played by the gene for HLA-B27 in ankylosing spondylitis is supported by the finding that, in Japan, where HLA-B27 is an extremely rare antigen in the normal population, approximately two thirds of patients with ankylosing spondylitis are HLA-B27–positive.

Most associations between HLA and disease are with the Class II antigens, and the HLA-DR2, -DR3, and -DR4 antigens have been most commonly implicated, in either a positive or negative association, with a wide variety of diseases. The association of a Class II antigen with a given disease can, in some cases, be as strong as that of HLA-B27 with ankylosing spondylitis; for instance, patients with gluten enteropathy are HLA-DR3 in almost 100 percent of cases.

Haplotypes containing HLA-B8 and -DR3 are more common in the normal population than expected, and therefore represent a genetic dysequilibrium between these two HLA antigens. The HLA-B8/DR3 haplotype is positively associated with multiple autoimmune diseases, e.g., systemic lupus erythematosus and Graves' disease.

In addition, the HLA-B8/DR3 haplotype has been associated with altered immunoreactivity in a normal population. Decreased antigen degradation and removal of immune complexes by the reticuloendothelial system is associated with normal individuals expressing the HLA-B8/DR3 haplotype. These abnormalities are also observed in the HLA-B8/DR3–associated disease, systemic lupus erythematosus.

Although there is a striking association between certain diseases and the frequency of given HLA antigens, such association is usually not absolute. There are many reasons why this may be so. Understanding the many reasons for these phenomena is important both in evaluating the meaning of these associations and in improving our ability to determine more significant associations.

First, the genes of the HLA that are associated in increased frequency with a given disease may not be the HLA antigens themselves but rather genes linked to those determining the disease susceptibility. Therefore, the association depends on the linkage disequilibrium or interactions between the disease susceptibility genes and HLA genes. To the extent that linkage disequilibrium is not absolute, any association will be less than complete.

Second, there is the problem of disease heterogeneity. The diseases that we classify under one name may actually be a collection of somewhat different entities, and any strong association between an HLA susceptibility gene and one of these disease entities will be obscured by the fact that a second entity included within this same general disease category may not be associated with the same disease susceptibility gene.

Third, the HLA molecules and their antigens are still being subdivided and redefined as new sera and other reagents become available. This heterogeneity will lead to the same difficulties of finding significant associations as will disease heterogeneity.

Finally, to the extent that genes segregating independently of HLA are important in the pathogenesis of a given disease process, the genetic complexity of different individuals will influence our ability to find significant associations between one of the genes (that linked to HLA) and the disease itself.

CONCLUDING REMARKS

The major histocompatibility complex was first defined by the role played by genes of that complex in graft rejection. Immune response genes are included within the complex, and are probably identical to the genes encoding the histocompatibility antigens, since those antigens determine restricted recognition and thus regulation of the immune response. This was of the greatest import in focusing further attention on the MHC.

Studies utilizing recombinant DNA technology as well as extensive investigations at the protein level of the Class I and Class II HLA products give promise that we will soon better understand how HLA functions in its many different roles.

Bibliography

Ameil, J. L.: Study of the leucocyte phenotypes in Hodgkin's disease. *In* Custoni, E. S., Mattiuz, P., and Tosi, R. (eds.): Histocompatibility Testing 1967. Copenhagen, Munksgaard, 1967, p. 79.

Blumenthal, M. N., and Bach, F. H.: Immunogenetics of atopic disease. *In* Middleton, E., Reed, C. E., and Ellis, E. F. (eds.): Allergy: Principles and Practices. St. Louis, C. V. Mosby Co., 1983, Vol. 1, pp. 11–17.

Bubbers, J. E., Blank, K. J., Freedman, H. A., et al.: Mechanisms of the H-2 effect on viral leukemogenesis. Scand. J. Immunol. 6:533, 1977.

Duquesnoy, R., Marrari, M., and Vierira, J.: Definition of MB and MT antigens by Eighth International Histocompatibility Workshop: B cell alloantiserum clusters. *In* Terasaki, P. I. (ed.): Histocompatibility Testing 1980. Los Angeles, UCLA Tissue Typing Laboratory, 1980, p. 861.

Hartzman, R. J., Pappas, F., Romano, P. J., et al.: Dissociation of HLA-DR using primed LD typing. Transplant. Proc. 10:809, 1978.

Reinsmoen, N. L., and Bach, F. H.: Five HLA-D clusters associated with HLA-DR4. Hum. Immunol. 4:249, 1982.

Ryder, L. P., Anderson, E., and Svejgaard, A. (ed.): HLA and disease registry. Third report. Copenhagen, Munksgaard, 1979.

Sheehy, M. J., Sondel, P. M., Bach, M. L., et al.: HLA LD (lymphocyte defined) typing: a rapid assay with primed lymphocytes. Science 188:1308, 1975.

Svejgaard, A., Platz, P., and Ryder, L.: Disease studies: insulin dependent diabetes mellitus. *In* Terasaki, P. I. (ed.): Histocompatibility Testing 1980. Los Angeles, UCLA Tissue Typing Laboratory, 1980, p. 638.

Terasaki, P. I. (ed.): Histocompatibility Testing 1980. Los Angeles, UCLA Tissue Typing Laboratory, 1980.

6

Primary and Acquired Immunodeficiency Diseases

REBECCA H. BUCKLEY, M.D.

Outline continued on following page

81

Other Primary Immunodeficiencies (Complement and Phagocytic Cells) Complement Component Deficiencies Phagocytic Cell Dysfunctions Acquired Immune Deficiencies Chronic Mucocutaneous Candidiasis	Acquired Immune Deficiency Syndrome (AIDS) **Treatment** Treatment of Antibody Deficiency Disorders Treatment of Cellular Immunodeficiency

INTRODUCTION

Since the discovery of the first human immunodeficiency disease, agammaglobulinemia, just over three decades ago, information regarding such defects has accrued at an enormous rate, and new abnormalities are being described each year. Immunodeficiency diseases may involve any of the components of the immune system, including lymphocytes, phagocytic cells and the complement proteins. Despite the increase in knowledge of functional derangements and cellular abnormalities in the various primary immunodeficiency disorders, the fundamental biologic errors for most of them remain unknown. Exceptions include two defects accompanied by purine salvage pathway enzyme deficiencies; adenosine deaminase (ADA) in some cases of autosomal recessive severe combined immunodeficiency disease (SCID), and purine nucleoside phosphorylase (PNP) in some patients with Nezelof's syndrome.

The genetic errors in many other immunodeficiencies must, by definition, be located on the X chromosome. None of the primary defects have associated deficiencies of particular HLA antigens; thus, it is unlikely they involve defects of HLA-linked immune response genes on chromosome 6. Trace amounts of immunoglobulins of all five isotypes can usually be found in the serum of even the most severely agammaglobulinemic patient. Therefore, immunoglobulin deficiency states are probably not due to deletions of genes encoding for immunoglobulin heavy chains. This does not exclude the possibility of other regulatory gene defects.

Primary, or congenital, immunodeficiency is rare. Agammaglobulinemia occurs with a frequency of 1:50,000 and severe combined immunodeficiency with a frequency of 1:100,000 to 1:500,000 live births. Selective absence of serum and secretory

IgA is the most common defect, with reported incidences ranging from 0.03 to 0.97 percent.

CLASSIFICATION OF IMMUNODEFICIENCY SYNDROMES

Classifications of immunodeficiency disorders have postulated the cellular levels at which the defects occur. Cells with mature differentiation markers of both T and B lymphocytes have, however, been found in most of the known defects, indicating that in most cases the suspect cell line is not missing but malfunctional (Table 6–1).

Antibody Deficiency Disorders

Antibody deficiency occurs clinically either as a congenital or an "acquired" abnormality, with deficiencies in all or selected classes of immunoglobulins. These patients are identified when they have recurrent infections with encapsulated bacteria or fail to respond to therapy.

X-Linked Agammaglobulinemia (Bruton's Agammaglobulinemia)

A majority of boys afflicted with this malady are well during the first 6 to 9 months of life, presumably protected by maternally transmitted immunoglobulin. Thereafter, unless treated with prophylactic antibiotics or immune serum globulin (ISG), they acquire repeated infections with virulent extracellular pyogenic organisms such as pneumococci, streptococci, and Haemophilus. The most common infections are sinusitis, pneumonia, otitis, furunculosis, meningitis, and septicemia. Patients with this disorder, however, usually grow normally unless they develop bronchiectasis or persistent enterovirus infections. Chronic fungal infections and *Pneumocystis carinii* pneumonia rarely occur unless there is an associated neutropenia. Responses to viral infections and live virus vaccines are normal, except for hepatitis virus and enterovirus infections. Paralysis following the administration of polio vaccine has occasionally occurred, presumably from mutations of the persisting live vaccine viruses. In addition, more than 30 such patients have developed chronic progressive and eventually fatal CNS infections with various echoviruses.

The diagnosis of X-linked agammaglobulinemia is suspected when serum concentrations of IgG, IgA, and IgM are far below

Table 6–1. Classification of Immunodeficiency Disorders

Disorders	Functional Deficiencies	Presumed Cellular Level of Defect
I. Antibody Deficiency Disorders		
A. X-linked agammaglobulinemia (Bruton's)	Antibody	Pre-B cell
B. Common variable immunodeficiency	Antibody	B lymphocyte
C. Selective IgA deficiency	IgA antibody	IgA B lymphocyte
D. Secretory component deficiency	Secretory IgA	Mucosal epithelium
E. Selective IgM deficiency	IgM antibody	T helper cells
F. Immunodeficiency with elevated IgM	IgG and IgA antibodies	IgG, IgA B lymphocytes
G. Transient hypogammaglobulinemia of infancy	None; immunoglobulins low but antibodies present	Unknown
H. Antibody deficiency with near-normal immunoglobulins	Antibody	Unknown; ?B cell
I. X-linked lymphoproliferative disease	Anti-EBNA antibody	B cell; ?also T cell
II. Cellular Immunodeficiency Disorders		
A. Thymic hypoplasia (DiGeorge's syndrome)	T-cellular; some antibody	Dysmorphogenesis of 3rd & 4th pharyngeal pouches
B. Cellular immunodeficiency with immunoglobulins (Nezelof's syndrome)	T-cellular; some antibody	Unknown; ?thymus; ?T cell
1. With purine nucleoside phosphorylase deficiency	T-cellular; some antibody	T cell
III. Severe Combined Immunodeficiency (SCID) Syndromes		
A. Autosomal recessive	Antibody and T-cellular	Unknown
B. Due to ADA deficiency	Antibody and T-cellular	T cell
C. X-linked recessive	Antibody and T-cellular	Unknown
D. Bare lymphocyte syndrome	Antibody and T-cellular	All cells with HLA-A, -B and -C antigens
E. SCID with leukopenia (reticular dysgenesis)	Antibody, T-cellular, and polymorphonuclear cells	Unknown

Table continued on opposite page

the 95 percent confidence limits for appropriate age and race-matched controls (Fig. 6–1). The demonstration of severe and persistent antibody deficiency in serum and external secretions is important to distinguish this disorder from transient hypogammaglobulinemia of infancy. Tests for natural antibodies to blood group substances and/or for antibodies responding to standard courses of immunizing antigens (diphtheria, tetanus and pneumococcal) are useful in this regard. Polymorphonuclear functions

Table 6–1. Classification of Immunodeficiency Disorders *Continued*

Disorders	Functional Deficiencies	Presumed Cellular Level of Defect
IV. Partial Combined Immunodeficiency Disorders		
A. Immunodeficiency with thrombocytopenia and eczema (Wiskott-Aldrich syndrome)	Antibody and T-cellular	Unknown
B. Ataxia telangiectasia	Antibody and T-cellular	B lymphocyte; helper T lymphocyte
C. Immunodeficiency with short-limbed dwarfism	T cellular	G1 cycle of many cells
D. Immunodeficiency with thymoma	Antibody; some T-cellular	B lymphocyte; excessive T suppressor cells
E. Hyperimmunoglobulinemia E syndrome	Specific immune responses; excessive IgE	Unknown
V. Other Primary Immunodeficiencies		
A. Complement component deficiencies	Depends on component; abnormal CH50 for all	Unknown
B. Phagocytic cell dysfunctions		
1. Chédiak-Higashi-Steinbrink syndrome	Defective NK, chemotaxis, and microbicidal function	Lysosomes of many cells
2. Chronic granulomatous disease of childhood	Impaired intracellular killing of bacteria and fungi	Membrane-bound NADPH oxidase of phagocytic cells
VI. Acquired Immune Deficiencies		
A. Chronic mucocutaneous candidiasis	Variable cellular	T, B cells; ?antigen overload
B. Acquired immune deficiency syndrome (AIDS)	Helper T-cellular, NK, B cellular	HTLV-III infected T helper cells

are usually normal if heat stable opsonins (e.g., IgG antibodies) are present, but some patients with this condition have had transient, persistent or cyclic neutropenia.

The total number of T cells is usually increased and the percentages of T-cell subsets are normal in most patients. In contrast, there is an absence or small number of blood lymphocytes bearing surface immunoglobulin, "Ia-like" antigens, the EBV receptor, or antigens reactive with specific anti–B-cell sera. Nevertheless, normal numbers of pre-B cells are found in the bone marrow. Hypoplasia of adenoids, tonsils, and peripheral lymph nodes is the rule; germinal centers are not found in lymph nodes, and plasma cells are rare. Cell-mediated immune responses are intact, and the thymus is morphologically normal.

The overall prognosis is reasonably good if antibody replace-

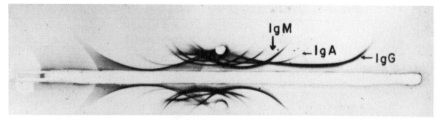

Figure 6–1. Immunoelectrophoretic analysis of normal human serum (upper well) and congenital agammaglobulinemic serum (lower well). Goat anti-whole human serum was used in the trough. Precipitin arcs for IgA, IgG, and IgM are not visible in the lower pattern. (From Buckley, R. H.: *In* Smith, D. T., Conant, N. F., and Willett, H. P. (eds.): Zinsser Microbiology, 14th ed. New York, Appleton-Century-Crofts, 1968, p. 291.)

ment therapy is instituted early, except in patients who develop polio, persistent enterovirus infection or lymphoreticular malignancy (of which an incidence as high as 6 percent has been reported). Many patients may develop crippling sinopulmonary disease despite antibody replacement, since it is not possible to replace secretory IgA at the mucosal surface.

Common Variable Immunodeficiency

Common variable immunodeficiency, or idiopathic late-onset immunoglobulin deficiency, may resemble X-linked agammaglobulinemia. The principal differences are a later age of onset, somewhat less severe infections, and an almost equal sex distribution. Patients with common variable immunodeficiency may have normal or enlarged tonsils and lymph nodes, and splenomegaly is common. The serum immunoglobulin and antibody deficiency may be as profound as in X-linked agammaglobulinemia (Fig. 6–1), and the kinds of infections and bacterial etiologic agents involved are the same. Thus far, only two cases of fatal echovirus meningoencephalitis have been documented in patients with common variable immunodeficiency.

This condition has been variably associated with a sprue-like syndrome, with or without nodular follicular lymphoid hyperplasia of the intestine; thymoma; alopecia areata; hemolytic anemia; gastric atrophy; achlorhydria; and pernicious anemia. Frequent complications include giardiasis (more often than in X-linked agammaglobulinemia), bronchiectasis, gastric carcinoma, lymphoreticular malignancy, and cholelithiasis. Lymphoid interstitial pneumonia, pseudolymphoma, amyloidosis, and noncaseating granulomata of the lungs, spleen, skin, and liver have also occurred.

There are normal numbers of circulating immunoglobulin-bearing B lymphocytes, and cortical follicles are present in the lymph nodes. The lymphocytes, however, do not differentiate in vivo into immunoglobulin-producing plasma cells nor in vitro even in the presence of the polyclonal B-cell activator, pokeweed mitogen. Thus, the defect in most patients is apparently due to abnormal terminal differentiation of the B-cell line. This disorder has occurred in first-degree relatives of some patients with selective IgA deficiency, and some patients with hyper IgM have later become panhypogammaglobulinemic (or vice versa). Accordingly, it is possible that all these diseases result from a defect leading to maturation arrests at various stages of B-cell development.

Selective IgA Deficiency

An isolated absence or near-absence (i.e., <10 mg/dl) of serum and secretory IgA is the most common immunodeficiency disorder. A recent study in Tennessee reported a frequency of 1:333 for IgA deficiency among putatively normal blood donors. While this disorder has been observed in apparently healthy individuals, it is commonly associated with ill health.

Infections occur predominantly in the respiratory, gastrointestinal, and urogenital tracts. Bacteria responsible are the same as in other types of antibody deficiency syndromes. Patients with this disorder do not have an undue susceptibility to viral agents. Children with IgA deficiency vaccinated with killed polio virus intranasally produced local IgM and IgG antibodies. Studies suggest that the IgM antibody is synthesized locally and combines with secretory piece for local secretion, as does IgA. Serum concentrations of other immunoglobulins are usually normal in patients with selective IgA deficiency, although an IgG_2 subclass deficiency has been reported in some and the usually elevated IgM may be of the low molecular weight variety. This can give artifactually high IgM levels with the agar diffusion technique due to faster diffusion secondary to lower molecular weight.

IgA antibodies against cow's milk and ruminant serum proteins are frequently found in IgA deficiency. Autoantibodies have also been found frequently, which may explain the association of IgA deficiency with collagen vascular and autoimmune diseases. Adults with this defect may develop a sprue-like syndrome that may or may not respond to a gluten-free diet.

The defect which accounts for selective IgA deficiency is unknown. More than 80 percent of the IgA-bearing B cells also coexpressed surface IgM and IgD (similar to cord blood B cells) in 10 of 11 IgA-deficient individuals. Normals have fewer than 10 percent triple isotype-bearing IgA B cells (IgA, IgD, IgM), suggesting a B-cell maturation arrest in the IgA-deficient patients. The occurrence of IgA deficiency in both males and females and in families suggests autosomal inheritance, which is apparently a recessive trait in some families and dominant, with variable expressivity, in others.

The presence of antibodies to IgA in the sera of 44 percent of patients with selective IgA deficiency is of great clinical significance. The intravenous administration of blood products or immune serum globulin (which contains a small amount of IgA) to IgA deficient patients is contraindicated, because they may develop severe or fatal anaphylactic reactions. Burks, Sampson, and Buckley (1986) have detected IgE antibodies to IgA in two patients with common variable immunodeficiency who had several episodes of anaphylaxis after infusions of IgA containing blood products. Additional circumstantial evidence implicates "IgE anti-IgA antibodies in the pathogenesis of anaphylactic reactions of IgA," but, as the authors also note, "it will be necessary to evaluate additional patients to confirm a general role for IgE antibodies in these reactions." The only treatment for IgA deficiency is appropriate antimicrobial therapy. The transport of IgA into the external secretions is an active process involving only locally produced IgA, therefore, even if passive replacement were possible (in the face of anti-IgA antibodies), injected IgA would not reach the mucosal surfaces.

Secretory Component Deficiency

One patient with chronic intestinal candidiasis and diarrhea has been described who lacked IgA in external secretions, despite having a normal serum IgA concentration. This was due to an absence of secretory piece, which prevented the normal transport of locally produced IgA onto mucous membrane surfaces.

Selective IgM Deficiency

There are few reported cases of selective IgM deficiency. Infections occurring in these patients include: septicemia due to meningococci and other gram-negative organisms, pneumococcal meningitis, tuberculosis, recurrent staphylococcal pyoderma, periorbital cellulitis, recurrent otitis, bronchiectasis, and other respiratory infections. There is no specific treatment; early and appropriate administration of antibiotics is recommended to avoid fatal septicemia.

Immunodeficiency with Elevated IgM

This disorder is characterized by very low serum concentrations of IgG and IgA, but either a normal or, more frequently, a markedly elevated concentration of polyclonal IgM. Patients with this defect, like patients with X-linked agammaglobulinemia, may develop recurrent pyogenic infections such as otitis media, sinusitis, pneumonia, and tonsillitis during the first or second year of life. Lymphoid hyperplasia, in contrast to the hypoplasia seen in X-linked agammaglobulinemia, is present in this disease and delays the diagnosis of immunodeficiency. There is also a greater frequency of autoimmune disorders than with some of the other antibody-deficiency syndromes. Hemolytic anemia and thrombocytopenia have occurred in several patients, and transient, persistent or cyclic neutropenia is common. Thymic-dependent lymphoid tissues and T-cell functions are usually normal, but several patients have had partial T-cell deficiencies. The occurrence of this disease in females makes it unlikely that this is always a sex-linked defect.

The precise defect in the hyper IgM syndrome is unknown. Normal or slightly reduced numbers of IgM and/or IgD B lymphocytes have been found in the blood of these patients. However, cultured B-cell lines from these patients synthesize only IgM, suggesting a B-cell maturation defect that prevents isotype switching. Treatment is the same as for agammaglobulinemia, because these patients are unable to make IgG antibodies.

Transient Hypogammaglobulinemia of Infancy

This condition results from a prolongation and exaggeration of the normal decline in serum immunoglobulin concentrations during the first 3 to 7 months of life. The finding of only 11 cases of transient hypogammaglobulinemia of infancy among more than 10,000 patients, whose sera were sent to the author for immunoglobulin studies over a 12-year period, indicates that this is not a common disorder. The 11 patients all could synthesize antibodies to human type A and B erythrocytes and to diphtheria and tetanus toxoids, usually by 6 to 11 months of age, and well before immunoglobulin concentrations became normal. There were no abnormalities in the percentages of lymphocyte subsets in these 11 patients. Gamma globulin replacement therapy is not indicated in this condition because passively administered IgG antibodies can suppress endogenous antibody formation, just as RhoGAM suppresses anti-D antibodies in Rh-negative mothers bearing Rh-positive infants.

Antibody Deficiency with Near-Normal Immunoglobulins

There have been a few reports describing patients with normal T-cell function and normal or near-normal immunoglobulin concentrations but with deficient antibody responses. Blood group antibody is frequently absent; diphtheria, tetanus, and pneumococcal antibody titers are significantly lower than normal; and primary immune responses to bacteriophage øX174 are far below normal. These patients are candidates for immune serum globulin replacement therapy because they do not have the ability to produce antibodies.

X-Linked Lymphoproliferative Disease

This condition, also referred to as Duncan's disease (after the original kindred in which it was described), is a recessive disorder and is characterized by an inadequate immune reaction to infection with Epstein-Barr virus (EBV). Affected males are apparently healthy until they contract infectious mononucleosis. Two thirds of the 100 patients studied have died of overwhelming EBV-induced B-cell proliferation during mononucleosis. Most patients surviving the primary infection developed hypogammaglobulinemia and/or a B-cell lymphoma. There is marked impairment of antibody synthesis to the EBV nuclear antigen (EBNA), but titers of antibodies to the viral capsid antigen are zero to markedly elevated. Antibody-dependent cell-mediated cytotoxicity (ADCC) against EBV-infected cells is impaired in many patients, natural killer (NK) function is depressed, and there is also a deficiency in long-lived T-cell immunity to EBV. Studies with monoclonal antibodies of lymphocyte subpopulations have revealed elevated percentages of T suppressor cells (T8). Immunoglobulin synthesis in response to polyclonal B-cell mitogen stimulation in vitro is markedly depressed. Thus, both EBV-specific and nonspecific immunologic abnomalities occur in these patients.

Cellular Immunodeficiency Disorders

Patients with defects in T-cell function have more severe and resistant infections and/or other clinical problems than do patients with antibody deficiency disorders. Some of these include: growth failure, susceptibility to graft-versus-host reactions, fatal infection with live virus vaccines, and increased risk of malignancy. Rarely do the T-cell–defective patients survive beyond infancy or childhood.

Cellular Immunodeficiency with Thymic Hypoplasia (DiGeorge's Syndrome)

This syndrome results from dysmorphogenesis of the third and fourth pharyngeal pouches early during embryonic life, resulting in hypoplasia or aplasia of the thymus and parathyroid glands. Other structures forming at the same age are frequently affected, with consequent anomalies of the great vessels (right- or left-sided interrupted aortic arch and aberrant subclavian arteries); esophageal atresia; bifid uvula; congenital heart disease (truncus arteriosus Type I, ventricular septal defects, tetralogy of Fallot); a short philtrum of the upper lip; hypertelorism; an antimongoloid slant to the eyes; mandibular hypoplasia; and low-set, often notched, ears. The diagnosis is usually first suggested by the presence of hypocalcemic seizures during the neonatal period. This condition, which occurs in both males and females, has rarely had a familial occurrence. It has been associated in two families with monosomy of chromosome 22.

A variable degree of hypoplasia is more frequent than total aplasia of the thymus and parathyroid glands in this syndrome. Such infants, who have little trouble with life-threatening infections and grow normally, are classified as having partial DiGeorge syndrome. Others, with more severe thymic hypoplasia, may resemble patients with severe combined immunodeficiency disorders (SCID) in their susceptibility to infection with low-grade or opportunistic pathogens (i.e., fungi, viruses, and *Pneumocystis carinii*) and to graft-versus-host disease (GVHD) from nonirradiated blood transfusions.

Concentrations of serum immunoglobulins are usually near normal, but some fractions, particularly IgA, may be decreased and IgE may be increased. The number of T cells is decreased and the number of B cells is increased. T-cell subset analysis with monoclonal antibodies demonstrates that there are normal proportions of cells with the helper (T4) and suppressor (T8) phenotypes. The synthesis of DNA by peripheral blood lymphocytes following mitogen stimulation and the delayed skin test response are absent, reduced, or normal, depending upon the degree of thymic deficiency. Thymic tissue, when present, contains Hassall's corpuscles and a normal number of thymocytes,

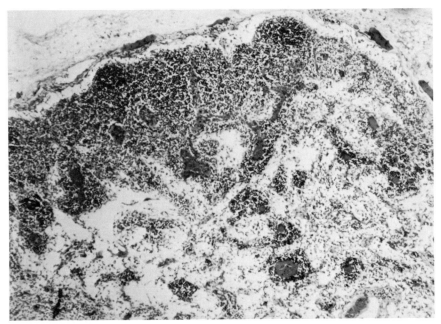

Figure 6–2. Photomicrograph of lymph node section from infant with DiGeorge's syndrome. Primary follicles are present in the cortex, but lymphocytes in the deep cortex (paracortical region) are extremely sparse.

and there is a sharp corticomedullary distinction. Lymphoid follicles usually appear normal, but the thymus-dependent regions of the spleen and paracortical areas of the lymph nodes show variable degrees of depletion (Fig. 6–2).

Cellular Immunodeficiency with Immunoglobulins (Nezelof's Syndrome)

This syndrome is characterized by lymphopenia, diminished lymphoid tissue, abnormal thymus architecture, and normal or increased serum levels of most of the five immunoglobulin classes. Patients present during infancy with recurrent or chronic pulmonary infections, failure to thrive, oral or cutaneous candidiasis, chronic diarrhea, recurrent skin infections, gram-negative sepsis, urinary tract infections, severe varicella, and/or progressive vaccinia, neutropenia, and eosinophilia. Selective IgA deficiency, markedly elevated IgE, and elevated IgD levels are found in some. The pattern of inheritance suggests autosomal recessive in some but an X-linked mode has seemed more likely in others.

The depression of cellular immune function is revealed by decreased or absent responses to intradermal injections of recall antigens in vivo and of lymphocyte responses to mitogens and allogeneic cells in vitro. These patients have profoundly decreased numbers of T cells and T-cell subsets. There is, however, usually a normal ratio of helper (T4) to suppressor (T8) cells, in contrast to patients with the acquired immunodeficiency syndrome (AIDS) in whom the ratio is markedly inverted due to a selective deficiency of T4 cells. Peripheral lymphoid tissues are hypoplastic and demonstrate paracortical lymphocyte depletion. The thymus is small, shows poor corticomedullary distinction, has few thymocytes, and usually has no Hassall's corpuscles. However, in contrast to AIDS, thymic epithelium is present. These differences can help distinguish Nezelof's syndrome from AIDS in pediatrics, since it is the immunodeficiency disorder most likely to be confused with AIDS.

Cellular Immunodeficiency with Purine Nucleoside Phosphorylase (PNP) Deficiency. This deficiency has been detected in more than a dozen patients with Nezelof's syndrome. In contrast to patients with ADA deficiency, serum and urinary uric acid are markedly decreased, and there are no characteristic physical or skeletal abnormalities. Unlike the majority of Nezelof patients, there may be a few Hassall's corpuscles in the thymus of PNP deficient patients. Analyses of lymphocyte subpopulations with monoclonal antibodies in two PNP deficient patients revealed a marked decrease in the numbers of total T cells and of T-cell subsets and an increased number and function of natural killer (NK) cells. Enzymatic replacement with normal erythrocyte transfusions has not been successful.

Severe Combined Immunodeficiency (SCID) Syndromes

The syndromes of SCID are distinguished by a congenital absence of all adaptive immune function. An absence or a failure of proliferation and/or differentiation of the "primordial" stem cell has been postulated to be the basis of these syndromes. However, this does not explain the diversity of genetic, enzymatic, hematologic, and immunologic features observed. Death usually occurs before the patient's first birthday, and invariably before the second, unless germ-free (gnotobiotic) isolation is instituted or immunologic reconstitution is achieved by bone marrow transplantation.

Autosomal Recessive

This form of SCID was first reported by Swiss workers in 1958. Affected infants developed, within the first few months of life, frequent episodes of otitis, pneumonia, sepsis, diarrhea, and cutaneous infections. Growth may be normal initially, but extreme wasting usually develops after onset of infections and diarrhea. Infections with *Candida albicans, Pneumocystis carinii,* vaccinia, varicella, measles, cytomegalovirus, and bacillus Calmette-Guérin (BCG) frequently are lethal because of delays in diagnosis and institution of adequate treatment. These infants not only are unduly susceptible to infection but they also are unable to reject foreign tissue, which makes them at risk for GVHD. Immunocompetent maternal lymphocytes capable of producing GVHD can cross the placenta while the infant is in utero, or viable incompatible lymphocytes can be introduced by administration of blood products.

Infants with SCID usually are profoundly lymphopenic and anergic. Serum immunoglobulin concentrations are diminished to absent, and antibody fails to develop following immunization. Analyses of lymphocyte subpopulations have demonstrated marked heterogeneity among SCID patients, even among those with similar inheritance patterns or with ADA deficiency. Despite the uniformly profound lack of T- and B-cell function, some patients have had low numbers of both B and T lymphocytes, whereas others have had elevated numbers of B cells; occasionally, even normal numbers of both T and B cells have been found. Cytofluorographic studies with monoclonal antibodies to mature T cells and subsets have generally revealed some, albeit low, percentages of cells reacting with all such reagents; however, no patients have had increased numbers of lymphocytes reacting with the monoclonal antibody to the T6 antigen, present on immature cortical thymocytes. Thus, the lymphocytes present appear to have acquired surface markers characteristic of mature T cells. In contrast to lymphopenic patients with AIDS, SCID patients rarely have an inverted ratio of helper (T4) to suppressor (T8) cells. The author characterized a phenotype of SCID in which virtually all lymphocytes of two infants with SCID were large granular lymphocytes with NK cell phenotype and function. NK function has been totally lacking in other SCID patients, further illustrating the striking cellular heterogeneity. Typically, SCID patients have a very small thymus (less than 2 gm) that fails to descend from the neck, contains few thymic lymphocytes, lacks corticomedullary distinction, and usually lacks Hassall's corpuscles. Despite the profound thymocyte depletion in SCID patients, thymic epithelium is present, in contrast to patients with AIDS, in whom there is marked thymic epithelial atrophy. Both follicular and paracortical areas of the peripheral lymph nodes of SCID patients are depleted of lymphocytes, and the tonsils, adenoids, and Peyer's patches are absent or extremely underdeveloped.

SCID due to Adenosine Deaminase (ADA) Deficiency

Absence of this enzyme has been observed in some, but not all, patients with the autosomal recessive form of SCID. Approximately 30 families have been identified in whom the enzyme deficiency was associated with severe immunodeficiency. In contrast to "classic" SCID, the thymuses of ADA deficient patients have a few Hassall's corpuscles and changes suggestive of early differentiation. Other distinguishing features of ADA-deficient SCIDs include radiologic evidence of rib cage abnormalities resembling a rachitic rosary and multiple skeletal abnormalities of chondroosseous dysplasia. Enzyme replacement therapy with 15 ml/kg of glycerol-frozen, irradiated, packed normal erythrocytes every 2 to 4 weeks has resulted in immunologic and/or clinical improvement in a few such patients. However, this treatment is ineffective in the majority.

X-Linked Recessive SCID

This is probably the most common form of SCID in the United States. Deficiencies of the purine salvage pathway enzymes ADA or PNP have not been encountered in pedigrees in which there has been a proven or putative X-linked mode of inheritance. Patients with the X-linked form usually are immunologically and histopathologically similar, if not identical, to those with the autosomal recessive form.

Bare Lymphocyte Syndrome

There is a lack of expression of HLA antigens and absence of β_2 microglobulin on lymphocytes in this combined immunodeficiency. The associated defects of immunity and of HLA expression support the concept of a biologic role of HLA determinants in the development of functional T lymphocytes.

SCID with Leukopenia (Reticular Dysgenesis)

Identical twin male infants exhibiting a total lack of both lymphocytes and granulocytes in peripheral blood and bone marrow were described in 1959. Seven of eight infants reported with this defect died of overwhelming infections at 3 to 119 days of age. The eighth underwent complete immunologic reconstitution following a bone marrow transplant. The few granulocytes present in three patients were mature and normal-appearing, and the percentage of E-rosetting T cells in the cord blood of a fourth patient was normal—evidence against a total failure of stem cell differentiation in this defect. The T cells in the cord blood of the fourth patient failed to give an in vitro proliferative response to mitogens. The thymus glands all weighed less than 1 gm, Hassall's corpuscles were absent, and there were few or no thymocytes. An autosomal mode of inheritance seems most likely.

Partial Combined Immunodeficiency Disorders

Immunodeficiency with Thrombocytopenia and Eczema (Wiskott-Aldrich Syndrome)

This X-linked recessive syndrome is characterized clinically by the triad of eczema, thrombocytopenic purpura with normal-appearing megakaryocytes, and marked susceptibility to infection. There is often prolonged bleeding from a circumcision site or bloody diarrhea during infancy. The thrombocytopenia appears to be due to an intrinsic platelet abnormality, since there are normal survival times of homologous but not autologous ^{51}Cr-labeled platelets in these patients.

Atopic dermatitis and recurrent infections usually develop during the first year of life. Pneumococci and other bacteria with polysaccharide capsules cause infections including otitis media, pneumonia, meningitis, and sepsis. Infections with agents such as *Pneumocystis carinii* and herpes viruses are more frequent in the older patient. Infections or bleeding are major causes of death, there is a 12 percent incidence of fatal malignancy, and survival beyond the teens is rare. There is an impaired humoral immune response to polysaccharide antigens as evidenced by an absence or markedly diminished titer of isohemagglutinins and poor or no response to immunization with polysaccharide antigens. Antibody titers to proteins also diminish with time, and anamnestic responses are often poor or absent. The synthesis of immunoglobulins and the catabolism of albumin, IgG, IgA, and

IgM are accelerated, resulting in highly variable immunoglobulin concentrations even within the same patient. The predominant pattern is a low serum IgM, elevated IgA and IgE, and a normal or slightly low IgG. The responses of lymphocytes from these patients to mitogens in vitro may be normal, but more often responses are moderately depressed, and anergy is frequently present. There are low percentages of lymphocytes reacting with monoclonal antibodies to all T cells and to the helper (T4) and suppressor (T8) subsets. However, as with the other primary cellular immunodeficiencies, there is usually a normal T4:T8 ratio.

Antibody replacement has become possible by intravenous infusion, because of the availability of safe intravenous immune serum globulin preparations. Several patients who had undergone splenectomy for uncontrollable bleeding subsequently exhibited impressive increases in platelet counts and improved clinically on chronic antibiotic and antibody replacement therapy. The platelet and immunologic abnormalities have been completely corrected in several patients with this disorder by transplants of matched sibling bone marrow after the patients had been conditioned with irradiation or busulfan and cyclophosphamide.

Ataxia Telangiectasia

This is a complex syndrome with neurologic, immunologic, endocrinologic, hepatic, and cutaneous abnormalities. The most prominent clinical features are progressive cerebellar ataxia, oculocutaneous telangiectasias, chronic sinopulmonary disease, a high incidence of malignancy, and variable humoral and cellular immunodeficiency. Ataxia typically becomes evident soon after the child begins to walk and progresses to confinement in a wheelchair, usually by the age of 10 to 12 years. The telangiectasias develop between 3 and 6 years of age. Recurrent, usually bacterial, sinopulmonary infections occur in roughly 80 percent of these patients, but common viral exanthems and smallpox vaccination have not usually resulted in untoward sequelae. However, fatal varicella occurred in one of the author's patients.

Lymphoreticular malignancies have been reported, but adenocarcinomas have also been described. There is also an increased incidence of malignancy in unaffected relatives of such patients. The patients' cells and the cells of heterozygous carriers of the defect have increased sensitivity to ionizing radiation, defective DNA repair, and frequent chromosomal abnormalities. An autosomal recessive mode of inheritance seems likely. The most frequent humoral immunologic abnormality is the selective absence of IgA in 50 to 80 percent of these patients, in some of whom catabolism of IgA is increased. IgE concentrations are usually low, IgM may be of the low-molecular-weight variety, and IgG_2 or total IgG may be decreased. Specific antibody titers may be decreased or normal. Cell-mediated immunity is present but impaired, as evidenced by reduced cutaneous responses to recall antigens and prolonged allograft survival. There are moderately depressed proliferative responses of lymphocytes in vitro to T- and B-cell mitogens. Analyses in five patients of T cells and subsets revealed reduced percentages of total T cells and T helper (T4) cells, with normal or increased percentages of T suppressor (T8) cells. The abnormality in immunoglobulin synthesis probably results from both helper T cell and intrinsic B cell defects. The thymus is very hypoplastic, exhibits poor organization, and lacks Hassall's corpuscles. No satisfactory treatment is known.

Immunodeficiency with Short-Limbed Dwarfism

An unusual form of short-limbed dwarfism, with frequent and severe infections, was reported among the Amish in 1964; non-Amish cases have since been described. Features include short and pudgy hands; redundant skin; hyperextensible joints of hands and feet but an inability to completely extend the elbows; and fine, sparse light hair and eyebrows. Radiographically, the bones show scalloping and sclerotic or cystic changes in the metaphyses and flaring of the costochondral junctions. Severe and often fatal varicella infections, progressive vaccinia, and vaccine-associated poliomyelitis have also been observed.

The severity of the immunodeficiency varies. There are three patterns of immune dysfunction: defective antibody mediated immunity, defective cellular immunity (most common form), and severe combined immunodeficiency. In vitro studies of lymphocytes have shown decreased total numbers of T cells and defective cell proliferation caused by an intrinsic defect related to the G1 phase. The trait is autosomal recessive with variable penetrance.

Immunodeficiency with Thymoma

These patients are adults who simultaneously develop recurrent infections, panhypogammaglobulinemia, deficits in cell-mediated immunity, and benign thymoma, predominantly of the spindle cell variety. There may be eosinophilia or eosinopenia, aregenerative or hemolytic anemia, agranulocytosis, thrombocytopenia, or pancytopenia. Antibody formation is deficient and there is progressive lymphopenia, although percentages of immunoglobulin bearing B lymphocytes are normal. Several patients have had excessive suppressor T cell activity.

Hyperimmunoglobulinemia E Syndrome

The hyper IgE syndrome is a primary immunodeficiency characterized by recurrent severe staphylococcal abscesses and markedly elevated levels of serum IgE (see Chapter 4). The disorder was first reported in two young boys in 1972 by the author and her coworkers. Since then a total of 22 patients have been evaluated by the author. These patients have staphylococcal abscesses from infancy involving the skin, lungs, joints, and other sites and persistent pneumatocoeles as a result of recurrent pneumonias (Figs. 6–3 and 6–4). The associated pruritic dermatitis is not typical atopic eczema and does not always persist; respiratory allergic symptoms are usually absent.

Laboratory features include exceptionally high serum IgE concentrations, elevated serum IgD concentrations, usually normal concentrations of IgG, IgA, and IgM, pronounced blood and sputum eosinophilia, abnormally low anamnestic antibody responses, and poor antibody and cell-mediated responses to neoantigens. In vitro studies have shown normal percentages of E-rosette forming and T3-, T4-, and T8-positive lymphocytes, and no increase in the percentage of IgE-bearing B lymphocytes.

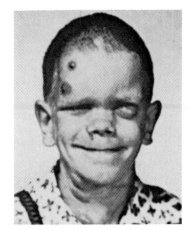

Figure 6–3. Patient with the hyper IgE syndrome, showing multiple abscesses of the face and neck and coarse facial features. (From Buckley, R. H., Wray, B. B., and Belmaker, E. Z.: Pediatrics 49:59, 1972.)

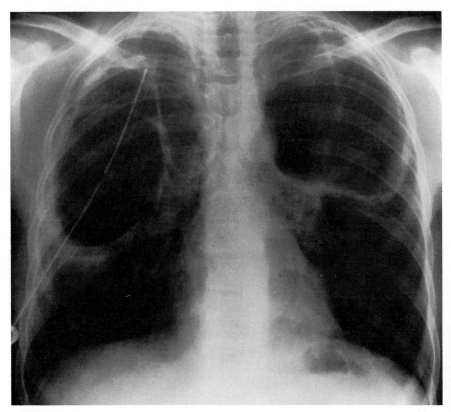

Figure 6–4. Chest roentgenogram of a 12-year-old boy with the hyper IgE syndrome. Giant pneumatocoeles were present for more than 1 year. A putrid abscess due to *Enterobacter cloacae* led to chest tube insertion on the right. The left cyst required emergency excision because of massive hemoptysis and was found to contain an aspergilloma. (From Buckley, R. H.: *In* Kodes, H., and Kagan, B. N. (eds.): Pediatric Immunology. New York, Science and Medicine Publishing Co., 1979, p. 221.)

Lymphocyte proliferative responses to mitogens are normal, but responses to antigens or allogeneic cells from family members are very low or absent. Blood, sputum, and histologic sections of lymph nodes, spleen, and lung cysts show striking eosinophilia. Hassall's corpuscles and normal thymic architecture were observed at postmortem examination of one patient.

Phagocytic cell ingestion, metabolism and killing, and total hemolytic complement activity are normal. Defects of mononuclear and/or polymorphonuclear chemotaxis are present in some but not all patients and, therefore, are not the basic defect in these patients.

Both males and females have been affected, as have members of succeeding generations, suggesting an autosomal dominant

form of inheritance with incomplete penetrance. The most effective management consists of chronic administration of a penicil-
linase-resistant penicillin with other antibiotics or antifungal
agents added as required for specific infections, and appropriate
thoracic surgery for infected pneumatocoeles or those persisting
beyond 6 months.

Other Primary Immunodeficiencies (Complement and Phagocytic Cells)

Complement Component Deficiencies (See Chapter 3)

There are several well-defined primary immune defects involving the complement system and phagocytic cells. There are
reports of genetically determined deficiencies for all of the components of complement, and undue susceptibility to infection is
a characteristic of certain of these, particularly C2, C3, C5, C6,
and C7 deficiencies. The types of infections experienced in C2,
C3, and some cases of C5 deficiency are similar to those of
patients with antibody deficiency syndromes, whereas infections
in patients with defects of the terminal components are usually
caused by meningococci or gonococci. A normal CH50 excludes
all heritable complement deficiencies.

Phagocytic Cell Dysfunctions (See Chapter 4)

Phagocytic cell deficiencies are grouped into disorders of
production (such as the various hereditary neutropenias) or
function. The latter category includes a variety of chemotactic
defects, opsonic defects, ingestion defects, and killing defects.
Only two of these will be discussed.

Chédiak-Higashi-Steinbrink Syndrome

This rare disorder is characterized by gigantism of cytoplasmic lysosomes in white cells, melanocytes, Schwann cells,
and possibly other cells. Affected individuals have partial albinism (oculocutaneous) with resultant photophobia; undue susceptibility to viral and enteric bacterial infections; hepatosplenomegaly, lymphadenopathy, anemia, and leukopenia; cutaneous
ulcers; and neurologic changes. Peripheral blood smears show
abnormally large peroxidase-positive granules in the neutrophils
and eosinophils. The response of polymorphonuclear cells to
normal chemotactic stimuli is depressed, and there is an intracellular microbicidal defect. All aspects of adaptive immunity
are normal, but there is a marked deficiency of lymphocyte

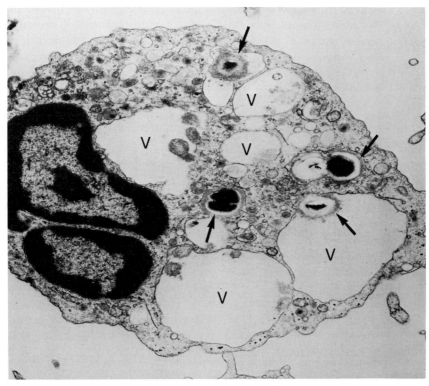

Figure 6–5. Polymorphonuclear leukocyte from a normal control patient incubated with staphylococci for 30 minutes. Many bacteria (arrows) in various stages of destruction are evident within the cell. Note cytoplasmic vacuoles (V) around or adjacent to the degenerating bacteria (×18,000). (From Quie, P. G., et al.: J. Clin. Invest. 46:668, 1967. Reproduced from *The Journal of Clinical Investigation* by copyright permission of the American Society for Clinical Investigation.)

natural killer cell function. Death from infection usually occurs before the fifth year of life. Heterozygous carriers of this autosomal recessive trait are identified by the presence of the granule anomaly in leukocytes.

Chronic Granulomatous Disease of Childhood (CGD)

This syndrome is characterized by chronic suppurative infections, draining adenopathy, pneumonia, hepatomegaly with liver abscesses, osteomyelitis, splenomegaly, hypergammaglobulinemia, and dermatitis, with infections usually beginning before the age of 1 year. Neutrophils can phagocytize but are defective in killing catalase positive bacteria *(Staphylococcus aureus,* klebsiella, aerobacter, or proteus organisms, and *Serratia marcescens)* and some fungi *(Candida* and *Aspergillus)* (Figs. 6–5 and 6–6). In contrast, catalase-negative organisms such as streptococci, pneumococci, meningococci, and *Haemophilus influenzae,* which generate their own peroxide, are killed normally by these cells. Leukocytes from CGD patients fail to show normal oxygen consumption, direct oxidation of glucose, or hydrogen peroxide formation. Leukocytes do not lyse bacteria, owing to an inability to stimulate the direct pathway of glucose metabolism to form hydrogen peroxide during phagocytosis. The myeloperoxidase, iodide (or other halide), hydrogen peroxide system is an important bactericidal system of human polymorphonuclear cells; hence, the failure of CGD cells to generate peroxide, the superoxide anion radical, and/or singlet oxygen explains their impaired microbicidal activity.

There appear to be several biochemical defects in CGD and more than one mechanism of genetic transmission. Stimulation of normal granulocytic membranes during phagocytosis activates the membrane-bound electron transport chain, NADPH-oxidase, which acts on NADPH to reduce molecular oxygen to the superoxide anion. The NADPH-oxidase system consists of at least two

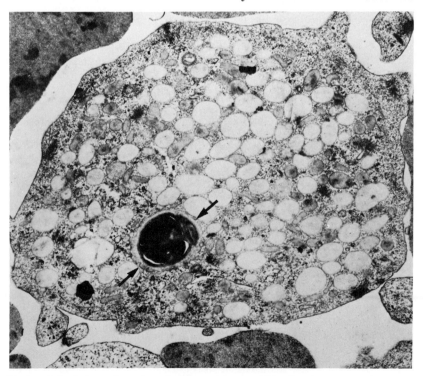

Figure 6–6. Polymorphonuclear leukocyte from a child with chronic granulomatous disease incubated with staphylococci for 1 hour. An intact bacterium is visible in the cytoplasm. (× 22,500). (From Quie, P. G., et al.: J. Clin. Invest. 46:668, 1967. Reproduced from *The Journal of Clinical Investigation* by copyright permission of the American Society for Clinical Investigation.)

components, a flavoprotein and cytochrome b. Failure of oxidase activity could result from defective transport chain activation, absence of any of the chain components, or lack of substrate, probable examples of each of which have been reported. A multicenter study of 27 CGD patients from Europe failed to detect the heme-containing protein cytochrome b-245 in any of the 19 males in whom the defect appeared to be located on the X chromosome. Female carriers had reduced cytochrome b-245 and a variable proportion of cells that were unable to generate superoxide. In all of the 8 patients with probable autosomal recessive inheritance, cytochrome b-245 was present but nonfunctional. The reason for the latter is not clear, but the mechanism for adding electrons or hydrogen to the cytochrome may be defective. The failure of polymorphonuclear cells from affected individuals to reduce the redox dye nitroblue tetrazolium (NBT) to purple formazan during phagocytosis serves as a simple screening test for this disorder.

Acquired Immune Deficiencies

There are many instances of acquired immune deficiency among patients given immunosuppressive agents. Two other conditions will be discussed.

Chronic Mucocutaneous Candidiasis

This possibly acquired clinical syndrome likely has multiple etiologies. There are chronic candidal infections of the skin and mucous membranes of the host, but only rarely is there a life-threatening systemic infection. *Candida* is often the only infectious agent to which these patients are markedly susceptible. Some patients have endocrinopathies involving the parathyroid, thyroid, adrenal, and/or pancreatic glands. However, many have neither associated endocrinopathy nor demonstrable immunological abnormalities. Serum immunoglobulins are usually normal or increased, but IgA deficiency has been reported. Precipitating or agglutinating antibodies to *Candida* are usually present. Some patients have in vivo and/or in vitro evidence of deficient cell-mediated immunity, but even in these patients it is not clear if this is a primary problem or secondary to extensive fungal disease (e.g., an antigen-overload mechanism). Reversal of the anergy has followed diminution of fungal lesions by high doses of intravenous amphotericin B. A majority of patients improve dramatically when treated with ketoconazole.

Acquired Immune Deficiency Syndrome (AIDS)

This disorder, first noted in male homosexuals in 1981, is a highly lethal epidemic infectious disease primarily affecting the T helper cells. Patients with this condition present with life-threatening opportunistic infections and/or Kaposi's sarcoma. The opportunistic infectious agents include most of the bacterial, fungal, and parasitic agents associated with cellular immuno-deficiency, e.g., *Pneumocystis carinii, Candida albicans, Myco-bacterium avium intracellare, Herpes simplex, Toxoplasma gon-dii,* hepatitis B, cytomegalovirus, and cryptococcus. The variety of agents infecting AIDS patients far exceeds that in infants with the most severe primary combined immunodeficiency dis-orders. Until recently, Kaposi's sarcoma was rarely encountered in North America or Europe, occurring only in persons aged 50 years or older and responding to chemotherapy or irradiation. Since 1979, many cases of Kaposi's sarcoma have been reported in the United States in young homosexual males. Epidemiologic, culture, and immunoserologic data have demonstrated that an infection with human T lymphocytotropic virus III (HTLV-III) causes the severe depression of immune function by infecting T4-positive lymphocytes. The mortality from AIDS is greater than 40 percent and probably close to 100 percent.

Major groups at risk for AIDS include: homosexual males (75 percent of cases), intravenous drug abusers with no history of homosexuality (13 percent of cases), and hemophiliacs (0.7 percent of cases). The disorder, primarily a sexually transmitted disorder among males, has also been reported in female sexual partners of affected males, in children born (primarily infected in utero) of affected females, and in men whose only risk factor appears to be heterosexual promiscuity, particularly with pros-titutes. Other contributing factors include promiscuity among homosexuals, treatment of hemophiliacs with lyophilized concen-trated factor VIII prepared from thousands of blood donors, and genetic factors, since the frequency of HLA-DR5 is increased in patients with Kaposi's sarcoma. The AIDS-related complex (ARC), consisting of generalized adenopathy, recurrent fever, weight loss, and leukopenia, is now frequently recognized among high-risk groups and may be a prodromal form of AIDS. The prodromal phase can last for many months or even years, which, together with other epidemiologic data, suggests that there may be a very prolonged incubation period (6 to 48 months).

AIDS patients have a severe and profound cellular immu-nodeficiency. This is characterized by the absence of delayed hypersensitivity, an absolute lymphopenia due to an absolute deficiency of T4 helper cells, reversal of the usual ratio of T helper (T4) to T suppressor (T8) cells, depressed lymphocyte responses to mitogens, and impaired natural killer cell function. There is usually hypergammaglobulinemia as well as high antibody titers to many antigens, but there is also evidence for a B-cell defect. There is usually a persistence of some lymphoid cells in the thymus glands of patients dying from AIDS, despite which there is marked thymic epithelial atrophy. The thymuses of SCID patients, in contrast, reveal preservation of the epithelium but marked depletion of thymocytes.

There is at present no known effective treatment for AIDS. Prevention based on the above epidemiologic information and treatment of opportunistic infections for which therapy is available are the principal approaches to management. Bone marrow transplantation has not been successful thus far, because of infection of the graft with the virus.

TREATMENT

Therapy of the primary immunodeficiency disorders includes use of antibiotics for the eradication and/or prevention of bacterial and fungal infections, protective isolation, and replacement of missing humoral or cellular immunologic functions. The complexities of the immunodeficiency diseases and their treatment necessitates that all such patients be evaluated in centers where detailed studies of immune function can be conducted before instituting treatment.

Treatment of Antibody Deficiency Disorders

Antibiotics and repeated administration of antibodies are the only effective treatments for these disorders. Patients with agammaglobulinemia, X-linked immunodeficiency with hyper IgM, antibody deficiency with near normal immunoglobulins, or the Wiskott-Aldrich syndrome are candidates for antibody replacement therapy. The latter is contraindicated in patients with selective absence of serum and secretory IgA or transient hypogammaglobulinemia of infancy. Patients with IgG subclass deficiency should not be given replacement therapy unless they are shown to have a profound antibody deficiency.

Immune serum globulin (ISG) for intramuscular use or modified for intravenous use, the antibody content of each of which is mainly IgG with traces of other classes, is the only commercially available form of such therapy. The recommended loading dose of 200 mg/kg and maintenance dose of 100 mg/kg/month of IgG are arbitrary and obsolete; studies are under way to establish guidelines for selecting the optimal doses for individual patients. There have been no reports of their transmission of either hepatitis antigens or AIDS. The use of random donor plasma carries the risk of transmission of hepatitis B and/or AIDS. Patients with severe defects in cellular immunity are at risk of GVHD unless such plasma is irradiated to inactivate viable lymphocytes of donor origin. Systemic reactions may occur but are uncommon, except in patients with selective IgA deficiency.

Treatment of Cellular Immunodeficiency

Immunologic reconstitution with an immunocompetent tissue transplant is the only adequate therapy for severe forms of cellular immunodeficiency. Three types of immunocompetent tissue have been used successfully. The tissue of choice is mature bone marrow that is major histocompatibility complex (MHC)–compatible or haplo-identical with the recipient, except in cases of complete DiGeorge syndrome, in which fetal thymic tissue is probably satisfactory. Neither fetal liver nor thymic tissue are as effective as bone marrow in the treatment of SCID. The major risk to the recipient from transplants of bone marrow or fetal tissues is GVH reaction. Fetal tissue transplants, even though incompatible, have a low risk of fatal GVH, for reasons that are not understood. The development of new techniques to deplete post-thymic T cells from donor marrow now allows haplo-identical (half-matched) bone marrow transplants without GVH, constituting a major advance in correcting the immunologic defect in SCID. Soybean lectin and sheep erythrocytes, which have an affinity for post-thymic T cells, completely remove these and other mature cells from bone marrow, leaving the stem cells intact (Chapter 9). More than 40 infants with SCID have been successfully treated in this manner with virtually no signs of GVHD. Patients with less severe forms of cellular immunodeficiency will reject bone marrow grafts unless they are treated with immunosuppressive agents prior to transplantation. Several patients with Wiskott-Aldrich syndrome and other forms of partial cellular immunodeficiency have been treated successfully with bone marrow transplants following immunosuppression.

Agents advocated as augmentors of existing cellular immunity include transfer factor, thymosin, and levamisole. Some clinical and less impressive immunologic improvements have been reported in individual cases; however, the natural variability of the less severe forms of cellular immunodeficiency treated with these substances precludes accurate assessment of these techniques. Controlled clinical trials are necessary with each of these agents before their usefulness can be established.

Bibliography

Bortin, M. M., and Rimm, A. A.: Severe combined immunodeficiency disease. Characterization of the disease and results of transplantation. JAMA 238:591, 1977.

Buckley, R. H.: Normal and abnormal development of the immune system. In Zinsser H. (ed.): Textbook of Microbiology and Immunology, 18th ed. New York, Appleton, Century, Crofts, 1984, pp. 318–339.

Buckley, R. H.: Primary immunodeficiency diseases. In Wyngaarden, J. B., and Smith, L. G. (eds.): Cecil Textbook of Medicine, 17th ed. Philadelphia, W. B. Saunders Co., 1985.

Buckley, R. H., and Sampson, H. A.: The hyperimmunoglobulinemia E syndrome. In Franklin, E. C. (ed.): Clinical Immunology Update. New York, Elsevier North-Holland, Inc., 1981, pp. 147–167.

Buckley, R. H., Schiff, S. E., Sampson, H. A., et al.: Development of immunity in human severe primary T cell deficiency following haploidentical bone marrow stem cell transplantation. J. Immunol. 136:2398, 1986.

Burks, A. W., Sampson, H. A., and Buckley, R. H.: Anaphylactoid reactions after gamma globulin administration in patients with hypogammaglobulinemia; detection of IgE antibodies to IgA. New Engl. J. Med. 314:560, 1986.

Centers for Disease Control Task Force on Kaposi's Sarcoma and Opportunistic Infections: Epidemic aspects of the current outbreak of Kaposi's sarcoma and opportunistic infections. N. Engl. J. Med. 306:248, 1982.

Harada, S., Sakamoto, K., Seeley, J. K., et al.: Immune deficiency in the X-linked lymphoproliferative syndrome. I. Epstein-Barr virus specific defects. J. Immunol. 129:2532, 1982.

Salvaggio, J. E. (ed.): Primer on allergic and immunologic diseases. JAMA 248:2579, 1982.

Stiehm, E. R., and Fulginiti, V. A. (eds.): Immunologic Disorders in Infants and Children, 2nd ed. Philadelphia, W. B. Saunders Co., 1980.

Webster, A. D. B.: Metabolic defects in immunodeficiency diseases. Clin. Exp. Immunol. 49:1, 1982.

Wedgwood, R., Rosen, F. S., and Paul, N. W. (eds.): Primary Immunodeficiency Diseases. New York, Alan R. Liss, 1983.

7

Immunologic Tolerance*

WILLIAM O. WEIGLE, Ph.D.

INTRODUCTION

Although immune reactivity can be nonspecifically manipulated by a number of reagents and procedures, antigen-specific immunologic tolerance requires interaction between antigen and its specific reactive lymphocytes. This type of tolerance is best defined as an immune refractory state to contact with antigen under conditions that would ordinarily result in an immune response. It is antigen-directed, since prior contact with the specific antigen is required, and it is specific in that animals tolerant to one antigen can make a normal immune response to

---

*This is publication No. 3361-IMM from the Department of Immunology, Scripps Clinic and Research Foundation, La Jolla, California.

a nonrelated antigen. Immunologic tolerance is important not only in the normal regulation of immune responses but also to our understanding of self-nonself recognition and autoimmunity. The immune mechanism must be able to discriminate between self and non-self in order for an animal to make an immune response to foreign substances, such as bacteria, viruses, and tumor antigens, and yet not respond to its own body constituents. Thus, during prenatal and/or neonatal life, before the immune mechanisms mature, animals develop a state of immunologic unresponsiveness to their own body constituents, but this does not interfere with their ability to respond, as adults, to foreign antigens.

BACKGROUND

During the past three decades, studies of the cellular mechanisms of acquired tolerance to foreign antigens have provided considerable insight into the cellular events involved in self-tolerance. That tolerance, as well as immunity, can be induced in animals was first predicted in 1959 by Burnet, who suggested that unresponsiveness to foreign antigens can be induced in animals by injecting the antigens during early life. This suggestion developed from the earlier work of Owen, who in 1945 first demonstrated that contact with foreign antigenic substances during early life results in immunologic tolerance. He observed that mature dizygotic twin cows tolerate each other's body tissues in that they do not reject mutual grafts. Undoubtedly, tolerance results from embryonic parabiosis in which blood is exchanged between the twins. Subsequently, Billingham and coworkers, in 1953, found that adult mice of an inbred strain tolerate skin grafts of a second inbred strain if, as newborns, animals of the first strain were injected with replicating cells of the second strain.

Since the prediction by Burnet, numerous experimental models of immunologic tolerance have been reported with cellular antigens, bacteria, viruses, polysaccharides and other bacterial products, synthetic peptides, and soluble serum proteins. Although all of these models are characterized by antigen specificity, requirement for previous antigen contact, and a refractory state to subsequent challenge with the specific antigen, the mechanisms responsible for the unresponsive state vary from model to model. The degree and duration of the unresponsive state is dependent on such conditions as the nature of the antigen, the immune status of the host, the dose of the antigen, and such other factors as the route of injection.

TYPES OF IMMUNOLOGIC TOLERANCE

Many of these models of tolerance result from regulatory mechanisms that operate in the normal control of the immune response after it has been initiated. It is quite understandable that, as important as are the events that are responsible for initiation of the immune response, so are too those events required for the regulation of that response once it is initiated. In contrast to models governed by these normal regulatory responses are other models in which a functional deletion of the antigen-reactive cells apparently occurs. Although it is difficult to establish the precise mechanism for immunologic tolerance in all of these models, one can divide the putative mechanisms into two general categories; (1) peripheral inhibition and (2) central unresponsiveness.

Peripheral Inhibition

In peripheral inhibition, cells of competent immune capacity are present, but their function is blocked. Lymphocytes of a tolerant host can bind antigen, and the tolerant state disappears when the cells are transferred to neutral hosts. Furthermore, the tolerant state may be associated with the transient appearance of antibody. This type of unresponsiveness probably does not represent a true tolerant state, but rather suppression induced by mechanisms that normally control the immune response, such as suppressor cells, antigen blockade, or antibody suppression. It is well accepted that a subpopulation of T lymphocytes that is capable of suppressing the immune response plays a major role in regulating various parameters of the immune response, once it is initiated. Once activated, the mature suppressor cells release suppressor factors that act on helper T cells and, to a lesser extent, B cells. Although this is part of a normal regulatory circuit that is active in almost all immune responses, there are some conditions in which suppression so dominates the immune response that an apparent tolerant state exists.

It is also well established that antibody itself feeds back on the immune response and is a potent regulatory factor, either suppressing or enhancing the response. As with suppressor cells, conditions can be selected in which suppression is dominant. Not only is antibody specific for the given antigen involved in such suppression but antibody directed to the antigen-reactive site of the antibody (idiotype) may also be involved. Antigen blockade can also result in an apparent tolerant state. This latter type of suppression is more often associated with B cells and thymus-independent responses. A model for B-cell tolerance has been described that is termed clonal anergy. In this model, antigen-reactive B cells are present but do not respond either to antigen or to mitogens and are not suppressed by any of the above mechanisms. It has been suggested that this latter model may also be partly responsible for tolerance enjoyed by our own body to self-constituents at the B-cell level.

Central Unresponsiveness

In contrast to peripheral inhibition, central unresponsiveness is characterized by an immune state in which the host is incapable of reacting specifically with the tolerated antigen. No antigen-specific binding cells are detectable, and antibody-producing cells do not appear even transiently. The cellular and subcellular events involved in this type of tolerance are probably identical to those at play in tolerance to self. Suppressor cell activity may be concomitant, but not responsible. Antigen blockade is not involved, and lymphocytes transferred from the tolerant donor to a neutral host remain unresponsive. Central unresponsiveness can be induced in adult animals with either nonimmunogenic forms of antigen or after temporary inhibition of the immune system, but it is more easily and effectively induced before the immune response matures.

Central unresponsiveness is more readily induced by simple serum protein antigens than by more complex antigens such as bacteria, viruses, microbial antigens, and mammalian cells (including red blood cells). The purified serum protein antigens equilibrate between the intra- and extravascular fluid spaces where they persist, being metabolized at a rate similar to the host's own serum proteins. Thus, these antigens come in contact with all the potential antigen-reactive cells and readily induce tolerance. On the other hand, antigens such as intact cells and microbial products are rapidly eliminated from the body fluids, do not equilibrate between the intra- and extravascular fluid spaces, and do not come in contact with potential antigen-reactive cells in the extravascular tissue. These latter antigens are more often associated with tolerance resulting from peripheral inhibition. Central unresponsiveness is also more readily induced in situations in which the immune response is minimized. Thus, it is more easily and effectively induced during either fetal or neonatal life, before the immune response has developed. It can be induced in adult animals with either nonimmunogenic forms of antigen or after temporary inhibition of the immune system. A tolerant state has been described with a few antigens in which tolerance was induced with both low and high doses of antigen, with intermediate doses causing immunity. However, it is not clear whether these models result from peripheral inhibition or central unresponsiveness. Central unresponsiveness is dose-dependent with most antigens, and, once a dose sufficient to induce tolerance is established, all higher doses also induce a tolerant state, with no intermediate dose resulting in immunity.

INDUCTION OF TOLERANCE AT THE CELLULAR LEVEL

Subpopulations of both thymus-derived (helper T) lymphocytes and bone marrow–derived lymphocytes (B cells) are required for antibody production to most antigens, and other subpopulations of T lymphocytes are required for cell-mediated lympholysis and delayed-type hypersensitivity. Macrophages are also a requisite and present the antigen to the T cells in a genetic-restricted fashion. Tolerance can be induced to specific antigens in all of these subpopulations of T cells and in B cells. Since macrophages are not antigen-specific, they are not rendered tolerant in the presence of antigen but may play an active role in the induction of tolerance in T cells.

In a classic model of central unresponsiveness, tolerance is induced in adult mice following the injection of preparations of deaggregated human gamma globulin (DHGG) tolerogen. Tolerance in this model may result from the failure of macrophages to deliver appropriate signals to the helper T cell (see tolerance in T cells). This unresponsive state is antigen-specific and persists, at least in part, for over 1 year, as evidenced by the failure of the tolerant mice to respond to a subsequent injection of heat-aggregated human gamma globulin (HGG) immunogen. Although both the helper T cells and B cells become tolerant, the duration of tolerance differs in the two cell types, and this tolerance is maintained in cells transferred to irradiated-syngeneic hosts (Table 7–1). Although suppressor cells are associated with this model of tolerance, they are not obligatory for either the induction or persistence of tolerance, and they are of rela-

Table 7–1. Temporal Patterns of Immunologic
Unresponsiveness to HGG in A/J Mice*

Site	Induction (days)	Maintenance (days)
Thymus	1	120–135
Bone marrow	8–15	40–50
Spleen		
T cells	1	100–150
B cells	2–4	50–60
Whole animal	1	130–150

*Injected with 2.5 mg of DHGG on day 0. DHGG = deaggregated human gamma globulin (tolerogen); HGG = heat-aggregated human gamma globulin (immunogen).

tively short duration. Furthermore, induction of tolerance in B cells requires 100 to 1000 times more antigen than that required for induction of tolerance in T cells. Deaggregated HGG rapidly equilibrates between intra- and extravascular fluid spaces following injection and persists in both the intra- and extravascular fluid spaces, with a half-life of approximately 7 days. Thus, the longer duration of tolerance in the T cells is most likely a reflection of the persistence of antigen and their requirements of low concentrations of antigen for tolerance.

Tolerance in B Cells

Tolerance of B cells induced in this manner is a form of central unresponsiveness resulting from the functional deletion of potential antibody-producing cells. Specific antigen-binding B cells cannot be detected in the HGG-mouse model. However, the B cell tolerance of other models, involving different antigens, has been attributed to clonal anergy rather than clonal deletion. As mentioned previously, although tolerance can be induced in adult animals, it is more readily induced in neonatal animals, in which immature B cells are predominant. Little is known concerning the cellular or subcellular events that determine whether immunity or tolerance is induced. It has been suggested that tolerance results if the B cell does not receive the required number of signals to drive it to differentiate into an antibody-producing cell. B cells are known to complete their differentiation through sequential interaction with antigen, T-cell–derived B-cell growth factors, a macrophage-derived lymphokine, and T-cell–derived differentiating factors. If the B cell receives only a portion of the appropriate signals, tolerance rather than antibody production may result. Nonspecific agents that cause B-cell differentiation interfere with the induction of tolerance. In line with the multiple signal hypothesis is the presence of two different receptors on B cells, both of which are required for thymus-dependent antibody responses. Since IgM appears first in the ontogeny of immunoglobulin receptors for antigen on B cells, and IgD does not appear until later, it has been suggested that IgM may initiate a limited number of signals that result in tolerance induction and that IgD then initiates the remaining signals that result in antibody production rather than tolerance. This concept is compatible with the ontogeny of thymus-dependent immune responses, since neonatal mice are immunoincompetent and optimal immune reactivity does not peak until early adult life, simultaneously with the appearance of IgD receptors. Thus, the dual receptor concept may explain the ability to induce tolerance of immature B cells in vitro but not of mature B cells; however, if mature B cells are treated so that the IgD receptors are preferentially removed from the B cells, tolerance can be as readily induced in these mature cells as in cells from newborn animals.

Tolerance in T Cells

The mechanisms for the induction of tolerance in helper T cells are not as clear. Before T cells can function in thymus-dependent responses, they must be activated by antigen-reactive macrophages. Antigen-pulsed macrophages, in the absence of any apparent cell-free antigen, can activate specific helper T cells. The antigen-pulsed macrophages present, to the helper T cell, a processed antigen that is recognized by the T cell where there is conformity of a major histocompatibility complex gene product on the two cells. This recognition apparently supplies the first signal to the T cell, and it has recently been shown that a second signal is required. The second signal is supplied by a lymphokine (interleukin-1) released from the activated macrophage and received by receptors on the helper T cell. However, like the B cell, insufficient signals to the T cell may also result in tolerance rather than immunity. (In any event, it would not be surprising if the subcellular mechanism responsible for inducing tolerance in T cells differs from that in B cells, since the concentration of antigen required to maintain tolerance in the two types of cells differs markedly.) Thus, if the T cells are appropriately presented with antigen by the macrophage but do not receive the interleukin-1 (IL-1) signal, tolerance rather than immunity may result. Recently, the use of antigen-specific T helper cell clones has lent support to this hypothesis. A tolerant-like state can be induced in these clones if they are appropriately presented with the antigen but do not receive the IL-1 signal. This contention is also compatible with the suggestion that nonspecific handling of antigen by macrophages plays a determining role in inducing tolerance to deaggregated gamma globulins. Genetically determined susceptibility to tolerance induction in different mouse strains has also been established as being dependent on macrophages. Thus, it may be that IL-1 is not released during the processing of deaggregated gamma globulins and T cells thus receive only one signal, resulting in tolerance rather than immunity. On the other hand, the processing of aggregated gamma globulin by macrophages may cause the release of IL-1, giving the second signal to the T cell and thus resulting in immunity.

Tolerance in Primed T and B Cells

Tolerance is more readily induced in immature B cells than in adult mature B cells and is extremely difficult to induce in memory B cells. However, under certain conditions, specific immunologic tolerance can also be induced in mature adult B cells. The conditions selected must temporarily inhibit the immune response sequence, thus interfering with delivery of the appropriate signals to the T and/or B cells. The deaggregated HGG mouse model is an example of tolerance in which appropriate signals are not given to the T cells resulting in tolerance in these cells. Since tolerant T cells cannot generate appropriate lymphokines to deliver the necessary complete set of signals to B cells, the B cells also become tolerant. Tolerance is also readily induced in memory B cells, provided they are resting cells and do not receive the appropriate T-cell signals. The ability to induce a tolerant-like state in cloned T cells that do not receive the complete set of antigen-generated signals also suggests that tolerance can be induced in memory T cells. Since cloned T cells are both specific for the antigen and are selected by reactivity with that antigen, they are obviously primed cells. However, it appears that further activation of these cells with macrophage lymphokines precludes the induction of tolerance. The in vivo activation of unprimed T and B cells by lymphocyte mitogens also precludes the induction of tolerance.

AUTOIMMUNITY

The relationship between experimentally induced tolerance to exogenous antigens and acquired tolerance to self has both practical and theoretical implications. Immunologic tolerance can develop through two different pathways and thus may play two major biologic roles in self-nonself recognition. Specific suppressor cell activity has been associated with numerous models of experimentally induced tolerance. This subset of T cells comprises a network of regulatory cells that control the normal immune response initiated by foreign antigens. As in the responses to exogenous antigens, such a regulatory network similarly monitors the various parameters of autoimmunity and may be instrumental in the clinical progression of autoimmune diseases. However, it is not clear what role, if any, suppressor-inducer, precursor-suppressor, or suppressor cells themselves play in initiating autoimmunity. This suppressor cell circuit may play a role as a failsafe mechanism after autoimmunity is initiated and be responsible for regulating self-nonself recognition, and thus autoimmunity. The available evidence would strongly support a second model of immunologic tolerance involving functional deletion of antigen-reactive T and/or B cells. Once this central unresponsive state to self is acquired during early life, it usually persists throughout the animal's life, since a concentration of self-antigen sufficient to maintain this state is constantly present. Tolerance is present in both T and B cells when self-antigens are in high concentrations in body fluids. T cells alone are tolerant when small concentrations of self-antigen are present, and the animal's B cells are capable of reacting with that self-antigen. The B cells, however, remain dormant in the absence of appropriate T-cell help. Under certain abnormal situations, these immunologically competent B cells can be stimulated to respond to self-antigens if they receive a combination of signals that bypass specific helper T cells. Depending on the target tissue, the nature of the antibody, and the duration of such B-cell activation, the autoantibody response could be accompanied by an autoimmune disease. If self-antigens are present in the body fluids in extremely small concentrations, neither T cells nor B cells would be expected to be tolerant. Appropriate stimulation by self-antigen could then activate self-specific T effector cells and immunologically competent B cells, resulting in an autoimmune response and subsequent disease initiated either by the effector T cells, by antibody, or by both.

Experimental Autoimmune Thyroiditis

One example of experimental autoimmune thyroiditis (EAT), a model for Hashimoto's thyroiditis, appears to involve tolerant T cells and competent B cells. The self-antigen of this model is thyroglobulin that persists in the body fluids at a concentration that results in tolerance in T cells but not in B cells; B cells reactive with autologous thyroglobulin can be detected. Thyroiditis and autoantibodies to thyroglobulin are readily induced in laboratory animals immunized with either heterologous or chemically altered homologous thyroglobulin injected in aqueous form. Following injection, altered portions of the homologous thyroglobulin, or determinants on the heterologous thyroglobulin unrelated to autologous thyroglobulin, activate their specific T cells. This allows the self-determinants to stimulate their immunologically competent B cells to produce antibody reactive with the animal's own thyroglobulin. The infiltration of inflammatory cells in the thyroid gland of this model is initiated by antibody to thyroglobulin. T cells are not activated in this model, but a limited activation of T cells can be induced when the thyroglobulin is incorporated into a potent adjuvant. Although only minimal T-cell activation occurs in the adjuvant model of EAT, it is accompanied by thyroid disease.

Experimental Allergic Encephalomyelitis

The concentration in the body fluids of other self-antigens may be so low that neither the T cells nor the B cells are tolerant. In this situation, appropriate challenge of such animals with the self-antigen activates B cells and both effector and helper T cells. The effector T cells are tissue-damaging in themselves, and the T helper cells collaborate with B cells in the production of autoantibodies. Experimental allergic encephalomyelitis is an example that has some features in common with multiple sclerosis in humans. This disease is induced experimentally by immunizing animals with basic protein of myelin incorporated into an adjuvant. Although both T and B cells are activated and antibody is produced, only T cells are required for the initiation of the clinical symptoms and the histologic lesions. What role antibody plays in the progression of the disease is not clear.

Myasthenia Gravis

Another model in which neither the T nor the B cell is tolerant to the self-antigen is myasthenia gravis (see Chapter 1 in *Principles of Immunology and Allergy*). This autoimmune disease results from antibody directed to the acetylcholine receptor of skeletal muscle, thus impairing neuromuscular transmission. This receptor is present in extremely small concentrations in the body fluids, allowing both T and B cells to escape self-tolerance. Injection of rats with acetylcholine receptor from the electric eel causes the rats to make antibody cross-reactive with their own receptor, resulting in a clinical disease that is similar to myasthenia in man. Although T cells are activated, they are not required for the initiation of the disease but may play some role in its progression.

These three models represent only one set of mechanisms that could lead to autoimmune reactivity. Other mechanisms involving abnormalities in regulatory circuits and networks may also be directly or indirectly responsible for many autoimmune disorders. Certainly these regulatory systems are involved in control of autoimmune disorders once they are initiated by whatever mechanism.

Bibliography

Billingham, R. E., Brent, L., and Medawar, P. B.: Actively acquired tolerance to foreign cells. Nature 172:603, 1953.

Burnet, F. M.: The clonal selection theory of acquired immunity. Cambridge, Cambridge University Press, 1959.

Howard, J. G., and Mitchison, N. A.: Immunologic tolerance. Prog. Allergy 18:43, 1975.

Kettman, J. R., Cambier, J., Uhr, J. W., et al.: The role of receptor IgM and IgD in determining triggering and induction of tolerance in murine B cells. Immunol. Rev. 43:69, 1979.

Lamb, J. R., Skidmore, B. J., Green, N., et al.: Induction of tolerance in influenza virus–immune T lymphocyte clones with synthetic peptides of influenza hemagglutinin. J. Exp. Med. 157:1434, 1983.

Metcalf, E. S., Schrater, A. F., and Klinman, N. R.: Murine models of tolerance induction in developing and mature B cells. Immunol. Rev. 43:143, 1979.

Nossal, G. J. V.: Cellular mechanisms of immunological tolerance. Ann. Rev. Immunol. 1:33, 1983.

Owens, R. D.: Immunogenetic consequence of vascular anastomoses between bovine twins. Science 102:400, 1945.

Weigle, W. O.: Immunological unresponsiveness. Adv. Immunol. 16:61, 1973.

Weigle, W. O.: Analysis of autoimmunity through experimental models of thyroiditis and allergic encephalomyelitis. Adv. Immunol. 30:159, 1980.

8

Transplantation Immunity

DAVID W. TALMAGE, M.D.,
and FRANCISCO G. LA ROSA, M.D.

Introduction	Mechanisms of Graft Rejection
Histocompatibility Antigens	Mechanism of Transplantation
Major and Minor Histocompati-	Tolerance
bility Loci	

INTRODUCTION

In 1953, Billingham, Brent, and Medawar astounded the immunologic community with the demonstration that inbred mice could be made tolerant of skin grafts from other strains of mice by the prior intrauterine injection of bone marrow cells from the graft donor (Fig. 8–1). These experiments were based on the findings of Owen that cattle twins possessed mixed blood (chimeras), and, in fact, the tolerant mice of Billingham and coworkers were stable blood and bone marrow chimeras. The other effects and uses of bone marrow transplantation are covered in Chapters 6 and 9.

The discovery of acquired immunologic tolerance by Owen and by Billingham, Brent, and Medawar played an important role in stimulating the development of a new and highly successful field of research, i.e., cellular immunology. Nevertheless,

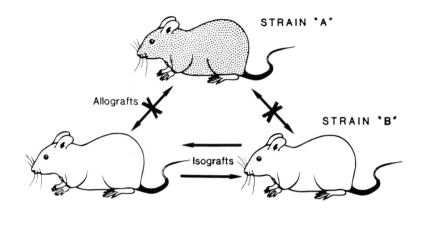

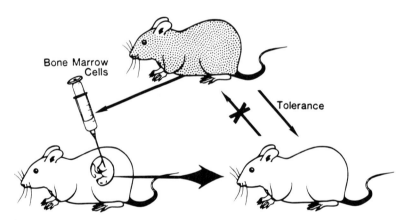

Figure 8–1. Billingham, Brent, and Medawar's experiment illustrating the induction of chimeric tolerance in the mouse by the intrauterine injection of bone marrow cells. (———indicates graft acceptance; ——indicates graft rejection.)

and somewhat paradoxically, the phenomena of graft rejection and its abrogation through chimeric tolerance are almost as puzzling today as they were 30 years ago.

The observations of transplantation immunity are fairly straightforward and consistent. Grafts from one individual to another individual of the same species *(allografts)* usually fail (Fig. 8–1), whereas *isografts* (between genetically identical individuals) are uniformly accepted. Second allografts are rejected more promptly if they are from the same or genetically identical donors. This so called "second set" immunity may be transferred by T lymphocytes and is highly specific. A second allograft from a different donor may show either a primary or accelerated rejection pattern depending on the genetic relationship between the two donors.

HISTOCOMPATIBILITY ANTIGENS

The development of inbred strains of mice, rats, and guinea pigs played an important role in elucidating the genetic basis of transplantation. The rejection of grafts and tumors was shown to depend on the existence of numerous histocompatibility genes. Thus, a hybrid animal (F_1), formed from the cross of two inbred strains, contains all the histocompatibility antigens of both strains. Such an F_1 hybrid will accept grafts from either parental strain, but a hybrid graft will be rejected by both parental strains (Fig. 8–2).

While F_1 hybrids uniformly accept grafts from both parental strains and from each other, mice of the F_2 generation (obtained by mating two identical F_1 hybrids) do so very rarely (Fig. 8–2). This is because of the random assortment of chromosomes. The minimum number of genetic loci responsible for graft rejection can be calculated from the frequency of rejection of parental strain grafts by F_2 mice. This minimum number of histocompatibility loci was calculated for mice in 1916 by Little and Tyzzer and was found to be 14 or 15, which is probably a gross underestimate. Their experiments involved the rejection of a carcinoma, which undoubtedly carried only a small percentage of all the tissue-specific antigens (see next paragraph). Furthermore, each genetic locus undoubtedly contains the genes for many antigens.

MAJOR AND MINOR HISTOCOMPATIBILITY LOCI

Among histocompatibility antigens in inbred mice, one antigen, called antigen II, received particular study for two reasons: (1) it was found on both normal and tumor cells and even on erythrocytes, and (2) differences between this antigen in two inbred strains correlated with rapidity of graft rejection. The genetic locus determining these antigens in mice was first called the H-2 locus. Subsequently it was called the *major histocompatibility complex* (MHC) when it was determined that more

STRAIN "A"   STRAIN "B"

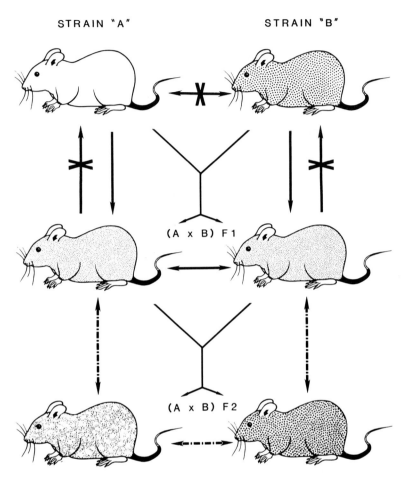

Figure 8–2. Tissue transplantation between parental, F1, and F2 mouse strains (see details in the text). (➡100 percent acceptance; ✗➡100 percent rejection; ⟶·➡ less than 5 percent acceptance.)

than one antigen was involved and that similar dominant loci existed in other species. In humans the MHC codes for the HLA proteins (see Chapter 5).

The MHC antigens play a dominant role in graft rejection because of their unique association with the recognition system of T cells. Unlike antibodies, T cells cannot recognize or react directly with non-MHC antigens (viruses, allergens, or minor histocompatibility antigens) but recognize these antigens only in association with or complexed to an MHC antigen.

There are two classes of MHC antigens. Class I MHC antigens are present on every cell in the body and for this reason

Figure 8–3. Distribution of major and minor antigens in different cells from the same individual. Class I MHC antigens (●) are present on all cells. Class II MHC antigens (►) are usually present on cells (S+) with the function of stimulating T helper cells, whereas minor antigens (⌐⊥⌐) 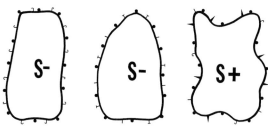 have an uneven distribution, showing, in some cases, organ specificity. Cells that lack the capacity to stimulate T lymphocytes are labeled S –

are important targets of the rejection reaction. Class II MHC antigens, which are present only on leukocytes, monocytes, and a few other cells, activate T helper lymphocytes (Th), which are thought to be necessary because of their production of lymphokines or helper factors.

There are probably hundreds of non-MHC or *minor* histocompatibility antigens. Many or most of these antigens are tissue-specific, and for that reason the total number can never be enumerated (Fig. 8–3). It seems likely that any alloantigen can serve as a minor histocompatibility antigen if it is capable of complexing with either the Class I or Class II MHC antigens.

MECHANISMS OF GRAFT REJECTION

The cytotoxic T cell (Tc) is the most likely *cause* of the highly specific and rapid destruction seen in a graft rejection. However, the participation of less specific cells, such as macrophages and natural killer (NK) cells, cannot be ruled out.

Prior to recognition of the distinction between T and B lymphocytes, Rosenau and Moon had noted that lymphoid cells from sensitized animals were able to destroy homologous cells in tissue culture. A few years later Friedman had noted inhibition of antibody-forming plaques, and Vainio had observed release of radioactive thymidine from labeled targets. In 1968, Brunner, Manuel, Cerrotini, and Chapuis first described the now standard ^{51}Cr release assay.

Two sets of observations have been cited to cast doubt on the role of Tc in graft rejection. First, Simpson and her colleagues have noted exceptions to a generally good correlation between the ability of a female mouse of an inbred strain to reject male skin grafts of the same strain and the capacity of the same mouse to produce Tc against isologous male target cells in vitro.

Second, Loveland and Mackenzie claimed to have demonstrated that Tc are not responsible for skin graft rejection and that a helper T cell was both necessary and sufficient. Adult mice, thymectomized, irradiated, and restored with T-cell depleted bone marrow (ATXBM) were unable to reject allografts unless repleted with Lyt-1 + immune spleen cells. In general, Tc and suppressor T cells are Lyt-2 +, whereas helper cells and cells responsible for delayed hypersensitivity are Lyt-1 + 2 − .

These two sets of experiments clearly show that cells other than Tc (probably helper cells) are required for graft rejection, but they do not rule out an essential role for Tc. These cells or their precursors, in Loveland's experiments, may have been present in the recipient ATXBM mice, since such cells have been found in athymic nude mice. A variability in the induction of tolerance in vivo, in Simpson's experiments, could also account for some of the observed lack of correlation of graft rejection with Tc production in vitro, and the conditions required for activation of helper cells may not be the same in vivo as in vitro.

A number of experiments have provided strong evidence favoring a role for Tc in graft rejection. Billingham and Silvers found a highly specific sparing of pigmented syngeneic cells embedded in nonpigmented allogeneic skin undergoing rejection in guinea pigs. These results indicate that the destructive mechanism is highly cell-specific and requires cell-to-cell contact. This absence of bystander effect indicates that the destruction is not the result of the nonspecific effects of an inflammatory reaction.

Experiments with endocrine allografts cultured in oxygen also support an essential role of Tc in allograft rejection but suggest that a cooperation between two types of T cells is required. The established prolongation of allograft survival after culture in oxygen is attributed to the destruction of the passenger leukocytes and endothelial cells capable of activating recipient lymphocytes. La Rosa and Talmage found that culturing thyroid grafts containing only MHC antigens completely abolished subsequent lymphocytic infiltration, whereas the same treatment had little effect on the infiltration of grafts containing minor antigens only. There was a synergism between the responses to the minor antigens (delayed hypersensitivity) and the major antigens (Tc response). Only in adequately cultured grafts containing both types of antigen did infiltration lead to destruction. A proposed mechanism of synergism is illustrated in Figure 8–4.

In the absence of passenger leukocytes, minor antigens from the graft are picked up and presented by host macrophages, inducing a form of delayed hypersensitivity. Within the focus of

A:

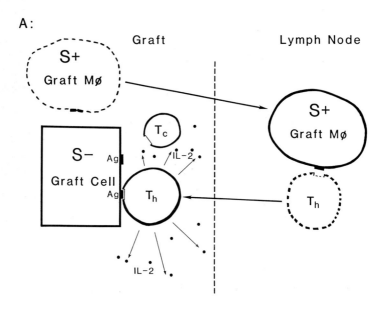

B:

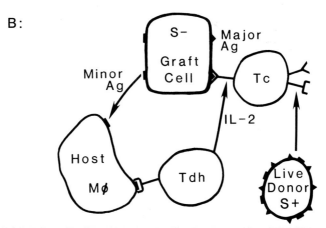

Figure 8–4. *A,* Proposed mechanism of rejection when the graft contains macrophages (Mφ). Mφ from the graft move to the lymph node, where they activate T helper cells (Th). Th move back to the graft and activate cytotoxic T cells (Tc). *B,* Proposed synergistic model of rejection in the absence of graft Mφ (after culture). Minor antigens from graft cells are taken up and presented by host Mφ, producing an inflammatory focus of delayed hypersensitivity (Tdh). In the presence of IL-2 accumulating in the focus, Tc against the major antigens of the graft are activated. Tc against both major and minor antigens may be activated by the injection of donor spleen cells (S+).

infiltration thus caused, a sufficient concentration of lymphokine (particularly IL-2) accumulates to activate Tc directly against the major antigens of the graft.

Destruction of all types of cultured grafts followed injection of spleen cells of the donor strain. Two requirements for this induced reaction indicated that the rejection was mainly due to activation of Tc. First, the donor spleen cells injected needed to be alive to be effective, and second, spleen cells containing only minor antigens induced the rejection of a completely syngeneic graft (same at minor and MHC loci) more rapidly than a graft that had the same minor antigens but differed at the MHC. The latter is evidence of MHC restriction in the response to the injected cells. The fact that an effective response occurred only when the injected cells and the graft had the same MHC indicates that a direct cell-to-cell contact of responding cell with the graft is required for destruction.

MECHANISM OF TRANSPLANTATION TOLERANCE

There are at least two types of tolerance (passive and active) that prevent the rejection of transplants. The chimeric tolerance of Billingham, Brent, and Medawar is probably largely passive, resulting from the deletion of clones of cells responsive to the passenger leukocytes of the graft. This type of tolerance is abrogated by the injection of normal spleen cells of the recipient's genotype. The effect of deleting the cells capable of responding to passenger leukocytes is the same as deleting passenger leukocytes from the graft by culture in oxygen. In both cases transplantation of organs is greatly prolonged, usually indefinitely, even though the graft may contain strong tissue-specific antigens. Since these tissue antigens are not present on stimulating cells, they are unable to activate responding lymphocytes directly. However, a chronic rejection reaction may take place as a result of the processing of these tissue-specific antigens on the macrophages of the host and the development of delayed hypersensitivity to the processed antigen.

Fortunately for the graft, a second type of tolerance develops slowly to the antigens of the graft. This tolerance is an active process and cannot be abrogated by normal spleen cells. It occurs as well in chimeric recipients and in nonchimeric recipients of cultured grafts.

The mechanism of the active transplantation tolerance is

unknown. It takes months to develop and is only partial and relative. However, it protects new grafts even if they contain new antigens. It may be due to antibody, to suppressor T cells, or to anti-idiotype responses. It probably accounts for the enhanced survival of organ grafts seen in humans after third party blood transfusions. Thus the elucidation of the mechanism of active transplantation tolerance may be important in the abrogation of the rejection of organ transplants in the human.

Since chimeras are difficult to produce in humans, a combination of active transplantation tolerance, immune suppression, and organ culture seems the most promising approach to successful human organ transplantation.

Bibliography

Anderson, C. B., Sicard, G. A., and Etheredge, E. E.: Pretreatment of renal allograft recipients with azathioprine and donor-specific blood products. Surgery 92:315, 1982.

Billingham, R., and Silvers, W.: The Immunology of Transplantation. Englewood Cliffs, NJ, Prentice-Hall, 1971.

Brunner, K. T., Manuel J., Cerottini, J. C., et al.: Quantitative assay of the lytic action of immune lymphoid cells on ^{51}Cr labelled allogeneic target cells in vitro; inhibition by isoantibody and by drugs. Immunology 14:181, 1968.

Dallman, M. J., and Mason, D. W.: Role of thymus-derived and thymus independent cells in murine skin allograft rejection. Transplantation 33:221, 1983.

Faustman, D., Lacy, P., Davie, J., et al.: Prevention of allograft rejection by immunization with donor blood depleted of Ia-bearing cells. Science 217:157, 1982.

Friedman, H.: Inhibition of antibody plaque formation by sensitized lymphoid cells: rapid indication of transplantation immunity. Science 145:607, 1964.

Hurme, M., Chandler, P. R., Hetherington, C. M., et al.: Cytotoxic T cell responses to H-Y: correlation with the rejection of syngeneic male skin grafts. J. Exp. Med. 147:768, 1978.

La Rosa, F. G., and Talmage, D. W.: The failure of a major histocompatibility antigen to stimulate a thyroid allograft reaction after culture in oxygen. J. Exp. Med. 157:898, 1983.

Loveland, B. E., and McKenzie, I. F. C.: Which T cells cause graft rejection? Transplantation 33:217, 1982.

Naji, A., Silvers, W. K., and Barker, C. F.: Influence of organ culture on the survival of major histocompatibility complex–compatible and incompatible parathyroid allografts in rats. Transplantation 32:296, 1981.

Oei, L. S., Thompson, J. S., and Corr, R. J.: Effect of blood transfusions on survival of cadaver and living related renal transplants. Transplantation 28:482, 1979.

Owen, R.: Immunogenetic consequences of vascular anastomoses between bovine twins. Science 102:400, 1945.

Persijn, G. G., Cohen, B., Lansbergen, Q., et al.: Retrospective and prospective studies on the effect of blood transfusions in renal transplantation in the Netherlands. Transplantation 28:396, 1979.

Persijn, G. G., Van Leeuwen, A., Parlevliet, J., et al.: Two major factors influencing kidney graft survival in eurotransplant: HLA-DR matching and blood transfusion(s). Transpl. Proc. 13:150, 1981.

Pimsler, M., Trial, J. A., and Forman, J.: Antigen-presenting cells that induce anti-H-2K T cell responses: differences in stimulator-cell requirements for induction of proliferation and cell-mediated lympholysis. Immunogenetics 12:297, 1981.

Rosenau, W., and Moon, H. D.: Lysis of homologous cells by sensitized lymphocytes in tissue culture. J. Natl. Cancer Inst. 27:471, 1961.

Silvers, W. K., Fleming, H. L., Naji, A., et al.: Evidence for major histocompatibility complex restriction in transplantation immunity. Proc. Natl. Acad. Sci. USA 79:171, 1982.

Vainio, T., Koskimies, O., Perlmann, P., et al.: In vitro cytotoxic effect of lymphoid cells from mice immunized with allogeneic tissue. Nature (London) 204:453, 1964.

9

Bone Marrow Transplantation*

ROBERT A. GOOD, M.D., Ph.D.

*Original studies described herein were supported by AI 22360, AG 05628, and the March of Dimes Birth Defects Foundation 1-789.

131

INTRODUCTION

Transplantation of bone marrow as a form of cellular engineering has been used as the sole or adjunct treatment for almost 50 otherwise lethal diseases (Table 9–1). Although bone marrow transplantation is already the treatment of choice for more than 40 of these, it is still at an early stage of development. The first successful allogeneic marrow transplant was carried out by our Minnesota group in 1968; since then approximately 5000 marrow transplants have been done throughout the world, and more than 5000 marrow transplants will be performed during the next 2 years. Marrow transplantation, once one of the most difficult of all therapeutic procedures, has been so simplified that it is now performed in at least 160 centers in the United States, Europe, and Japan.

In addition to its successful use in immunodeficiency and hematopoietic abnormalities, marrow transplantation is now used for some generalized malignancies, e.g., neuroblastoma, oat cell lung cancer, and other radiosensitive cancers. It has been effectively used to treat certain inborn errors of metabolism that cannot be classified as either primary immunodeficiencies or congenital hematopoietic abnormalities.

HISTORY

Bone marrow transplantation dates from the late 1940s when Jacobson demonstrated that there was often complete hematologic and lymphoid recovery by rabbits subjected to lethal total body irradiation, provided their spleen or bone marrow was shielded to protect them from the cellular destruction that otherwise follows total body ionizing irradiation. The shielded rabbits replenished all of their hematopoietic and lymphoid cells and tissues from the splenic or marrow stem cells that had been protected from injury. These cells migrated through the circulating blood to set up hematopoietic and lymphoid centers in the depleted bone marrow and lymphoid sites. Hematopoietic reconstruction was later achieved by cells from such other cell sources as fetal liver, blood, and even from thymus precursors.

A series of subsequent investigations with mice indicated that stem cells, among cells aspirated from the bone marrow, could entirely replenish the complex hematopoietic and lymphoid systems. Donor marrow cells, injected intraperitoneally or intravenously into lethally irradiated syngeneic recipients, regularly

Table 9–1. Otherwise Lethal Diseases Treated
by Bone Marrow Transplantation (1986)

1. Severe combined immunodeficiency (SCID), autosomal recessive—deficient T and B cells
2. SCID, X-linked recessive—deficient T and B cells
3. SCID, autosomal recessive—deficient T and deficient or normal B cells
4. SCID with adenosine deaminase (ADA) deficiency
5. SCID with nucleoside phosphorylase deficiency (NPD)
6. SCID with TP40 deficiency and abnormal T and B cell functions
7. SCID with deficient T cells and normal B cells
8. Wiskott-Aldrich syndrome
9. Common variable immunodeficiency
10. Bare leukocyte syndrome
11. T helper cell deficiency, autosomal recessive
12. Chédiak-Higashi syndrome
13. Chronic granulomatous disease of childhood
14. Severe neutrophil dysfunction
15. Osteopetrosis infantile, autosomal recessive
16. Osteopetrosis tardive, autosomal recessive
17. X-linked infantile agammaglobulinemia
18. P150,95,CR-3, M-1 deficiency with monocyte and granulocyte malfunction
19. Maroteaux-Lamy syndrome, arylsulfatase B deficiency
20. Pure red cell aplasia (Blackfan-Diamond syndrome)
21. Thalassemia major
22. Sickle cell anemia
23. Paroxysmal nocturnal hemoglobinuria
24. Myelofibrosis
25. Idiopathic aplastic anemia—immunologically based
26. Idiopathic aplastic anemia—nonimmunologically based
27. Aplastic anemia—postviral
28. Aplastic anemia—toxic or drug induced
29. Aplastic anemia associated with Fanconi syndrome
30. Mucopolysaccharidosis other than Maroteaux-Lamy syndrome
31. Acute undifferentiated leukemia M-1
32. Acute myelogenous leukemia M-2
33. Acute pregranulocytic leukemia M-3
34. Acute myelomonocytic leukemia M-4
35. Acute monocytic leukemia M-5
36. Acute erythroleukemia M-6
37. Acute lymphoblastic or lymphocytic leukemia (ALL), T cell leukemia
38. ALL B cell leukemia
39. ALL Non T-Non B
40. ALL CALLA—after first exacerbation
41. ALL Pre B cell
42. ALL L_1
43. ALL L_2
44. ALL L_3
45. Neuroblastoma
46. Small cell carcinoma of the lung
47. Disseminated radiosensitive cancers

restored all hematopoietic and lymphoid structures that had been destroyed by lethal or supralethal total body irradiation. Whereas syngeneic marrow transplants were successful, allogeneic marrow transplants often failed completely, because they gave rise to a wasting or runting disorder called secondary disease or graft-versus-host disease (GVHD). This often fatal disease could be attributed to graft-versus-host reactions (GVHR) that were due to recognition by the donor lymphoid cells of the foreignness of the recipient cells, resulting in the allograft "attack."

A leukemic patient who received a bone marrow transplantation at the University of Minnesota in 1959 died several weeks following the irradiation and transplantation. At autopsy no evidence of leukemia was found, and the donor's (father's) lymphoid cells had infiltrated the liver, skin, and bowel of the recipient child, producing a GVHR that was thought to have been the cause of death.

Between 1959 and 1968, efforts in animals were made experimentally to use allogeneic marrow grafts to correct immunologic and hematologic defects. The results were always disastrous, usually attributable to GVHR and GVHD. During this period the Minnesota system was developed for studying transplantation immunity. Donors of transplants were matched with recipient mice at the major histocompatibility complex (H-2). Among a number of dramatic results of such experiments was regular induction of immunologic tolerance in neonates, frequent induction of immunologic tolerance during adult life, successful performance of fully functional pituitary transplants, successful fully functional adrenal transplants, and even ovarian transplants that produced eggs that could be fertilized. The state of tolerance was transferred from one animal to another by either parabiosis or spleen cell injection, providing early evidence of the specific suppressive immunologic function of lymphoid cells. Tolerant states were also induced by injection of material from disrupted donor cells during the neonatal period or during adult life. This series of studies in mice revealed the importance for tissue transplantation of matching donor and recipient. The separate roles of the thymus and bursa in chickens were defined as central lymphoid organs for two major immunologic systems. It seemed clear, from both clinical and experimental studies in mice, chickens, rats, and hamsters, that the bone marrow and fetal liver stem cells could be considered precursors of both the thymus-derived T lymphocytes and the bursa- or bone marrow–derived B lymphocytes and plasma cells. The pathogeneti bases for the primary immunodeficiency diseases could thus be postulated in terms of development of T cells, B cells, or both. X-linked infantile immunodeficiency became, for us, the prototype of faulty B-cell development; DiGeorge's athymic syndrome, the prototype of deficient T-cell development; and severe combined immunodeficiency (SCID), the prototype of faulty development of both lymphoid systems, which we reasoned must reside in the bone marrow.

In subsequent experiments the lymphoid system of neonatally thymectomized mice was reconstructed by transplants of neonatal thymus, of epithelial thymus anlagen, or of spleen cells containing large numbers of mature peripheral lymphoid cells from intact donors that were either syngeneic with the recipients or had been matched with recipients at the MHC–H-2 determinants. If the spleen cells were from donors mismatched at the MHC, the transplanted mice regularly died as a consequence of GVHR. These studies formed the basis of our approach to the use of cellular engineering for the treatment of some of the primary immunodeficiency syndromes in man, e.g., DiGeorge's, T-cell deficient athymic syndrome (by thymus transplantation), and SCID with deficiency of both T and B cells (by bone marrow transplantation).

It was essential that we find human donor matches equivalent to those found useful for mice, in order that a safe and successful hematopoietic transplant be possible in man. It seemed possible to match a donor perfectly one fourth of the time at the MHC if a sibling were used who was identical to the recipient at the A and B loci and by MLC matching. An initial attempt with fetal liver plus thymus transplants from an embryonic donor corrected the immunodeficiency disease of one patient with SCID. The patient did not, however, do well, because transfusion with blood mismatched by MHC caused a devastating GVHR.

MATCHED SIBLING ALLOGENEIC BONE MARROW TRANSPLANTATION

Severe Combined Immunodeficiency Disease (SCID) with Aplastic Anemia

Attempts to cure SCID by bone marrow transplantation would require use of an MHC-matched sibling donor as a source of lymphoid cell precursors. Patients with SCID would probably require no further preparation as recipients for a marrow transplant, since SCID results from an inborn error of development of the lymphoid system with profound deficiencies of T, B, and plasma cell populations. A patient with X-linked SCID was given a marrow transplant in 1968 and became the first patient cured of this primary immunodeficiency disease. A complicating GVHR resulted in aplastic anemia, which was treated successfully by a second bone marrow transplant from the same donor.

Wiskott-Aldrich (WA) Syndrome

Also in 1968, Bach and coworkers in Wisconsin transplanted marrow in a child with the complex immunodeficiency and hematopoietic abnormality called the Wiskott-Aldrich syndrome (WA). In this instance, lethal doses of cyclophosphamide were first given to inhibit an allograft rejection potential by the child and to facilitate the acceptance of the hematopoietic precursor cells. Although not cured completely of WA by the marrow transplant, the immunodeficiencies associated with the WA syndrome were corrected. This child, the first patient with WA treated successfully by bone marrow transplantation, has remained a mixed chimera with a lymphoid system and immunologic functions attributable to the HLA-matched sibling donor. At present writing, this patient and our initial case of SCID live in good health. Our patient is a full chimera, since all of his lymphoid cells, hematopoietic cells of his marrow, red cells, white blood cells, and cells of his lymphoid tissues have the karyotype and other distinctive markers of the sister who was the original bone marrow donor. Nearly 100 SCID patients have now been cured using *matched sibling donors,* and complete correction of at least eight different, otherwise lethal, forms of SCID has been accomplished. Similarly, all of the hematopoietic abnormalities and immunologic deficiencies associated with the Wiskott-Aldrich syndrome have regularly been corrected in 30 instances.

The best results, with fewest complications, have been achieved by preliminary myeloablation with Busulfan and cyclophosphamide, a method adapted from studies of successful marrow transplantation in rats. A combination of lethal total body irradiation coupled with antithymocyte globulin plus procarbazine as a conditioning regimen has also been successful. Curative correction of the highly lethal WA syndrome should be attempted as early in life as it is discovered. We have, therefore, advocated the Busulfan-cyclophosphamide conditioning regimen to avoid damage to growth centers in bone and other complications that can result from total body irradiation.

Prevention of Malignancies in SCID and WA Syndrome

Patients with untreated SCID and WA syndrome are prone to malignancies, which occur, for the most part, among residual lymphoid cells or tissues. The frequency of such malignancies in patients with SCID may be 4 to 5 percent or higher per year. During the past 17 years, none of the fully reconstituted patients with SCID have developed lymphoid or other malignancies. As many as 50 percent of untreated patients or patients with marrow transplants from HLA-mismatched donors who have achieved incomplete immunologic reconstruction have developed a malignancy of the lymphoid system. Similarly, among the 30 fully reconstructed WA patients to date, none have experienced lymphoid or other malignancies, while, by contrast, 12 to 20 percent of untreated WA patients did develop them.

Malignancies of the B lymphocytes or of the plasma cell series are the most frequent in patients with SCID. The malignant cells can often be shown to result from a monoclonal expansion of lymphoid cells infected by the Epstein-Barr virus (EBV). These findings, noted in both SCID and WA, suggest that a deficiency of immunosurveillance against certain cancers prior to treatment is fully restored by bone marrow transplantation.

SCID due to ADA Deficiency

The first defined inborn error of metabolism to be cured by marrow transplantation was SCID due to lack of the enzyme adenosine deaminase (ADA). This enzyme of the purine salvage pathway of metabolism catalyzes conversion of adenosine and 2-deoxyadenosine to inosine. The toxic metabolites (adenosine, 2-deoxyadenosine, and 2-deoxy ATP) that accumulate behind this metabolic block interfere first with development of T lymphocytes and then with development of B lymphocytes. Several of our patients with this deficiency have been cured by bone marrow transplantation. The first patient successfully treated was a 1-year-old child whose sister was perfectly matched at the HLA ACB D/Dr loci. Unlike those of the patient, the sister's red, white, and lymphoid cells possessed normal amounts of ADA. The patient's RBCs, leukocytes, and bone marrow cells, by contrast, were strikingly deficient in this enzyme. Repeated marrow transplantation, without any preliminary myeloablation, fully corrected the immunodeficiency. To this day, 15 years later, this patient is completely normal immunologically and is a stable chimera. Her red blood cells, white blood cells, and monocytes still lack the enzyme ADA, whereas her lymphoid cells possess normal amounts of this enzyme. The lymphocytes are thus entirely attributable to the marrow precursors, transplanted from her sister, that can produce the enzyme ADA. They are responsible for her good health. These findings suggest that at least sometimes the correction of an enzyme defect does not require that all of the cells of the body that normally possess an enzyme need to be replaced to correct the consequences of the enzyme deficiency.

Osteopetrosis

Bone marrow transplantation is now used to treat many more forms of such highly lethal primary immunodeficiency diseases as X-linked agammaglobulinemia, combined immunodeficiency diseases, and hematopoietic deficiencies like thalassemia major or even sickle cell anemia. A dramatic correction of such a disease has been achieved repeatedly by bone marrow transplantation in cases of severe osteopetrosis, a highly morbid, ultimately lethal, disease resulting from failure of function of osteoclastic cells. The function of these cells, of the phagocyte lineage, is essential for normal bone growth to maintain them as major sites of hematopoiesis. Blindness and deafness regularly occur because the failure of the normal function of osteoclasts to remodel bone may result in the impingement of bone on the optic and acoustic nerves. The osteoclasts, like all cells of the monocyte macrophage line, are derived from bone marrow precursors. There are at least two separate genetic, autosomal recessive forms of osteopetrosis in which osteoclasts do not develop and do not function normally. The cure of this disease requires employment of high-dose Busulfan plus cyclophosphamide as preparation before marrow transplantation. Table 9–2 lists the changes that followed successful bone marrow transplantation and full correction of the osteopetrosis syndrome. It is essential to achieve a sustained hematopoietic marrow transplantation and persistent acceptance of the hematopoietic precursors of the osteoclasts for treatment to succeed. A peripheral graft of osteoclasts of donor origin, achieved without a persistent central marrow graft, yields only a transient correction of the metabolic abnormality that only temporarily corrects some of the abnormal physiology, and the disease recurs. It is important to achieve a full and sustained acceptance of the bone marrow grafts for this and for most of the other diseases in which marrow transplantation is useful.

Mucopolysaccharidoses

Maroteaux-Lamy Syndrome

Bone marrow transplantation has been used with impressive partial success to treat the metabolic abnormality of the Maroteaux-Lamy syndrome. This disease is characterized by an absence of the enzyme arylsulfatase B from all tissues. This deficiency results in accumulation in the tissues of the mucopolysaccharide dermatin sulfate, which causes hepatosplenomegaly, defective cardiopulmonary function, clouding of the lens and cornea with progressive failure of vision, and decreased joint mobility.

Storage of the mucopolysaccharide seemed to be pathogenic for the progressive abnormalities of the spleen, liver, eyes, and joints, and central nervous system malfunction is not present. It therefore seemed likely that marrow transplantation could be used as a treatment for the Maroteaux-Lamy syndrome. Furthermore, mucopolysaccharidosis type VI occurs in cats and can be corrected by bone marrow transplantation. The Busulfan-cyclophosphamide preparation plus bone marrow transplantation was then used to treat a 13-year-old patient with the Maroteaux-Lamy arylsulfatase B deficiency. Therapy was instituted relatively late in life, after irreversible damage had already been done by the deposited mucopolysaccharide. Nevertheless, the transplantation from the healthy donor led to an increase to normal levels of arylsulfatase B in peripheral leukocytes and granulocytes. There was also an increase of the ratio of liver arylsulfatase B to arylsulfatase A from 3 to 16 percent of normal while urinary excretion of the acid mucopolysaccharide decreased. Other shifts toward normal occurred and 24 months after transplantation, hepatosplenomegaly had markedly de-

Table 9–2. Osteopetrosis Syndrome Response
to Bone Marrow Transplantation

---

1. Extensive bone reabsorption
2. Augmentation of osteoclastic function attributable to donor osteoclasts
3. Remodeling of the bones
4. Expansion of intramedullary hematopoiesis
5. Decrease in the extramedullary hematopoiesis
6. Increase in linear growth
7. Correction of associated deficiency of thymulin function
8. Correction of NK deficiency
9. Permanent reconstitution necessitates sustained engraftment of marrow precursors of osteoclasts—peripheral reconstitution with osteoclasts alone does not yield sustained cure

---

Table 9–3. Changes Made by Bone Marrow Transplantation as Treatment of Mucopolysaccharidosis Type VI (Maroteaux-Lamy Syndrome) with Arylsulfatase B Deficiency

1. Successful hematologic and immunologic reconstitution by bone marrow transplantation in HLA/MLC-matched sibling sister with normal arylsulfatase B activity
2. Full engraftment over 24 months
3. Normal arylsulfatase B activity in peripheral lymphocytes and granulocytes
4. Liver biopsy showed increase in the ratio of arylsulfatase B to arylsulfatase A from 3 percent of normal to 16 percent of normal
5. Urinary excretion of acid mucopolysaccharide decreased
6. Ultrastructural evidence of accumulation of arylsulfatase B in marrow cells, peripheral blood lymphocytes, granulocytes, and platelets disappeared
7. Mucopolysaccharide accumulation in ITO cells of liver disappeared
8. Hepatosplenomegaly greatly decreased
9. Cardiopulmonary function remained normal
10. Visual acuity improved
11. Joint mobility improved
12. Child returned to school and performed well in academic subjects

creased, cardiopulmonary function was normal, and visual acuity and joint mobility had improved (Table 9–3).

Other Mucopolysaccharidoses

Efforts to treat other forms of mucopolysaccharidosis have been reported with somewhat less detail, but encouraging evidence of decreased progression of the connective tissue component of some of the diseases has been described. Careful investigations of bone marrow transplantation of these other forms of mucopolysaccharidosis are needed. Marrow transplantation, though progressively improved and simplified, is very costly and hazardous. It has been too hazardous to use for diseases that are not promptly fatal when untreated. Bone marrow transplantation offers very little if toxic metabolites are derived intrinsically (i.e., in CNS cells) rather than by intercellular transfer. However, as marrow transplantation becomes more successful, and as morbidity and mortality decline, other highly morbid and ultimately fatal or grossly disfiguring diseases will be treated by bone marrow transplantation. This is especially true when there is available a sibling with normal metabolic functions who matches the patient at the MHC.

Hematopoietic Diseases

Aplastic Anemia

There are many causes of aplastic anemia (Table 9–4); bone marrow transplantation seems likely to be the treatment of choice for each of these when an MHC-matched sibling is available. The patients with aplastic anemia who do best with bone marrow transplantation are those who have severe forms of the disease, who are treated early in the course, who have had few transfusions, and who have matched sibling donors. Laminar air flow isolation, decontamination, and provision of nonabsorbable antibiotics and sterilized food and fluids are of significant value in reducing both morbidity and mortality in patients with aplastic anemia treated by bone marrow transplantation. Occasionally, large doses of cyclophosphamide alone cure patients with aplastic anemia, but this is not predictable. Large doses of antithymus gammaglobulin or antilymphocyte globulin from horses have been effective; approximately 50 percent of patients have been cured or helped greatly by antithymocyte globulin treatment.

Leukemias

Marrow transplantation for leukemia had to compete with chemotherapy regimens, which had become quite successful in treatment of some forms of leukemia and lymphoma. At first, transplantation could be used only as treatment for end-stage leukemia, after all efforts at chemotherapy had already failed. Thomas and colleagues showed that long-term survival and some probable cures could be achieved in 10 to 20 percent of acute myeloid leukemia patients in whom all other forms of available treatment had been tried and failed. Once it was established

Table 9–4. Aplastic Anemias

1. Aplastic anemia with Fanconi's syndrome
2. Aplastic anemia due to toxic chemicals or drugs
3. Aplastic anemia after irradiation accident (e.g., Chernobyl incident)
4. Aplastic anemia due to immunosuppression of RBC, granulocyte, and platelet development
5. Aplastic anemia following viral infection, e.g., hepatitis B virus infection
6. Aplastic anemia, idiopathic
7. Other constitutional or inherited aplastic anemias

that marrow transplantation could achieve a goal not yet accomplished by any form of chemotherapy, marrow transplantation, using HLA-matched sibling donors, became the treatment of choice for acute myelogenous leukemia in first remission. If a matched sibling donor is available, marrow transplantation, following intense ablation of residual leukemia, complete myeloablation, and sufficient immunosuppression, has become an accepted means of treatment for patients having one of the many different forms of high-risk leukemias listed in Table 9–1.

OBSTACLES TO MARROW TRANSPLANTATION

The following are some of the problems that limit extensive application of marrow transplantation for treatment of leukemia and for the many inborn errors of metabolism, aplastic anemias, and certain immunodeficiencies: (1) the occurrence of idiopathic interstitial pneumonitis; (2) infections with opportunistic viruses, bacteria, and fungi; (3) the occurrence of GVHR and GVHD, even when marrow transplantation has been carried out using an HLA D/Dr–matched sibling as donor; and (4) lack of availability of a suitably matched sibling donor. In the United States, a matched sibling donor is available only 20 to 40 percent of the time. With noninherited diseases, the availability of a matched sibling approaches 40 percent. With inherited diseases a suitable matched sibling without the disease is available as a donor no more frequently than 20 to 25 percent of the time. Thus, if marrow transplantation is to be used more frequently to cure many otherwise lethal or highly morbid diseases, these four major problems must be overcome. Fortunately, progress is being made both clinically and experimentally toward solution of each of these major problems.

Opportunistic Infections

Infections with High-Grade Encapsulated Pathogens

A persistent and profound immunodeficiency is present in every patient subjected to the preparative regimens necessary to accomplish bone marrow transplantation. These deficiencies include, among many immunologic defects, the inability to make antibodies normally in response to many different antigens. A profound deficiency of cell-mediated immunologic response is also present in these patients for prolonged periods. The occurrence of a GVHR greatly prolongs and intensifies the immunodeficiency and its consequent hazard of an infectious complication. The availability of intravenous IgG (IVIG), prepared from large pools of donors, has greatly improved management of antibody deficiency. The preparations of IVIG must contain each of the IgG subclasses as well as antibody against many common encapsulated bacterial pathogens, such as pneumococci of various types, streptococci, *Haemophilus influenzae, Pseudomonas aeruginosa,* and other bacteria. They must also contain antibody against most of the common viruses and against fungi. Reactions, even to large doses of IVIG, have been minimal. Regular administration of IVIG in doses sufficient to maintain IgG levels in the normal range, even in patients with agammaglobulinemia following marrow transplantation, appears to have effectively inhibited development of infections with many microorganisms. IVIG has been particularly effective in preventing infections with encapsulated bacteria (pneumococci, streptococci, *Haemophilus influenzae,* and *Pseudomonas aeruginosa),* which had occurred frequently in immunodeficient patients who had profound failure of antibody production. Our bone marrow transplant recipients are given 300 mg/kg of either the Cutter Laboratories or the Sandoglobulin IVIG every 3 to 4 weeks. This is continued until antibody producing capacity has returned to normal, 6 months or so after transplantation. This has almost completely eliminated the sometimes overwhelming infections with the encapsulated bacterial pathogens mentioned above.

Pneumocystis carinii Pneumonia

This disease, a major problem in all immunocompromised hosts, usually occurs in marrow-transplanted patients during the period of leukopenia or during the first 8 weeks following marrow transplantation, when both T and B cell immunologic functions are most profoundly depressed. Fortunately, effective treatment is available with trimethoprim and sulfamethoxazole (TMP-SMZ), and alternatively with pentamadine isothionate. An even greater advantage is obtained by the regular prophylactic use of a smaller dose of the chemotherapeutic combination. The interstitial pneumonitis caused by *Pneumocystis carinii* accompanying bone marrow transplantation is now almost an experience of the past. The complication of overwhelming *Pneumocystis* pneumonia may develop from a mild persistent interstitial pneumonia attributable to *Pneumocystis carinii.* This is now almost always avoided by first treating all patients, e.g., those with SCID, with TMP-SMZ prior to bone marrow transplantation. A transformation of persistent, relatively mild pneumonitis into an overwhelming pneumonia has sometimes also occurred when certain viruses, e.g., adenovirus, parainfluenza, or respiratory syncytial virus, infect children with SCID at the time of accomplishing bone marrow transplantation from a matched sibling donor.

Gelfand suggested the use of antiviral therapy prior to the transplant, which we have also found to be an effective prevention. Administration of ribovirin by inhalation to patients with persistent parainfluenza or respiratory syncytial virus infection may avoid the production of overwhelming pneumonia and make a successful bone marrow transplantation possible.

Cytomegalovirus (CMV) Infection

Infections by either exogenous or endogenous CMV may complicate marrow transplantation. Such an infection, by any route, has often spelled disaster. The CMV infections can produce fever, arthritis, hepatitis, retinitis, gastrointestinal disease and dysfunction, or interstitial pneumonitis. The incidence and mortality from CMV infections has been very high in patients receiving bone marrow transplants. Interstitial pneumonitis due to CMV infections occurred in approximately 16 percent of the large number of recipients of bone marrow transplants in Seattle, and the fatality rate was approximately 80 percent.

In the United States, CMV infections have complicated marrow transplantations in 69 percent of patients who were seropositive for CMV prior to marrow transplantation and in 33 percent of those who were seronegative. The complicating infections occur between 30 and 100 days after marrow transplantation.

There is no specific therapy for CMV infections, but the complication can be prevented by: use of CMV negative blood products when treating bone marrow transplant patients, prophylactic use of very high doses (300 mg/kg) every 3 weeks of IVIG containing significant anti-CMV antibody titers, or prophylactic use of hyperimmune CMV gamma globulin prepared from patients recently recovered from CMV infections.

Bone marrow transplantation recipients should be given blood and blood products certified to be free of CMV virus and also free of evidence of HTLV III/LAV (AIDS virus) contamination.

Herpes Simplex Infection

Herpes simplex virus infections have also complicated bone marrow transplantation. Reactivation of herpes simplex virus infections usually occurs during the first 6 weeks following marrow transplantation and frequently involves the mouth, lips, and genitalia. Herpes simplex infections may cause a severe pneumonia that may also be complicated by infections with other viruses, bacteria, or fungi. Herpes complications have occurred in 70 to 80 percent of herpes-seropositive bone marrow transplantation recipients and in 20 to 25 percent of seronegative patients. Acyclovir, given intravenously in a dose of 1500 mg/m^2/day for 7 days, has effectively reduced symptoms and shortened the time to healing. Acyclovir, given by either the oral or the intravenous route, appears to protect against this complication, and it is now our custom to give acyclovir to all seropositive patients for at least 7 weeks, 1 week before and 6 weeks after marrow transplantation.

Varicella-Zoster Virus Infections

Varicella-zoster infections, which occur in 40 to 50 percent of bone marrow transplant recipients, are usually localized, but in approximately 30 percent of patients there is cutaneous spread beyond a single dermatome, and in 10 percent there is visceral involvement. When the disease is manifested as clinical varicella, 33 percent develop visceral as well as skin infections. The mortality rate of this complication is approximately 10 percent, higher in the varicella form than in the zoster form. This complication often occurs rather late, 4 to 5 months after marrow transplantation, and chronic GVHR or GVHD appears to provoke this complication. Either acyclovir or ara-A (vidarabine) have proven useful in treatment, reducing pain, lesion formation, and rescarring.

Epstein-Barr Virus (EBV) Infections

In bone marrow transplant recipients, as in other organ transplant recipients subjected to immunosuppression, EBV infection or reactivation can cause infectious mononucleosis and sometimes malignant proliferation of transformed cells of the B-lymphocyte series. The EBV-induced lymphoproliferative disorders and malignancies appear to arise when T lymphocytes are functionally deficient. Preliminary observations suggest that the frequency of these EBV-induced lymphoproliferative and malignant disorders may also be prevented or reduced by treatment with acyclovir. This is especially true when the marrow used for transplantation is from a partially mismatched donor and has been purged of lymphocytes by monoclonal antibody or lectins (see section on Prevention of GVHD, below).

Table 9–5. Virus Infections that Occur as Complicating
Infection in Bone Marrow Transplantation Recipients

1. Rotavirus
2. Enteroviruses
3. Papovavirus
4. Adenovirus
5. Parainfluenza viruses
6. Influenza viruses
7. Respiratory syncytial virus
8. Other respiratory viruses
9. Hepatitis B
10. Non-A, non-B hepatitis
11. Epstein-Barr virus (EBV)
12. Herpes simplex
13. Herpes zoster–varicella
14. Cytomegalovirus
15. Others

High-Dose IVIG to Prevent Virus Infections

The usefulness of high-dose IVIG to prevent infections due
to other viruses, listed in Table 9–5, will have to be ascertained
by subsequent study.

Graft-versus-Host Reactions

GVHR and GVHD (which often complicate the therapy)
constitute the greatest barrier to extension of the use of bone
marrow transplantation for other than highly lethal disease.
GVHR occurs when the recipient cannot reject T lymphoid cells
present in the graft or cannot eliminate the cells that are
committed to develop into T lymphocytes. The latter are incompletely differentiated cells that have already developed their
immunologic repertoire. These T lymphocytes recognize the antigens of host cells as foreign, and the GVHR ensues. GVHR is
not observed with marrow transplants from identical twins but
may occur when HLA-D/Dr matched sibling donors or haplo-
identical donors are used for marrow transplantation. The severity of GVHR is a function of the degree of genetic disparity
between donor and host.

As many as 60 percent of bone marrow transplant patients
still experience some degree of GVHR or GVHD, with an overall
mortality of 15 to 20 percent, even when HLA-matched siblings
are used as donors. Prophylaxis of GVHD has been accomplished
using methotrexate for the first 100 days following the marrow
transplant, and combinations of methotrexate and glucocorticosteroids have been more effective than methotrexate alone.

Controlled trials with cyclosporin A indicate it to have advantages over methotrexate in prophylaxis of GVHD. The removal of all T cells from the marrow used for transplantation is the most effective means of preventing GVHD. Unfortunately, this highly effective maneuver reduces the success of graft takes. The number of recurrences of leukemia may also be increased when the T-cell–deprived bone marrow has been transplanted in the treatment of leukemias.

An acute GVHR or GVHD must be treated promptly, initially with moderate doses of glucocorticosteroids. If the response is not prompt, larger doses of glucocorticosteroids must be given together with an immunosuppressive agent, such as azathioprine (Imuran); other immunosuppressive regimes such as cyclosporin A may also be effective. Severe graft-versus-host reactions are very difficult to treat, and GVHD and complications related to GVHD remain major obstacles to lowering the morbidity and mortality of bone marrow transplantation. GVHD is designated as chronic when acute GVHD extends beyond 100 days post transplant (Table 9–6). The treatment of chronic GVHD, still far from satisfactory, includes persistent gentle treatment with glucocorticosteroids, moderate doses of azathioprine, attention to nutritional needs, prophylactic antibacterial and antiviral therapies, and the careful detection and early treatment of complicating fungal, bacterial, or viral infections.

Table 9–6. Chronic GVHD—Nature and Manifestations

1. From 20 to 30 percent of patients are long-term survivors of matched sibling donor marrow transplants; incidence increases with age of recipient
2. Chronic when it persists more than 100 days post transplant
3. Involves skin and many organs and tissues
4. Malar erythema, reticulosis, hyperpigmentation, atrophy, ulceration, fibrous alopecia, and photosensitivity of skin
5. May have similarity to dermatomyositis with limitation of joint movement
6. Oral ulcerations
7. Polyserositis
8. Scleroderma-like picture may emerge
9. Liver disease with development of cholestasis in some
10. Restrictive or obstructive pulmonary disease
11. Desquamating esophagitis; sometimes esophageal strictures
12. Myositis, tendinitis, synovitis
13. Autoimmune manifestations; autoimmune hemolytic anemia
14. Aplastic anemia
15. Hypergammaglobulinemia, paraproteinemia
16. Elevated circulating immune complexes
17. Delayed return of immunocompetence–antibody deficiency syndrome
18. Greatly increased susceptibility to infection

Availability of a Donor

Progress is being made toward successful marrow transplantation when no matched sibling donor is available. As many as 10 percent of extensive studies of the tissue types of family members will yield a non-sibling relative sufficiently well matched with the patient at the MHC to permit successful marrow transplantation. Subsequent studies have shown that relatives mismatched at only a single HLA-D/Dr locus can also serve as marrow donors. Marrow transplants from such mismatched donors produce a greater frequency and severity of GVHR and, therefore, greater morbidity, but do not cause an increased mortality rate. Skillful use of immunosuppressive measures, in both prophylaxis and treatment, has probably minimized the morbidity and mortality of these complications.

PREVENTION OF GVHD USING HEMATOPOIETIC CELLS FREE OF T LYMPHOCYTES AND FREE OF IMMEDIATE T-CELL PRECURSORS

Uphoff, and her colleagues at the National Cancer Institute, discovered that stem cells from fetal liver in mice could sometimes be used to correct hematopoietic deficits and to achieve lymphoid reconstruction of recipients that had been subjected to total body irradiation without producing a fatal GVHR. This occurred even when donor and recipient differed from one another at the MHC. Our investigations revealed that a fetal liver, which was a safe source of stem cells and did not cause GVHR, contained hematopoietic cells that were free, or virtually free, of either post-thymic T cells or committed post-thymic precursors of T cells. It was thus possible in mice, and later in man, to employ fetal liver transplants plus thymus transplants to correct the immunologic defects in children with SCID. We were able to cure a few patients with this otherwise fatal disease despite the unavailability of a matched sibling donor. The use of fetal liver instead of bone marrow as a source of stem cells, however, resulted in immunologic corrections that were often incomplete and were also often too slow to develop.

Touraine also reported several successful treatments of SCID using fetal liver from donors younger than 12 weeks as a source of stem cells. Fetal liver is difficult to obtain, and the numbers of stem cells in suitably immature fetuses were too few to permit satisfactory corrections of hematologic deficits in treatment of aplastic anemia or of leukemia following myeloablation, cytoreduction, and appropriate immunosuppression. A source of stem cells was needed which, like fetal liver, would not induce GVHR or GVHD but would fully reconstitute the hematopoietic system and the lymphoid systems. Investigations in mice had established that GVHD could be avoided even in marrow transplants that crossed MHC barriers, or in parents to F_1 model system marrow transplant after total body irradiation, if the donor marrow had first been purged of T cells by treatment with an anti–T-cell antibody (anti–thy 1) plus complement.

Other investigations with rats established that removal of all T cells from the bone marrow was not sufficient. Removal of both T cells and T-cell precursors prevented GVHR and bone marrow transplantation after lethal or near lethal total body irradiation yielded a stable mixed chimerism featured by full immunocompetence. Extensive studies in our laboratory have shown that transplantation can be achieved in mice across major histocompatibility barriers without GVHR or GVHD. This required either purging marrow of post-thymic T cells or pre- and post-thymic precursors, tolerizing donors plus purging marrow of T cells, or use of nude athymic mice as donors.

These models have also been used to investigate bone marrow transplantation as a means of introducing resistance genes against virus-induced cancers, preventing and treating life-threatening autoimmune disease, treating and preventing juvenile type diabetes, and treating other diseases and disorders in mice. Haplo-identical marrow is more effective than is completely mismatched (fully allogeneic) marrow, because full chimeras that cross MHC barriers sometimes have had immunologic deficits and also may develop a late wasting and immunodeficiency syndrome that can be attributed to a subtle GVHD. Polyclonal or monoclonal antibodies used in vitro either with or without complement proved to be the best means of purging marrow cells for this purpose in the mice.

Similarly, human marrow has been purged of unwanted T cells with a lectin agglutination–centrifugation method or using monoclonal antibodies as single antibodies or in cocktails of a number of monoclonal antibodies. With this approach, we could approximate in man what has been accomplished in mice.

Several investigators have treated a few children with SCID or other diseases using haplo-identical donors whose marrow, prior to transplantation, had been purged of most of the unwanted T cells by treatment in vitro with an appropriate monoclonal antibody.

Reisner, Sharon, and colleagues had reconstituted lethally irradiated mice with either spleen cells or marrow cells purged of T cells and of T-cell precursors by differential agglutination and centrifugation following treatment with soybean and peanut lectins. The lectin separation method developed for mice did not prove directly applicable to human cells, but a modification was used successfully. Reisner and Kapoor developed, in our laboratory, a different, but also lectin-based, method to purge human marrow of the unwanted T lymphocytes and T-cell precursors.

This method involves an initial step of treatment with soy bean agglutinin plus differential sedimentation followed by rosetting the T cells with sheep RBC plus differential centrifugation. This method has now made possible full correction of immunologic defects in 30 of 60 patients with SCID, using purged parental marrow. An additional 15 patients have shown T-cell but not full B-cell immunorestoration. The method has permitted virtually complete prevention of GVHR and GVHD. Marrow from a haplo-identical donor, purged by the lectin procedure, has also been used successfully for treatment of leukemias, a few cases of congenital hematologic disorders, and to correct the immunodeficiency, platelet abnormality, and other hematologic-immunologic abnormalities of the Wiskott-Aldrich syndrome. Marrows from haplo-identical parental donors treated by lectin-purging or use of the monoclonal antibody have not made transplantation completely successful. Reconstitution of immunologic systems by hematopoietic stem cells and committed precursors occurs more slowly than when perfectly matched donors are used. Further, these grafts are more precarious than the grafts from matched siblings. T-cell–depleted marrow transplants from matched sibling donors are less effective in treatment of leukemia than are bone marrow transplantations from a matched sibling donor without depletion of T cells. Leukemias appear to return more frequently and more promptly when T-cell–purged marrow is used. This is because a certain amount of GVHD may be helpful as a graft-versus-leukemia reaction for the bone marrow graft to provide effective resistance against the leukemic cells.

SUMMARY AND CONCLUSIONS

Bone marrow transplantation has developed progressively as an increasingly effective means of treating many diseases. These include an extensive group of immunodeficiency diseases, a variety of congenital hematologic abnormalities, increasingly complex inborn errors of metabolism, seven different forms of aplastic anemia, and many different forms of high-risk leukemias plus an increasing array of nonleukemic cancers. The success of marrow transplants has been facilitated by the application of effective microbiologic decontamination, the chronic use of non-absorbable antibiotics, and the treatment of patients in protective environments, especially those that use laminar air flow isolation. Chemotherapy and prophylaxis against *Pneumocystis carinii* have been helpful in reducing complicating infections with these parasites. Protection against infections with encapsulated, bacterial pathogens, and with CMV have been afforded by intravenous gamma globulin prophylaxis. Prevention and effective treatment of herpes simplex virus infection and improved treatment and prevention of infections by other herpes viruses, including the varicella-zoster group, also have been achieved. The EBV infections, as complications that induce malignancy of the lymphoid cells, can probably also be prevented by chemotherapy with acyclovir. Each of these improvements has contributed greatly to the continued progress in applying bone marrow transplantation to the treatment of an increasing number of patients and diseases. Further improvements in the treatment and prevention of GVHR and progress toward making possible haplo-identical marrow transplantation are encouraging, but the improvements are as yet incomplete. Many experimental studies now indicate that bone marrow transplantation can be extended as a therapeutic modality far beyond its current impressive beginning. As the problems of using haplo-identical donors are overcome and marrow transplantation becomes a safer treatment, bone marrow transplantation will become the treatment of choice for many diseases in addition to the numerous otherwise lethal diseases for which marrow transplantation has already been found to be effective.

One other consideration must be mentioned, as it assumes increasing likelihood of success very soon. The approaches to bone marrow transplantation soon will be considered safe enough to use for much more common diseases that are not so rapidly lethal. During treatment of leukemia in a child who also suffered from sickle cell disease, it was found possible to cure sickle cell disease by marrow transplantation. But marrow transplantation has not been used to treat sickle cell disease *per se,* because it is still too hazardous a procedure. As the adversities of marrow transplantation are progressively eliminated (as is occurring in most transplantation units throughout the world) the use of marrow transplantation for the highly morbid thalassemias and sickle cell disease will be reevaluated and probably put to use.

A final word concerns the likelihood that gene therapy will shortly be used for the first time. The initial application of gene therapy, will, I believe, employ the same basic techniques being perfected for autologous bone marrow transplantation. The correcting genes, however, will be introduced into the cells to be transplanted. This is an exciting possibility to consider, and it will grow out of the experiences with bone marrow transplantation.

Bibliography

Anasetti, C., Doney, K. C., Storb, R., et al.: Marrow transplantation for severe aplastic anemia. Ann. Intern. Med. 104:461, 1986.

Blume, K. G., Beutler, E., Bross, K. J., et al.: Bone marrow ablation and allogeneic marrow transplantation in acute leukemia. N. Engl. J. Med. 302:1041, 1980.

Coccia, P. F., Krivit, W., Cervenka, J., et al.: Successful bone marrow transplantation for infantile malignant osteopetrosis. N. Engl. J. Med. 302:701, 1980.

Good, R. A., and Bach, F. H.: Bone marrow and thymus transplants: cellular engineering to correct primary immunodeficiency. In Bach, F. H., and Good, R. A. (eds.): Clinical Immunobiology, Vol. 2. New York, Academic Press, 1974.

Jacobson, L. O., Marks, E. K., Robson, M. J., et al.: The effect of spleen protection on mortality following x-irradiation. J. Lab. Clin. Med. 34:1638, 1949.

Kapoor, N., Kirkpatrick, D., Blaese, R. M., et al.: Reconstitution of normal megakaryocytopoiesis and immunologic function in Wiskott-Aldrich syndrome by marrow transplantation following myeloablation and immunosuppression with Busulfan and cyclophosphamide. Blood 57:692, 1981.

Krivit, W., Pierpont, M. E., Ayaz, K., et al.: Bone marrow transplantation in the Maroteaux-Lamy syndrome (mucopolysaccharidosis type VI). Biochemical and clinical status 24 months after transplantation. N. Engl. J. Med. 311:1606, 1984.

Lorenz, E., Congdon, C. C., and Uphoff, D. E.: Modification of acute irradiation injury in mice and guinea pigs by bone marrow injections. Radiology 58:863, 1952.

O'Reilly, R. J., Dupont, B., Pahwa, S., et al.: Reconstitution in severe combined immunodeficiency by transplantation of marrow from an unrelated donor. N. Engl. J. Med. 297:1311, 1977.

Reisner, Y., Kapoor, N., Pollack, S., et al.: Use of lectins in bone marrow transplantation. Advances in Bone Marrow Transplantation, UCLA Symposia 7:355, 1983.

Sorrell, M., Kapoor, N., Kirkpatrick, D., et al.: Marrow transplantation for juvenile osteopetrosis. Am. J. Med. 70:1280, 1981.

Thomas, E. D.: Bone marrow transplantation. In Burchenal, J. H., and Oettgen, H. F. (eds.): Cancer: Achievements, Challenges and Prospects for the 1980's, Vol. 2. New York, Grune and Stratton, 1981, p. 625.

Tutschka, P. J., and Santos, G. W.: Bone marrow transplantation in the Busulfan-treated rat. III. Relationship between myelosuppression and immunosuppression for conditioning bone marrow recipients. Transplantation 24:52, 1977.

10

Mechanisms of Allergic Injury

CHARLES H. KIRKPATRICK, M.D.

INTRODUCTION

Allergy may be defined as an altered state of specific reactivity comprising a broad spectrum of untoward physiologic events mediated by a variety of immunologic mechanisms. In 1963, Professors P. G. H. Gell and R. R. A. Coombs presented, in the first edition of their book *Clinical Aspects of Immunology* (see Bibliography), a classification (G.C.) of mechanisms of allergic and immunologic injury. Four basic types of reactions were described. Antibody molecules played essential roles in three of

Table 10–1. Mechanisms of Allergic Injury

Class 1: Reagin-dependent injury (G.C. Type I)
a. Anaphylaxis
b. Late-phase reactions
Class 2: Cytotoxic reactions (G.C. Type II)
a. Antibody-dependent; complement-mediated
b. Antibody-dependent; cell-mediated (ADCC)
c. T-lymphocyte–mediated (CTL)
d. Natural killer (NK) cells
Class 3: Immune-complex–mediated reactions (G.C. Type III)
Class 4: Anti-receptor antibodies
Class 5: Delayed hypersensitivity (G.C. Type IV)

G. C. = Gell & Coombs.

these: *G.C. Type I,* immediate hypersensitivity; *G.C. Type II,* antibody-mediated cytolysis; and *G.C. Type III,* immune-complex–dependent tissue injury. The fourth, *G.C. Type IV,* delayed hypersensitivity, is mediated by antibody-independent effects of lymphocytes upon target cells. This classification is valuable to both clinicians and investigators because it emphasizes the importance of determining the etiology of an allergic or immunologic disease and points out that certain disorders have common pathways that lead to tissue injury even though they differ in etiology.

Since the publication of this classification, much has been learned of the molecular mechanisms of allergic and immunologic inflammation. New techniques have identified the phenotypes of effector cells, defined the biologic activities of cell products, and uncovered additional forms of immunologic injury. This chapter will reconsider the mechanisms of allergic and immunologic tissue injury in the light of these developments.

A modified classification for these reactions is shown in Table 10–1.

CLASS 1: REAGIN-DEPENDENT ALLERGIC INJURY (G.C. TYPE I)

Definition and Mechanisms. These reactions occur when antigens interact with a unique class of immunoglobulins called reagins, which are homocytotropic antibodies bound to the membranes of mast cells, basophils, macrophages, and lymphocytes. The antigen-reagin interaction at the cell surface causes these sensitized cells to release biologically active substances (mediators) that produce the physiologic changes of allergic injury.

Reagins. Reagins have the unique property of binding to mast cells and baosphils through specific receptors for the Fc portion of the reagin molecule. Most of the reaginic activity in man and vertebrates is found in IgE molecules (see Chapters 11 and 12). Lower animals, such as mice, rats, guinea pigs, and rabbits, also have IgG molecules with a lesser degree of reaginic activity, because the molecules bind less avidly to mediator-containing cells. There is some evidence that similar IgG reagins are present in man, but they are relatively unimportant mediators of reagin-dependent reactions.

Reagins are bound at tissue sites for many hours after local injection. This was first recognized in 1921 by Prausnitz and Küstner when they injected serum from Küstner, who was allergic to fish, into the skin of non–fish-sensitive Prausnitz. Subsequent challenging of the injected site with an allergenic extract of fish produced a wheal and flare reaction. The property of stable binding of IgE molecules to receptors on tissue mast cells forms the basis for skin testing in the diagnosis of immediate hypersensitivity. Reagins are denatured by heating at 56°C for several hours.

Mechanisms of Mediator Release. Cross-linking of IgE molecules bound to mast cells or basophils by the specific interaction of allergens with the Fab portion of two IgE molecules, or by the interaction of anti-IgE with the Fc portion of bound IgE molecules, initiates a series of biochemical reactions that culminate in the release of granule-associated substances that produce the physiologic changes that characterize immediate-type hypersensitivity (Fig. 10–1). These mediators include vasoactive agents that constrict or dilate small blood vessels and increase the permeability of vessel walls (Table 10–2), chemotactic factors that attract other inflammatory cells into the site of the reaction (Table 10–3), and enzymes and proteoglycans that produce tissue injury and may provide important mechanisms for limiting the extent of the injurious process (Table 10–4). The complex biochemical events that are initiated by cross-linking of membrane-bound IgE are being studied. Current evidence indicates that changes in membrane phospholipids are early events. Activation of cells to secrete mediators requires energy, and the process is regulated, in part, by cyclic nucleotides. Release of the mediators from mast cells and basophils is a secretory rather than a cytolytic event. The biologic properties of many mast cell–derived mediators have been identified, but the individual roles and interactions of other mediators in the pathogenesis of acute allergic reactions are under investigation.

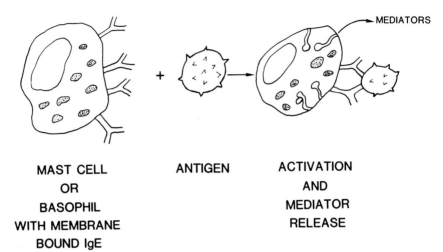

MAST CELL   ANTIGEN   ACTIVATION
OR   AND
BASOPHIL   MEDIATOR
WITH MEMBRANE   RELEASE
BOUND IgE

Figure 10–1. Antigen-mediated release of mediators of immediate hypersensitivity. Mast cells and basophils are sensitized by IgE molecules attached to Fc receptors on the cell membrane. Upon contact with the appropriate antigen, the cells secrete granule-associated substances into the extracellular environment.

Histamine. Histamine is the prototypic mediator of immediate-type hypersensitivity reactions. It is preformed in mast cells and basophils, where it is bound to the protein and proteoglycan of the granule matrix, comprising about 5 to 10 percent of the weight of the granules. The role of histamine in producing the physiologic changes of immediate-type allergic reactions has been revealed by the addition of histamine to isolated tissues and injection into experimental animals. Provocation tests in patients with disorders such as physical urticarias have reproduced allergic lesions and caused increased histamine levels in the affected tissues and the blood draining the affected sites.

The physiologic effects of histamine are initiated through two classes of receptors on the target tissues (Table 10–2). Activation of H_1 receptors causes contraction of the smooth muscle of bronchioles and the intestinal tract, increased permeability of venules, constriction of pulmonary blood vessels, and stimulation of nasal mucus production. Histamine is also a potent chemoattractant for eosinophils. Activation of H_2 receptors stimulates production of mucus in the lower airways, increase of vascular permeability, and increased secretion of gastric acid.

Histamine also produces biochemical events that affect the metabolism of other cells. Activation of H_1 receptors causes accumulation of cyclic guanosine monophosphate (cGMP), an

Table 10–2. Mediators of Immediate Hypersensitivity

Mediator (and Source)	Preformed or Generated	Function	Human Disease Association
Vasoactive Substances			

Histamine (mast cells/ basophils)	Preformed	Via H$_1$ receptors:
		  Contract smooth muscle
		  Increase vascular permeability
		  Induce pulmonary vasoconstriction
		  Increase nasal mucus production
		  Increase cGMP
		  Generate prostaglandins
		Via H$_2$ receptors:
		  Increase airway mucus production
		  Increase gastric acid secretion
		  Increase cAMP
		  Stimulate suppressor lymphocytes
		  Inhibit skin and basophil histamine release
		  Cause bronchodilation
		Via both H$_1$ and H$_2$ receptors:
		  Pruritus
		  Vasodilatation
		  Reduce threshold for ventricular fibrillation
			Asthma
			Anaphylaxis
			Urticaria
			Rhinitis

Platelet-activating factor [PAF] (monocytes, macrophages, alveolar macrophages, neutrophils, endothelial cells, platelets, possibly mast cells and basophils)	Generated	Aggregate platelets Release platelet amines and generate platelet thromboxane Sequester platelets in tissue Increase vascular permeability Vasodepression Vasoconstriction Bronchoconstriction Induce neutropenia, basopenia, thrombocytopenia	Possibly cold urticaria
Arachidonic Acid Metabolites			
LTC$_4$, LTD$_4$, LTE$_4$ [SRS-A] (mast cells, neutrophils, eosinophils, macrophages)	Generated	Constrict smooth muscle Increase vascular permeability Decrease peripheral blood flow Vasodepression Synergistic with histamine Generate prostaglandins Increase airway mucus production Cardiac depressants Coronary vasoconstrictors Inhibit lymphocyte response to mitogen	Anaphylaxis Asthma (?)
Prostaglandin D$_2$ [PGD$_2$] (mast cells)	Generated	Increase cAMP level Contract smooth muscle Increase vascular permeability	Mastocytosis Rhinitis
Prostaglandin-generating factor	Generated	Induce production of prostaglandins	

Modified from Wasserman, S. I.: J. Allergy Clin. Immunol. 72:101, 1983.

Table 10–3. Chemotactic Factors

Mediator (and Source)	Preformed or Generated	Function	Human Disease Association
Eosinophilic chemotactic factor of anaphylaxis [ECF-A] (mast cells)	Preformed	Attract and deactivate eosinophils Increase eosinophil complement receptors	Physical urticaria Asthma
ECF oligopeptides (mast cells)	Preformed	Attract and deactivate eosinophils and mononuclear leukocytes (more acidic peptide)	Physical urticaria Asthma
High-molecular-weight neutrophil chemotactic factor [HMW-NCF] (mast cells?)	Preformed	Attract and deactivate neutrophils	Physical urticaria Asthma
T-lymphocyte chemotactic factor (mast cells)		Activate T-lymphocyte–directed migration	
B-lymphocyte chemotactic factor (mast cells)		Activate B-lymphocyte–directed migration	
Lymphocyte chemotactic factor (mast cells)		Activate T- and B-lymphocyte random migration	
Inflammatory factor(s) of anaphylaxis (mast cells)	Preformed	Induce cutaneous neutrophil (early) and mononuclear (late) cellular infiltrate	
Histamine (mast cell, basophil)	Preformed	Via H_1 receptor: Activate directed and random migration of eosinophils and neutrophils Via H_2 receptor: Inhibit directed and random migration of eosinophils and neutrophils	Asthma Anaphylaxis Urticaria
Cyclooxygenase products [HHT*] (many cell types)	Generated	Activate directed and random migration of neutrophils and eosinophils	
Lipoxygenase products	Generated		
Hydroxyeicosatetraenoic acid [HETE] (many cell types)		Augment random and directed migration of neutrophils and eosinophils	
Leukotriene B_4 [LTB$_4$] (atypical mast cells)		Augment random and directed migration of neutrophils and eosinophils Increase neutrophil granule release and oxidative metabolism	
Platelet-activating factor [PAF]	Generated	Augment neutrophil-directed migration, enzyme release, and oxidative metabolism	

Modified from Wasserman, S. I.: J. Allergy Clin. Immunol. 72:101, 1983.
*HHT = 12-hydroxy heptadecatrienoic acid.

Table 10–4. Biologically Active Factors

Mediators (and Source)	Preformed or Generated	Function	Human Disease Association
Enzymes			
Tryptase (mast cell)	Preformed	Generate C3a	Mastocytosis
	MW 140,000	Proteolysis Degrade kininogen	
Basophil kallikrein	MW 400,000	Generate kinins	Anaphylaxis (?)
Basophil Hageman factor activator	MW 13,000	Activate Hageman factor	
Basophil prekallikrein activator	MW 80,000	Activate prekallikrein	
Myeloperoxidase (mast cell)	Preformed	Degrade peroxide	
Superoxide dismutase (mast cell)	Preformed	Degrade superoxide	
Lysosomal Hydrolases			
Beta-glucuronidase (mast cell)	Preformed	Cleave glucuronide residues	
Beta-hexosaminidase (mast cell, basophil)	Preformed	Cleave hexosamines	
Arylsulfatase (mast cell, basophil)	Preformed	Cleave sulfate esters	
Proteoglycans			
Heparin (mast cell)	Preformed	Bind histamine Inhibit complement activation Anticoagulant Bind platelet factor 4 Bind and activate tryptase	Mastocytosis
Chondroitin 4 and 6 sulfate (basophil)	Preformed	Bind histamine Bind platelet factor 4	
Chondroitin sulfates D and E (atypical mast cells)	Preformed	Bind histamine (?)	

Modified from Wasserman, S. I.: J. Allergy Clin. Immunol. 72:101, 1983.

event that enhances many lymphocyte-dependent immune responses, while activation of H_2 receptors causes accumulation of cyclic adenosine monophosphate (cAMP), which inhibits expression of these responses.

Clinically, histamine release is a major cause of the pruritus, flushing, hypotension, wheezing, mucus production, and shock that accompany systemic reagin-mediated allergic reactions.

Platelet Activating Factor (PAF). PAF is the most potent aggregator of platelets known. It is also possibly the most potent cell-derived mediator of bronchoconstriction and inflammation. It causes accumulation of platelets in the lung that is accompanied by local release of platelet factor 4 and thromboxanes. It also aggregates neutrophils and monocytes, and, when given intravenously to rabbits or baboons, produces profound peripheral pancytopenia. Injected intradermally, PAF causes an intense wheal and flare reaction, and moderately large doses may cause erythematous responses to develop at 3 to 6 hours. The bronchoconstricting activity following inhalation of PAF by rhesus monkeys is 20,000 times greater than that produced by histamine inhalation, and 600 times greater than that of leukotriene D_4. Systemically, PAF causes severe hypotension and cardiovascular collapse. Thus, PAF has many biologic properties that mimic changes in acute anaphylaxis. Its role in the pathogenesis of these reactions in man is under study; one investigator has already observed that PAF was released into the venous blood of the arms of patients with cold urticaria when their arms were immersed in ice water.

Arachidonic Acid Metabolites. The interaction of mast cell–bound or basophil-bound IgE and the specific allergen or anti-IgE results in release of arachidonic acid by phospholipases acting on phospholipids of the cell membrane. The arachidonic acid, in turn, undergoes a series of enzymatic conversions to mediators of allergic inflammation (Fig. 10–2).

The lipoxygenase pathway produces 5-hydroxyeicosatetraenoic acid (5-HETE) and leukotriene B_4 (LTB_4), which have potent chemotactic activities, and a group of compounds known as leukotrienes (LT) that are responsible for activities that have been attributed to the slow-reacting substance of anaphylaxis (SRS-A). These substances and PAF are the leading candidates for the mediators of the sustained constriction of smooth muscle that accompanies some immediate-type allergic reactions, including asthma.

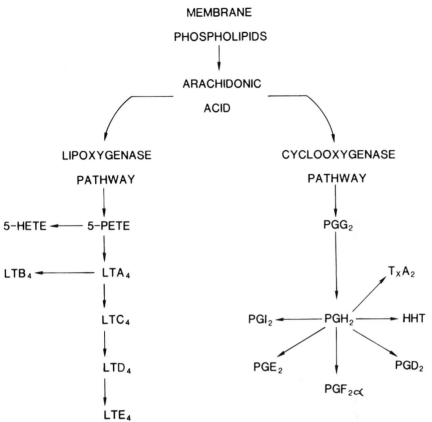

Figure 10–2. Metabolism of arachidonic acid into mediators of immediate hypersensitivity. The lipoxygenase pathway yields 5-HETE and LTB_4, which have potent chemotactic activities, and leukotrienes (LTC_4, LTD_4, and LTE_4). The cyclooxygenase pathway products include PGH_2, which is the parent of biologically active substances such as prostacyclins (PGI_2), prostaglandins (PGE_2, $PGE_{2\alpha}$), PGD_2, a chemotactic factor (HHT), and thromboxanes (TxA_2). HHT = 12-hydroxy heptadecatrienoic acid.

The other major pathway for conversion of arachidonic acid involves the enzyme cyclooxygenase and results in production of prostaglandins (PG), prostacyclins, and thromboxanes (Fig. 10–2). PGE_1, PGE_2, and $PGF_{2\alpha}$ increase vascular permeability. PGD_2 not only increases vascular permeability but also causes contraction of smooth muscle. The wheal and flare reaction produced by intradermal injection of PGD_2 lasts for several hours, and PGD_2 is believed to be responsible for the flushing and hypotensive episodes experienced by patients with mastocytosis. Thromboxane A_2 (TxA_2) causes bronchoconstriction, and increased amounts of thromboxane metabolites appear in the urine after episodes of bronchospasm.

There are many interactions among basophil- and mast cell–derived mediators. Histamine causes increased production of PGE_2, PGD_2, $PGF_{2\alpha}$, TxA_2 and PGI_2; leukotrienes also enhance thromboxane production. Thus, the physiologic changes that follow interactions between antigens and reagin-sensitized cells may be due to direct effects of some mediators and indirect effects of other mediators that are produced in response to the primary mediators.

Clinical Expressions of Reagin-Induced Reactions

Immediate-Type Reactions

Once the biochemical events are initiated, release of mediators occurs very rapidly. The reactions may vary from the localized wheal and flare responses to prick tests with allergens to the life-threatening systemic anaphylactic responses following insect sting, drug reaction, or food ingestion by the sensitive person, with hypotension, generalized urticaria, and death that may result from release of large amounts of mediators. This immediate mechanism is responsible for most common allergic reactions, including allergic rhinitis, allergic asthma, and many urticarias.

Late-Phase Reactions

Many allergic patients develop respiratory symptoms within minutes of, and again several hours after, exposure to an allergen. Interest in the mechanism and significance of these dual reactions was stimulated by the reports of Pepys and associates that patients with allergic bronchopulmonary aspergillosis often exhibited dual responses to skin tests with *Aspergillus* antigens. First there was a classic immediate-type wheal and flare response that faded after a few minutes, and secondly, an erythematous, pruritic, indurated response occurring 4 to 6 hours later. Immunopathologic studies showed that the late reacting tissues contained immunoglobulins and complement, findings that were similar to those of the Arthus reaction.

Subsequent studies have revealed an additional mechanism for late-phase cutaneous responses to a variety of substances, including extracts of molds, pollens, *Bacillus subtilis*, insect venoms, and drugs such as insulin. The typical response to allergen challenge includes an immediate-type wheal and flare reaction that subsides in 15 to 30 minutes. During the next hour or two the site shows some edema and erythema but is not symptomatic. After 4 to 5 hours the test site again becomes pruritic, and during the next few hours it becomes warm, more edematous and erythematous, and may be tender. The reaction becomes considerably larger than the original wheal and flare, but then subsides after 24 hours, although discoloration due to extravasation of erythrocytes may persist at the sites of severe reactions.

Late-phase reactions are dependent upon IgE antibodies and mediator release from mast cells at the site of the provocative test. Late-phase responses have been provoked by anti-IgE antibodies and by 48/80, a compound that causes nonimmunologic release of mediators from mast cells. Late-phase responses may be transferred to nonatopic subjects with serum from sensitive subjects; when the transferred site is repeatedly challenged, the intensity of the response diminishes, which indicates development of a local refractory state.

Histologically, late-phase lesions show edema and perivascular infiltration, first with mononuclear cells and later with neutrophils and eosinophils; basophils and mast cells are infrequent. In contrast to the Arthus-like reactions studied by Pepys and coworkers, immunoreactants such as immunoglobulins or complement are not found in the lesions of these late-phase reactions.

Most evidence indicates that late-phase responses are not affected by pretreatment with either H_1 or H_2 antihistamines, but the combination of H_1 and H_2 blockers completely inhibits the development of late-phase reactions. Pretreatment with glucocorticosteroids may reduce—but does not eliminate—late-phase reactions.

The clinical significance of late-phase reactions is still being defined. They may explain the persisting and progressive local responses to insect venoms and to drugs such as insulin, and there is growing evidence that these reactions may contribute to late-onset symptoms in patients with allergic asthma or allergic rhinitis. A recently developed rabbit model for late-phase allergic reactions to *Aspergillus* antigens should enhance understanding of these reactions.

CLASS 2: CYTOTOXIC REACTIONS (G.C. TYPE II)

Definition and Mechanisms. Cytotoxicity refers to reactions that disrupt cell membranes. Such cells are susceptible to osmotic lysis or are rapidly cleared by phagocytic cells of the reticuloendothelial system. A variety of mechanisms for production of the initial injury have been identified. For example, lytic injury of mismatched erythrocytes or drug-coated leukocytes or platelets, has a two-stage mechanism, with cells first sensitized by specific antibodies and membrane injury then mediated by proteins of the complement system (Chapter 3). Other reactions, such as cell-mediated cytolytic injury, require direct contact between effector cell and target cell, and there is no demonstrable role for such soluble factors as antibodies or complement proteins.

Antibody-Dependent, Complement-Mediated Cytotoxicity

These classic reactions, which produce lytic injury of foreign erythrocytes or bacteria, require two families of soluble factors. One is the family of antibody molecules that are specifically directed against antigenic determinants of the target cell or bacteria. The second is the complement system, which is nonspecifically activated by the complex of antibody and cell-associated antigenic determinants. The complement proteins interact with one another in sequence to disrupt the cell membrane. Three complement-mediated events occur: (1) recognition, during which C1q binds to the antibody molecules; (2) activation, during which activated proteolytic enzymes amplify the reactions; and (3) lytic injury, during which sequential activation of complement components C5 through C9, with eventual polymerization of C9, produces the final membrane attack complex.

IgG and IgM antibodies both form complexes that activate the classic complement system. A doublet of two IgG molecules is required for activation of the complement cascade, but a single molecule of IgM is sufficient. However, a much larger number of IgG antibody molecules is probably required on a cell membrane to achieve the proximity of two antibody molecules required for reaction.

Antibody-dependent, complement-mediated injury is most strikingly demonstrated in transfusions of mismatched erythrocytes. Intravascular lysis may occur when the mismatch involves major erythrocyte antigens. When the mismatch involves minor determinants, the sensitized cells show accelerated clearance from the circulation by the reticuloendothelial organs, especially the spleen. Acquired hemolytic anemias caused by drugs may occur through one of several mechanisms. Drugs such as quinine may interact with antiquinine serum antibodies and form immune complexes that attach to the erythrocyte. The erythrocyte is an "innocent bystander," but is damaged nonetheless. In other

Figure 10–3. In Class 2, antitissue antibodies (IgG or IgM) attach linearly to antigenic determinants along the alveolar basement membrane and initiate a variety of cytolytic events, including activation of complement, by either the classical (C1) or alternative (C3) pathways. (Reprinted, with permission, from Fink, J. N.: Immunologic lung disease. Hosp. Pract. 16(5):61, 1981. Drawing by Nancy Lou Gahan Makris.)

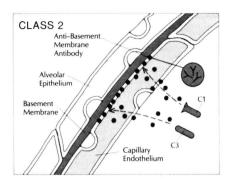

reactions, the drugs bind to erythrocyte membranes and serve as haptens that become the target of antibody-dependent, complement-mediated injury. Neutrophils and platelets may also be targets of antibody-dependent, complement-mediated lysis in disorders such as sedormid or quinidine-induced thrombocytopenia and levamisole-induced neutropenia.

Cytotoxic antibodies can also injure parenchymal organs. Heterologus anti-kidney antibodies promptly produce renal injury that is expressed within a few hours as proteinuria and reduced glomerular filtration. This subsides and is followed, within a few days, by a second stage of renal injury that is due to the host production of antibody, which reacts with antigenic determinants of the first (heterologous) antibody that had fixed to kidney cells (Masugi nephritis). A classic example of antibody-dependent tissue injury in man is Goodpasture's syndrome, in which the host's autoantibodies react with the basement membranes of the lung and the glomeruli (Figs. 10–3 and 10–4).

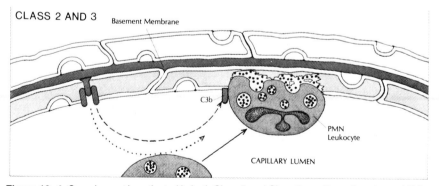

Figure 10–4. Complement is activated in both Class 2 and Class 3 reactions, thereby mobilizing inflammatory cells such as the polymorphonuclear leukocyte. (Reprinted, with permission, from Fink, J. N.: Immunologic lung disease. Hosp. Pract. 16(5):61, 1981. Drawing by Nancy Lou Gahan Makris.)

Antibody-Dependent, Cell-Mediated Cytotoxicity (ADCC)

This activity was first described as a mechanism for in vitro lysis of fibrosarcoma cells, but subsequently it has been demonstrated with many systems. For ADCC to occur, the target cell must first be coated with specific antibody of the IgG class. All subclasses of IgG appear to be equally effective, but IgM and IgA antibodies of the same specificity are not active. The effector cells of ADCC have receptors for the Fc portion of the IgG. Thus, the immunoglobulin molecule serves as a bridge between the target cell attached to the Fab portion and the effector cell on the Fc portion.

Many cells serve as effector cells for ADCC. These include polymorphonuclear neutrophils, macrophages, fetal liver cells, platelets, and a lymphoid cell termed a killer cell (K cell), which has Fc receptors but does not have phenotypic markers that identify it as a T cell or a B cell.

ADCC-mediated cytolysis requires living cells and energy, but does not require protein synthesis or the complement system. The activity of the effector cell may be modulated by cyclic nucleotides.

Although ADCC is a widely recognized in vitro phenomenon, its in vivo role is uncertain. This form of cytotoxic activity could occur in any setting in which sensitization by the target cell resulted in production of IgG antibodies that coated the target and the presence of effector cells with Fc receptors for IgG.

T-Lymphocyte–Mediated Cytotoxicity

This form of cell-mediated cytolysis has been studied extensively. The effector cells are thymus-derived lymphocytes that, in mice, have the Lyt-2$^+$, Lyt-3$^+$ phenotype and, in humans, have the OKT-8 or Leu-2a phenotype. They become activated to cytotoxicity by exposure to antigenic determinants—including viral antigens and tumor-associated antigens—that are expressed on the target cell membrane in association with antigens encoded by the major histocompatibility complex. The cytolytic activity of cytotoxic T cells is highly specific and, in the case of virus-infected target cells, the effector cell must simultaneously "recognize" both the antigenic determinants that resulted from the viral infection and Class I major histocompatibility antigens of the target cell membrane.

The cytolytic activity of cytotoxic T cells does not require antibodies or complement. Some workers have argued that lymphotoxin, a lymphokine, is a soluble mediator that effects cytolytic injury, but there is strong evidence against this, and cytolytic injury appears to require direct contact between the effector T cell and the target cell.* A single hit by the effector cell is sufficient to initiate membrane injury in the target, and there is evidence that a single effector cell may "recycle" to inflict cytolytic injury on multiple target cells.

T-cell–mediated lytic activity requires viable, metabolically active effector cells. The reactions are dependent upon Mg^{++} and Ca^{++} and integration of the microtubule and microfilament systems, but they do not require synthesis of DNA or RNA and probably do not require synthesis of proteins. Metabolic activity is not required for cells to be targets of cytolytic activity.

The initial contact between effector cells and target cells is highly specific and depends upon a specific antigen receptor on the effector cell. Following cell-to-cell contact, membrane injury occurs, but its molecular basis is unknown. Focal changes such as cytoplasmic bridges have not been found in the target cell membranes. Once injured, the target cell loses the ability to regulate salt and water flux and undergoes osmotic lysis.

The biologic role of cytotoxic T-cell activity is most clearly demonstrated by lytic injury of virus-infected cells. However, in the case of animal models such as murine lymphocytic chorio-meningitis, the activity of cytotoxic T cells against virus-infected targets has lethal consequences for the host. Cytotoxic T cells may also contribute to rejection of skin or other organ grafts, but this is not firmly established, and there is evidence that T cells of another phenotype (L3T4) are more active in allograft rejection.

Natural Killer (NK) Cells

The cytolytic activity of this cell population is unique, since there is no requirement for prior sensitization with antigens of the target cells; hence the name "natural" killer cells. The lineage of the effector cells is not well understood, but they appear to derive from bone marrow and are found in large numbers in the peripheral blood and spleen, but usually in small numbers in other lymphoid organs. They lack membrane-associated immunoglobulins, receptors for C3, and the phenotypic markers of T cells (L3T4, Lyt-2, Lyt-3). They do have receptors for the Fc portion of IgG and form rosettes with ovine erythrocytes, although weakly. Human NK cells have phenotypic markers (HNK-1, Leu-7, Leu-11) that can be identified with mono-

*See D.-E. Young et al., under Class 2: Cytotoxic Reactions in bibliography at end of chapter.

clonal antibodies. NK cells are not thymus-derived, since they are found in large numbers in athymic nude mice. Some, if not all, NK cells have cytoplasmic granules that have given rise to the term large granular lymphocytes (LGL).

The cytolytic activity of NK cells resembles T-cell–mediated lysis. The activity is independent of complement or antibodies, and cytolysis occurs in three stages: attachment, membrane injury, and lysis. NK cells can bind to NK-susceptible target cells, and their cytolytic activity is not restricted by the MHC or exclusively to target cells from the same species. It has therefore been argued that the portion of the target cell that is recognized by the NK cell has been widely conserved in nature. The mechanism of injury to the cell membrane is not completely known, but after attachment to the target cell the NK cells show a rapid increase in superoxide anion. After approximately 1 hour there is methylation of phospholipids and increased activity of phospholipase A_2 in the NK cell. The cytolytic attack is probably mediated by a secreted factor, and eventual lysis of the cell is probably osmotic.

Pharmacologic modulation of NK activity is similar to CTL. Agents that cause increases in cellular cyclic guanosine monophosphate (cGMP) increase activity, while agents that increase cyclic adenosine monophosphate (cAMP) decrease activity. The interferons are potent enhancers of NK-cell activity.

Most studies of NK activity employ tumor cells as targets, and it is argued that NK cells provide an important first line of nonspecific defense against tumors. However, there is even stronger evidence that NK cells may be important in host defenses against infectious agents such as virus-infected cells and parasites. It has also been argued that NK cells may provide regulatory activity in the differentiation of hematopoietic cells and the activation of B lymphocytes. For example, rejection of parental bone marrow by F_1 hybrid mice is due to NK-like cells.

NK activity is defective in a number of disorders, and in most cases this appears to result from a reduction in activity of the cells rather than from ablation of the cells themselves. NK-cell activity is reduced in many malignant diseases, in some patients with autoimmune diseases such as rheumatoid arthritis, lupus erythematosus, or thyroiditis, in chronic renal failure, in the acquired immune deficiency syndrome (AIDS), in the X-linked lymphoproliferative syndrome, and in the Chédiak-Higashi syndrome. Increased NK activity is found in association with renal graft rejection, graft-versus-host disease, and a variety of viral and parasitic infections.

The cytotoxic activity of activated macrophages is similar to

NK-mediated cytotoxicity. It does not require complement or antibodies and is regulated by soluble factors. This is a potent mechanism of cytotoxic activity against tumor cells.

CLASS 3: IMMUNE-COMPLEX–MEDIATED REACTIONS (G.C. TYPE III)

Definition and Mechanisms. Immune complexes are formed by the interaction of one or more antibody molecules with one or more molecules of antigen. In parenchymal tissues the antigen may be an integral part of the organ, such as the glomerular basement membrane; a secreted material, such as thyroglobulin; or a foreign substance, such as mycobacterial antigens, in pulmonary tuberculosis. In these disorders, circulating antibodies diffuse from the vascular system and interact with antigen in tissues. In other disorders, circulating antigens and antibodies interact within the vascular system. The circulating complexes deposit within tissues such as the kidneys, choroid plexus, joints, skin, and lungs (Fig. 10–5). The site of deposition of circulating complexes is a function of the size of the complex. Small complexes may not be deposited in tissues and may be harmless; very large complexes are rapidly cleared by cells of the reticuloendothelial system and also fail to produce inflammation. Thus, only complexes of intermediate size produce tissue injury.

There is experimental evidence that a change in vascular permeability is essential to produce immune-complex-mediated inflammation. In some species, IgE-mediated reactions or anaphylatoxins from complement proteins cause release of vasoactive factors such as histamine from mast cells and basophils, and these mediators produce changes in vascular permeability that allow complexes to leave the circulation and deposit in tissues.

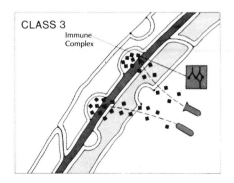

Figure 10–5. Class 3 reactions share many effector phenomena with Class 2, except that the initiation is by antigen-antibody complexes. These immune complexes are formed in the circulation and then pass through the capillary wall into the subendothelial structures of the alveolar basement membrane. They then form nodular lesions and are capable of activating complement and mobilizing inflammatory cells. (Reprinted, with permission, from Fink, J. N.: Immunologic lung disease. Hosp. Pract. 16(5):61, 1981. Drawing by Nancy Lou Gahan Makris.)

The Fc portion of the immunoglobulin component of the complex is essential for initiation of inflammation. Interaction of the Fc portion with Fc receptors on phagocytic cells activates the cells to secrete granule constituents such as proteases. Ward has suggested that these cells may also release toxic oxygen metabolites such as superoxide anion (O_2^-), hydroxyl radical (OH^-), hydrogen peroxide (H_2O_2), and halide derivates such as hypochlorous acid (HOCl), and that a significant portion of tissue injury may be due to these materials.

The Fc portion of immune complexes may also activate the classical pathway of the complement system, which, in turn, leads to production of anaphylatoxins and chemotactic factors. Thus, production of injury by immune complexes may involve both the complement system and phagocytic cells.

The prototypic model of immune-complex–mediated tissue injury is the Arthus reaction, which is initiated by injection of a depot of antigen into a subject whose serum contains circulating antibodies against the antigen. Formation of the antigen-antibody complex occurs in the walls of blood vessels. After activation of the complement system, there is an influx of neutrophils and damage to the vessel walls, with edema and extravasation of erythrocytes and plasma proteins. The reaction reaches a peak at 6 to 12 hours and subsides over the next few days. Other probable examples of immune-complex–mediated injury occur in serum sickness, systemic lupus erythematosus, acute and chronic glomerulonephritis, rheumatoid arthritis, certain forms of vasculitis and interstitial lung disease, and tissue injury associated with many infectious diseases.

CLASS 4: ANTI-RECEPTOR ANTIBODIES (NO PREVIOUS G.C. TYPE)

Definition and Mechanisms. Some syndromes of unknown etiology are associated with antibodies against the receptors for various hormones or mediators (Table 10–5). The best recognized among these syndromes are myasthenia gravis, in which the antibodies are directed against acetylcholine receptors; Graves' disease, in which the antibodies are directed against TSH receptors; insulin-dependent diabetes mellitus, in which antibodies are directed against insulin receptors; and, perhaps, some allergic disorders in which antibodies are directed against β-adrenergic receptors. Other studies will undoubtedly result in additional disorders to the list.

Table 10–5. Diseases That May Be Mediated by Antireceptor Antibodies

Target Cell	Hormone or Neurotransmitter Involved	Disease or Dysfunction
Motor end-plate	Acetylcholine	Myasthenia gravis
Thyroid epithelial cells	Thyroxin stimulation blockade	Thyrotoxicosis; hypothyroidism
Pancreatic islet cell	Gut hormone; glucose	Diabetes
Adipocytes	Insulin	Diabetes (insulin-resistant)
Gastric parietal cell	Gastrin	Hypochlorhydria
Adrenal cortical cells	Adrenocorticotropic hormone	Adrenocortical insufficiency
Graafian follicle; corpus luteum	Follicle-stimulating hormone; luteinizing hormone	Infertility; premature menopause
Parathyroid chief cell; renal tubule	Parathormone	Primary hypoparathyroidism; pseudohypoparathyroidism
Melanocyte	Melanocyte-stimulating hormone	Vitiligo
Central neurones	5-Hydroxytryptamine	Defects in function in experimental autoimmune encephalomyelitis

From Fink, J. N.: JAMA 248:2699, 1982.

Several possible consequences of antibody-receptor interaction have been demonstrated or proposed. These include complement-mediated lysis of the receptor, accelerated degradation of receptors, negative modulation of expression of receptors on the membranes, and blocking of the binding sites on the receptor for the hormone or agonist. Each of these effects interferes with interaction between the agonist and its receptor and could impair cell function. Myasthenia gravis and insulin-dependent diabetes may involve one or more of these mechanisms.

In thyrotoxicosis, the anti-receptor antibodies stimulate the receptors, increase cyclic adenosine monophosphate, cause cell growth, and increase production of thyroid hormones. In certain allergic diseases, antibodies against β-adrenergic receptors may block the effect of the agonist and contribute to the disease.

The unique situation in which the antibody against the receptor serves to activate the cells and produce disease justifies its inclusion as a separate mechanism.

CLASS 5: DELAYED HYPERSENSITIVITY (G.C. TYPE IV)

Definition and Mechanisms. These reactions are the consequence of interactions between antigens and antigen-responsive

T lymphocytes, with subsequent release of soluble factors (lymphokines) that produce inflammation and tissue injury. There is no role for antibodies or complement. The reactions are usually well localized, a feature that is clearly demonstrated by the responses of sensitive subjects to intradermal tests with tuberculin or *Candida* extracts or to patch tests with poison ivy (Fig. 10–6). However, delayed hypersensitivity reactions may be more extensive in rejection of tissue allografts or production of granulomatous reactions, and may even have systemic effects such as graft-versus-host disease.

Delayed hypersensitivity was observed by Koch, who injected tuberculin into the skin of tuberculous patients and animals. Many attempts to transfer these reactions to insensitive recipients with serum from sensitive donors were unsuccessful, and it was not until the early 1940s, when Merrill Chase and Karl Landsteiner performed the classic experiments, that the "cell-mediated" basis of delayed hypersensitivity was established. They showed that reactions such as contact allergy and delayed hypersensitivity could be transferred from sensitive guinea pigs to insensitive recipients with lymphoid cells, even when immune serum was unsuccessful.

Subsequent experiments have established that these responses are due to a unique subclass of T lymphocytes (Tdh

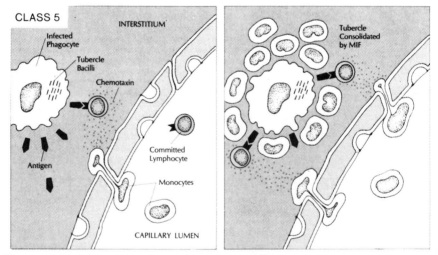

Figure 10–6. Class 5 reactions are entirely cell mediated and are entrained by antigenic sensitization of lymphocytes and macrophages in the circulation. The committed lymphocytes, in turn, migrate to a site of infection (e.g., tuberculosis) and chemotactically attract monocytes, which envelop the infected cells and activate macrophages to greater microbicidal activity. (Reprinted and modified, with permission, from Fink, J. N.: Immunologic lung disease. Hosp. Pract. 16(5):61, 1981. Drawing by Nancy Lou Gahan Makris.)

cells), maturation of which occurs in the thymus. Presumably, restriction of the repertoire of antigenic determinants to which each cell can respond occurs at the same time, but this has not been conclusively shown. In mice, most antigen-responsive T lymphocytes have the L3T4 phenotype, but there is some evidence that Lyt-2$^+$ may also be involved. Activation of antigen-responsive T cells by antigen requires participation of antigen-presenting cells such as macrophages, Langerhans' cells of the epidermis, or vascular endothelial cells. These interactions are restricted both by the antigenic determinant that is recognized by the T lymphocyte and by the genetically defined interactions between the antigen-presenting cells and the responding cells. In the case of T cells that proliferate in response to antigen, the genetic interactions with antigen-presenting cells are defined by Class II antigens of the major histocompatibility complex (MHC); growth of these cells also requires a hormone-like factor known as interleukin-2. Cytolytic activities are restricted by Class I antigens.

Once activated, the Tdh cells secrete molecules called lymphokines, which serve as inflammatory mediators (Table 10–6).

Table 10–6. Partial List of Lymphokines and Monokines

I. Factors that affect macrophage function
   1. γ-interferon—probably responsible for previously identified activities, such as:
     a. Migration inhibitory factor (MIF)
     b. Macrophage activating factor (MAF)
     c. Macrophage aggregation factor
     d. Factor that causes disappearance of macrophages from peritoneal cavity
   2. Macrophage chemotactic factor (MCF)
   3. Factors that alter surface tension
   4. Antigen-dependent MIF
II. Factors that affect neutrophil function
   1. Chemotactic factor
   2. Leukocyte inhibitory factor (LIF)
III. Factors that affect lymphocyte function
   1. Interleukin-1 (lymphocyte activating factor)
   2. Interleukin-2 (T-cell growth factor)
   3. Interleukin-3
   4. B-cell growth factor
   5. Chemotactic factor
   6. E-rosette augmenting factor (E-RAF)
   7. Transfer factor (TF)
   8. Antigen-dependent helper factor
   9. Antigen-independent helper factor
   10. Antigen-dependent suppressor factor
   11. Antigen-independent suppressor factor
IV. Factors that affect eosinophil function
   1. Immune complex–dependent chemotactic factor
   2. Eosinophil stimulation promoter (ESP)

The exact number of lymphokine molecules is unknown, but approximately 100 activities are attributed to lymphokines. Some activities, such as macrophage activation, may actually be due to immune interferon (γ-IFN). Nonetheless, the lymphokines, through chemotactic, cytotoxic, and cell-activating effects, produce local accumulations of inflammatory cells and injury to tissues.

Delayed cutaneous hypersensitivity is a well-known method for detection of prior exposure to microbiologic antigens. In addition, observations in patients and animals with impaired cellular immunity have demonstrated the importance of these mechanisms in defense against infections with certain parasites, fungi, and viruses. These observations were supported by studies in which restoration of immune competence had greatly increased resistance to infections with these agents. In addition, cell-mediated immune mechanisms are operative in certain forms of interstitial lung disease, granuloma formation, rejection of allogeneic tissues, and probably in resistance to certain tumors.

Cutaneous Basophil Hypersensitivity. This form of delayed-in-time cutaneous reaction was first noted by Jones and Mote in recipients of vaccines. Like classic delayed hypersensitivity, the cutaneous responses appear at 16 to 24 hours and then subside. In contrast, the responses are more erythematous and lack the induration that is usually associated with classic delayed cutaneous hypersensitivity. Histologic studies have shown that these responses contain larger numbers of basophils; these cells are not prominent in classic delayed reactions.

A number of other properties distinguish these reactions from classic delayed hypersensitivity. Cutaneous basophil hypersensitivity may be induced in guinea pigs with protein antigens in incomplete Freund's adjuvant; classic delayed hypersensitivity requires complete Freund's adjuvant. Cutaneous basophil hypersensitivity may be transferred to insensitive recipients with B lymphocytes and serum from immune donors; these modalities will not transfer classic delayed hypersensitivity.

The clinical significance of basophilic infiltrations is still unclear. The fact that basophilic infiltrations are found in contact allergic reactions, in rejecting allografts, and in cutaneous fungal infections in guinea pigs suggests a significant, but undetermined, role.

CONCLUSIONS

Advances in allergy and clinical immunology during the past two decades have defined several mechanisms of tissue injury that were previously unrecognized. These include IgE-mediated late-phase reactions that are probably important in the pathogenesis of certain cases of asthma, allergic rhinitis, and reactions to venoms. Natural killer cells have been well studied and are probably primarily involved in homeostatic and protective rather than pathogenic roles. The clinical consequences of defective natural killer cell activity in disorders such as the Chédiak-Higashi syndrome or the acquired immune deficiency syndrome (AIDS) are, however, probably very important. Indeed, some therapeutic strategies, such as use of interferons, are directed toward amplification of natural killer cell activity.

Certain effects of antibodies against receptors are mediated by previously described mechanisms such as complement-mediated lysis. However, the observation that antibodies against receptors may serve as agonists and modulate cell functions may be important in a number of autoimmune diseases.

The relationship of other processes to tissue injury is less clear. Antibody-dependent cellular cytotoxicity (ADCC) may be a fortuitous in vitro phenomenon, but additional information about the possible role of this reaction is needed. The same concerns surround cutaneous basophil hypersensitivity and the determination of the significance of accumulation of these mediator-rich cells at sites of inflammatory reactions.

The biochemistry of allergic injury continues to become more complex. The list of mediators continues to grow, and the networks of interaction become more complex and intriguing. The task of assigning specific roles to mediators like the lymphokines in the pathogenesis of allergic and immunologic injury is just beginning.

Bibliography

GENERAL

Coombs, R. R. A., and Gell, P. G. H.: Classification of allergic reactions responsible for clinical hypersensitivity and disease. In Gell, P. G. H., Coombs, R. R. A., and Lachmann, P. J. (eds.): Clinical Aspects of Immunology, 3rd ed. London, Blackwell, 1975, p. 761.
Paul, W. E.: Fundamental Immunology. New York, Raven Press, 1984, pp. 1–795.

CLASS 1: REAGIN-DEPENDENT ALLERGIC INJURY

Cox, C. P., Wardlow, M. L., Meng, K. E., et al.: Substrate specificity of the phosphatide 2-acylhydrolase that inactivates AGEPC. *In* Benveniste, B., and Arnoux, B. (eds.): Platelet Activating Factor. Amsterdam, Elsevier Science Publishers, 1983, p. 299.

de Shazo, R. D., Levinson, A. I., and Dvorak, H. F.: The late phase skin reaction: paradigm or epiphenomena? Ann. Allergy 51:166, 1983.

Gleich, G. J.: The late phase of an immunoglobulin E–mediated reaction: a link between anaphylaxis and common allergic disease. J. Allergy Clin. Immunol. 70:160, 1982.

Wasserman, S. I.: Mediators of immediate hypersensitivity. J. Allergy Clin. Immunol. 72:101, 1983.

CLASS 2: CYTOTOXIC REACTIONS

*D.-E. Young, J., Cohn, Z. A., and Podack, E. R.: The ninth component of complement and pore-forming protein from cytotoxic T cells: structural, immunologic and functional similarities. Science 233:184, 1986.

Henney, C. S., and Gillis, S.: Cell-mediated cytotoxicity. *In* Paul, W. E., (ed.): Fundamental Immunology. New York, Raven Press, 1984, p. 669.

Podack, E. R., Tschopp, J., and Muller-Eberhard, H. G.: Molecular organization of C9 within the membrane attack complex of complement. Induction of circular C9 polymerization by the C5b-8 assembly. J. Exp. Med. 156:268, 1982.

Roder, J. C., and Pross, H. F.: The biology of the natural killer cell. J. Clin. Immunol. 2:249, 1982.

CLASS 3: IMMUNE-COMPLEX–MEDIATED REACTIONS

Wiggins, R. C., and Cochrane, C. G.: Immune-complex–mediated biologic effects. New Engl. J. Med. 304:518, 1981.

CLASS 4: ANTI-RECEPTOR ANTIBODIES

Couraud, P. O., Lu, B. Z., Schmutz, A., et al.: Immunological studies of β-adrenergic receptors. J. Cell Biochem. 21:187, 1983.

Drachman, D. B., Adams, R. N., Josifek, L. F., et al.: Functional activities of autoantibodies to acetylcholine receptors and the clinical severity of myasthenia gravis. New Engl. J. Med. 207:769, 1982.

Flier, J. S., Kahn, C. R., and Roth, J.: Receptors, antireceptor antibodies and mechanisms of insulin resistance. New Engl. J. Med. 300:413, 1979.

CLASS 5: DELAYED HYPERSENSITIVITY

Waksman, B. H.: Cellular hypersensitivity and immunity: inflammation and cytotoxicity. *In* Parker, C. W., (ed.): Clinical Immunology. Philadelphia, W. B. Saunders Co., 1980, p. 173.

---

*Provides evidence for injury to target cell by soluble factors from cytotoxic T cells.

11

The Biology of the Mast Cell

K. FRANK AUSTEN, M.D.,
and DAVID W. FISHER

INTRODUCTION

Tissue mast cells are the primary effectors of immediate hypersensitivity reactions, and among the populations of immunologically active cells they uniquely possess a recognition system that is already in situ. Thus, IgE-bearing ("sensitized")

177

mast cells can recognize "non-self" cells without recruitment of other cells from the blood or lymphatic circulations. Furthermore, mast cells are located at cutaneous and mucosal surfaces and perivenularly, a localization that is ideal for protection of the host against exogenous organisms or toxic substances. Paradoxically, however, the "sentinel" function of the mast cells more often than not subserves an immunopathologic rather than an immunoprotective role. The medical community thinks of mast cell responses in the context of allergy to bee stings, to penicillin, or to pollens, rather than in the context of defense against helminthic infections, although there is good reason to believe that, in an evolutionary sense, it is the latter that led to their biologic development.

Although the outlines of the immunologic responses of mast cells and their initiation by the surface binding of immunoglobulin E (IgE) have long been understood, it was recognized only a few years ago that mast cell function was not limited to the release into the microenvironment of granules containing histamine and other preformed mediators such as proteoglycan and neutral proteases. We now know that in addition to the secretion of granules ("degranulation"), there is a parallel response sequential to the perturbation of the mast cell membrane. This membrane alteration leads to the oxidative metabolism of arachidonic acid, with resulting elaboration of two classes of highly potent mediators of inflammation and of immediate hypersensitivity—the prostaglandins and the leukotrienes.

Even more recent is the recognition of the heterogeneity of the mast cell population. There are at least two biochemically and biologically distinctive subclasses, varying in their mediator products and in their interaction with different receptors on target cells. This heterogeneity and its implications for our understanding of allergic diseases and their treatment will be a major focus of this chapter.

HISTORICAL PERSPECTIVES

In Vivo Studies

Before turning to these newer developments in our understanding, and to the explosive expansion of biologic investigation that produced them, it is useful to review the biology of the mast cell from an historical perspective. One can delineate three phases in research starting from the period during which all studies were essentially carried out on whole animals. At that time the participation of the mast cell in pathobiologic processes could only be appreciated by the effect on the animal in which the reaction was elicited. Thus, when the reaction involved the administration of antigen to the whole animal, the response was systemic anaphylaxis; when the reaction was restricted to injection of antigen into the skin, the response of skin mast cells was cutaneous anaphylaxis, perceived as an alteration in venular permeability; and when the antigen was given by aerosol and the tissue response studied was that of nonvascular smooth muscle, such as that of lung tissue, a constrictor response could be observed. In such "crude" systems, it was impossible to differentiate among different subclasses of mast cells and various mediators that might have been involved. Nevertheless, these early whole animal studies were immensely useful in establishing the role of the mast cell in immediate-type hypersensitivity. It was through these systems that immunologists and allergists came to a realization that the biologic amplification system required to make any immediate-type hypersensitivity response was effectively self-contained within the mast cell. Phenomena elucidated included the sensitization of mast cells by IgE binding and the activation of the mast cell by the bridging of the bound immunoglobulin by antigen (Fig. 11–1).

In Vitro Studies

The transfer of mast cell studies to in vitro systems, the second phase, was facilitated by the discovery that various rodent species, including rats, mice, and hamsters, harbor mast cell-rich cell populations free within their peritoneal cavities. Using peritoneal rat mast cells, it was feasible to obtain highly purified preparations for studies of the biochemical events that are involved in the immediate-hypersensitivity response, which we now know as the activation-secretion response. It was discovered that the membrane IgE receptors are linked to an adenylcyclase that is activated by the antigen-antibody combination. The substrate for the adenylcyclase is adenosine triphosphate (ATP); there is formation of cyclic AMP, with the resultant activation of a cyclic AMP-dependent protein kinase. This leads to a series of biochemical events, still not completely characterized, that causes the cytoplasmic granules of the mast cell to migrate to the cell surface. In the process, the granules fuse first with each other and then with the cell membrane; finally, the granules are extruded to the microenvironment of the cell. These events provide the first of the soluble mediators of immediate hypersensitivity, histamine (Fig. 11–2).

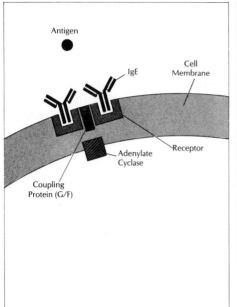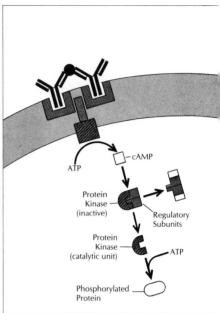

Figure 11-1. Mast cell membrane structures involved in the initial steps of the activation-secreti͏ response include the IgE receptors linked to a transmembrane coupling protein (G/F) and the cataly͏ unit of adenylate cyclase (left). When two IgE molecules are bridged by a specific antigen, the G͏ unit activates the adenylate cyclase (right) and cytoplasmic ATP is used to produce cAMP, whi͏ then recruits a cytoplasmic, cAMP-dependent protein kinase. This it does by binding to the t͏ regulatory units of the inactive kinase, liberating a catalytic unit that phosphorylates another, s͏ undefined protein, using additional ATP in the process. It is noteworthy that the biochemistry clos͏ parallels that of endocrine hormonal release. (Reprinted, with permission, from Austen, K. F.: Tiss͏ mast cells in immediate hypersensitivity. Hosp. Pract. 17(11):98, 1982. Artwork by Bunji Tagawa.)

MAST CELL AND DERIVED MEDIATORS

Rat and Human Mast Cells

For a number of years it was presumed that histamine was the exclusive mediator of the immediate-hypersensitivity response. However, as studies progressed, additional mediators were recognized as residing with histamine in the secretory granules and arising de novo from membrane fatty acids. A number of mediators were recognized through the in vitro studies on rat peritoneal mast cells and on human mast cells, most commonly pulmonary mast cells derived from lung biopsies. In both rats (and other rodent species) and humans, the mast cell granules contain amines; in addition to the histamine found in all mast cells, the rat granules contain serotonin. A second class of molecules was also identified in mast cells, termed proteoglycans, in which a peptide core is surrounded by side chains made up of highly charged, sulfated repeating sugar units. The proteoglycans effectively provide the granules with their relatively rigid skeletal structure. In the connective tissue mast cells the proteoglycan is heparin, while in the mucosal mast cells it is "oversulfated" chondroitin sulfate. Proteins constitute the third major component of the secretory granule. Interestingly, these proteins are almost all neutral proteases, enzymes with trypsin, chymotrypsin, or carboxypeptidase activity. These enzymes are

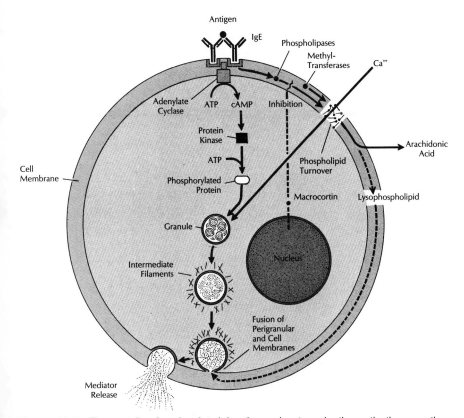

Figure 11–2. The protein phosphorylated by the early steps in the activation-secretion sequence (see Fig. 11–1) initiates movement of the granules toward the cell surface. This movement is facilitated by the action of intermediate filaments. At the cell surface, there is fusion between the perigranular and cell membranes, and the granules secrete their contents into the extracellular space. In parallel with degranulation, there is perturbation of the phospholipids of the cell membrane, also initiated by antigen bridging of IgE pairs. Phospholipases and methyltransferases catalyze phospholipid breakdown and the release of arachidonic acid. Another product, a lysophospholipid, facilitates membrane fusion and therefore degranulation. Also shown is the suggestion that steroids act in allergic diseases by generating macrocortin, which in turn inhibits phospholipid turnover. (Reprinted, with permission, from Austen, K. F.: Tissue mast cells in immediate hypersensitivity. Hosp. Pract. 17(11):98, 1982. Artwork by Bunji Tagawa.)

capable of digesting proteins in surrounding tissues including in all probability the peptide core of extracellular proteoglycans. Proteases in rat serosal (connective tissue) mast cells are present in a concentration of close to 40 μg per 10^6 cells. In human pulmonary mast cells the neutral protease is a tryptase with a concentration of 20 μg per 10^6 cells. From a pathophysiologic perspective this means that we have a set of cells in our tissues with a remarkable proteolytic destructive capacity. Although biologists have tended to think that the neutral protease contribution to the inflammatory response is imported with the influx of neutrophils, in fact there are already mast cells at the site of tissue reactions that have a proteolytic activity on a cell-for-cell basis far greater than that of neutrophils.

Similarities and Differences

A new dimension in the development of mast cell biology was made possible by a shift in focus from studies on rat peritoneal mast cells to studies on human mast cells obtained from the enzymatic digestion of lung tissue. Such processing yields cell suspensions that are 5 to 8 percent mast cells. This high percentage probably derives from the fact that the lung tissue is obtained on biopsy, and therefore the specimens are almost always from smokers, usually cancer or emphysema patients. These cell suspensions were further purified to yield mast cell preparations of greater than 60 percent purity. The human mast cell differed from that of the rat in that it had granules with a crystalline structure when examined by electron microscopy (Fig. 11–3). Within seconds of membrane activation by interaction of antigen and specific IgE, there was evidence of a change in the permeability of the perigranular membrane. The crystalline structure of the granule degenerated, the material within the perigranular membrane solubilized, and the granule swelled to about twice its preactivation size. The solubilized granule became surrounded by organelles, known as intermediate filaments, and migrated toward the cell surface. Finally, the granules merged with the cell membrane and extruded their contents into the extracellular environment.

The studies of the chemistry of the human mast cell revealed a number of similarities to that of the rat mast cell, but also some interesting differences. As in the rat mast cell, heparin proteoglycan was present, as was histamine, but serotonin was absent. The human mast cell protease is trypsin-like, rather than chymotryptic, in activity and proved to be structurally

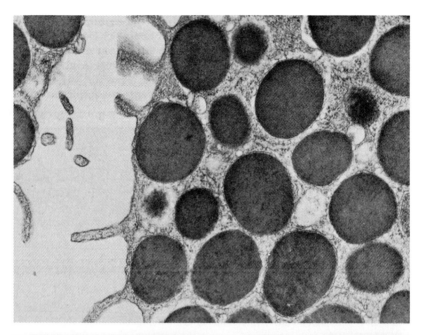

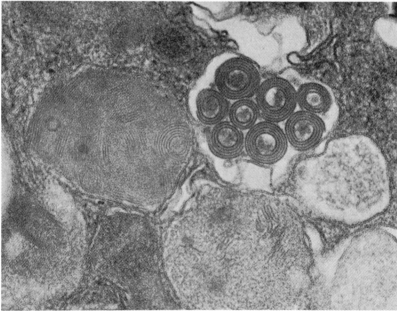

Figure 11–3. The amorphous internal structure of rat peritoneal mast cells (top, ×50,000) is in sharp contrast to the scroll-like crystalline structure of human mast cells (bottom, ×174,000). (Reprinted, with permission, from Austen, K. F.: Tissue mast cells in immediate hypersensitivity. Hosp. Pract. 17(11):98, 1982. Photomicrographs courtesy of Drs. John P. Caulfield and Ann Hein.)

unique. Rather than being composed of a single polypeptide chain, as are the neutral proteases of rat mast cells and other mammalian tissues, human mast cell tryptase is a four-chain molecule with two α chains (35,000 molecular weight) and two β chains (37,000). The fact that it has tryptic activity led to an examination of its activity in relationship to the third component of the complement system and it was demonstrated that the tryptase could cleave human C3 so as to release its anaphylatoxic C3a fragment. This was the first demonstration that mast cell activation in the human could lead to a recruitment of a biologically active complement fragment and, of course, had obvious implications for the known vascular effects of immediate hypersensitivity responses. As in any physiologic system, there is also a down regulation capacity; specifically it was found that the heparin product of degranulation accelerates the degradation of C3a by tryptase and inhibits any generation of C3a via the activation of the alternative complement pathway.

MEMBRANE-DERIVED PRODUCTS OF ARACHIDONIC ACID METABOLISM

Prostaglandins and Leukotrienes (LTB$_4$:SRS-A [LTC$_4$, D$_4$, E$_4$])

The next aspect of the human mast cell studies focused on exploration of the membrane-derived products of arachidonic acid metabolism. As with the rat connective tissue/serosal mast cell, the dominant product was found to be prostaglandin D$_2$ (PGD$_2$) as defined by correlation with IgE-Fc mediated histamine release. This was surprising, since the presumption had been that, in humans, the most likely candidate for production from the membrane would be slow reacting substance of anaphylaxis (SRS-A), i.e., leukotrienes. At this point, a clinical study of systemic mastocytosis proved most informative because it involved patients who not only had hives and also recurrent abdominal pain and diarrhea, but, interestingly, recurrent tachycardia with marked hypotension. Two of the patients with severe hypotensive episodes that proved refractory to treatment with antihistamines of both the H1 and H2 classes had markedly elevated levels of urinary metabolites of PGD$_2$. The clinical problem was solved by administering aspirin as a prostaglandin inhibitor along with H1 and H2 antihistamines. Thus it was possible to confirm clinically the in vitro observation that human mast cells synthesize PGD$_2$, and to show that in some individuals with mastocytosis the contribution of the prostaglandin to the disease may be as great or greater than that of histamine. This does *not* mean that human mast cells do not also generate leukotrienes, but rather that some cells, possibly representing different subclasses, produce PGD_2 and others preferentially produce LTC_4 (Table 11–1).

MAST CELL HETEROGENEITY

Subclasses (Differentiation of Serosal [Connective Tissue] and Mucosal Mast Cells)

The third major phase in the understanding of mast cell biology, and the current one, came with the recognition that mast cell heterogeneity goes far beyond differences in neutral proteases that are species specific. It has been recognized for about 20 years that mast cells in the gastrointestinal tissues have different staining properties from those associated with

Table 11–1. Biochemical Heterogeneity of Mast Cells

Biochemical Mediators	Cell Sources			
	Rat Serosal	Rat Mucosal	Human Pulmonary	Mouse Bone Marrow– Derived
Histamine Content ($\mu g/10^6$ cells)	8–24	0.16	1.7	0.1–0.45
Proteoglycan Content ($\mu g/10^6$ cells)				
Heparin	25–50	ND	4.0	–
Chondroitin sulfate	–	+	ND	2
Neutral Protease Content ($\mu g/10^6$ cells)				
Neutral protease type I (chymase)	24	–	–	*
Neutral protease type II	–	+	–	*
Carboxypeptidase A	~10	ND	–	ND
Tryptase	–	ND	20	ND
Arachidonic Acid Metabolites Generated by IgE-dependent Mechanisms ($ng/10^6$ cells)				
LTB_4	ND	ND	ND	4.5
LTC_4	ND	ND	25**	23
PGD_2	13	ND	39	1–2

ND, Not determined
–, Undetectable
+, Detected but not quantitated
*, Uncharacterized DFP binding serine proteins, most likely serine proteases
**, Does not correlate with histamine release

connective tissue. In this context, the term "atypical" or mucosal mast cell had been introduced to apply to the gastrointestinal mast cells. These observations have taken on new significance in the last five years with culture of mast cells from bone marrow and other tissues of the mouse and chemical differentiation of such cells from those of the mouse and rat serosal cavity (connective tissue). In at least four different laboratories that were harvesting murine bone marrow cells and studying their subsequent differentiation in culture, it was found that under certain conditions, one could derive homogeneous populations of granulated cells. In general, this was done by mitogenic stimulation of spleen tissue to generate lymphokines and then adding these soluble factors to bone marrow cells that had been cultured in conventional media that included fetal calf serum. The granulated cells could be increasingly concentrated by serial removal of adherent cells. The remaining nonadherent cells were rich in metachromatic granules and had IgE receptors. Heparin was not found in these cells; instead another charged and sulfated proteoglycan, unique at least in mammalian tissues, termed proteoglycan chondroitin sulfate E, was present. It was structurally markedly different from heparin (Fig. 11–4) and had a molecular weight of 225,000 as compared with heparin's 750,000. The murine serosal mast cell and bone marrow-derived, putative mucosal mast cell could also be distinguished phenotypically with monoclonal antibodies, i.e., they expressed both common and different epitopes. Another major difference between the two mast cell populations was particularly intriguing, both historically and in terms of continuing research. When the bone marrow–derived mast cells were sensitized with an IgE monoclonal antibody and activated with a hapten-specific antigen, their arachidonic acid was processed not to PGD_2, as occurred with rat serosal mast cells, but to leukotriene C_4 (LTC_4), a major constituent of SRS-A. In addition to LTC_4, the putative mucosal mast cell was also found to elaborate LTB_4 and a structurally distinct membrane-derived lipid mediator, platelet activating factor (PAF).

In further studies of the T cell influence on differentiation of the murine bone marrow–derived mast cells it was demonstrated that a specific lymphokine, interleukin 3, was responsible. Interleukin 3 is a product of a subset of helper T lymphocytes. This in vitro demonstration is compatible with in vivo findings that T cell–deficient rats and mice are impaired in their ability to proliferate intestinal mast cells and to clear helminthic parasites from their tissues. There is compelling evidence for the existence of two different mast cell populations in rats, and there is strong evidence for such heterogeneity in mice. But one also has to address the question at the human level. Atypical, putative mucosal mast cells have been described in human gastrointestinal tissues based upon fixation but not staining characteristics similar to those observed in rat and mouse intestine. It is known that human lung mast cells release PGD_2 in a correlative relationship with histamine in vitro and that some patients with systemic mastocytosis produce excessive amounts of PGD_2 as well as histamine, as assessed by urinary metabolites. However, mast cell–enriched populations of human lung cells also elaborate SRS-A and its constituent sulfidopeptide leukotrienes but without a direct correlative relationship to histamine release.

Furthermore, the sulfidopeptide leukotrienes are released from human nasal mucosa on inhalation challenge. That human nasal polyps produce less SRS-A relative to histamine than do human lung fragments in response to IgE-dependent activation was recognized more than a decade ago, and the likelihood of mast cell heterogeneity in the human seems quite evident from both functional and histochemical studies.

In addition to the heterogeneity of mast cells in terms of subclasses, there is another level of heterogeneity that has important implications for clinical allergic disease, namely, subclasses of cellular receptors for the products of mast cell activation. However, before discussing this aspect, it is necessary to briefly review the leukotrienes.

The biologic activity of one of the two major classes of leukotrienes has been studied for more than 40 years. The

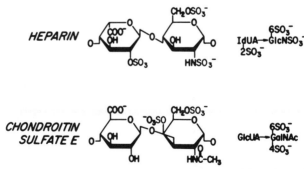

Figure 11–4. Major repeating disaccharide units of heparin and chondroitin sulfate E proteoglycan. (Reprinted, with permission, from Wilson, J. G., Fearon, D. T., Stevens, R. L., et al.: Inhibition of the function of activated properdin by squid chondroitin sulfate E glycosaminoglycan and murine bone marrow–derived mast cell chondroitin sulfate E proteoglycan. J. Immunol. 132:3058, 1984.)

leukotriene class was, as has been noted, originally designated SRS-A. We now know that SRS-A is composed of three distinct sulfidopeptide leukotrienes, the distinction arising from a sequential cleavage of the peptide side chain of the "parent" molecule, LTC_4 (Fig. 11–5). The diagram schematizes the derivation of the leukotrienes from arachidonic acid and notes the cleavage sequence and the enzymes responsible for producing from LTC_4, the other two molecules of this series, LTD_4 and LTE_4. The sulfidopeptide leukotrienes (LTC_4, LTD_4, and LTE_4), which form one major class of products of the 5-lipoxygenase pathway of arachidonic acid metabolism, exhibit remarkable vasoactive and spasmogenic activities. The other major class is composed of a dihydroxy leukotriene, LTB_4. Functionally, LTB_4 adds potent chemotactic activity and endothelial cell adherence activity to the vasoactivity of the sulfidopeptide leukotrienes.

Although there are 10 or more products with substantial biologic activity derived from the metabolism of arachidonic acid from membrane-associated phospholipids, namely, the prostaglandins and thromboxanes from the cyclooxygenase pathway, and the leukotrienes from the 5-lipoxygenase pathway, each cell type has a characteristic profile with respect to its products. Platelets, for example, make predominantly thromboxane A_2, which facilitates aggregation, whereas vascular endothelial cells produce PGI_2, which attenuates or inhibits the platelet aggregation response. Human eosinophils preferentially metabolize arachidonic acid to LTC_4, while human neutrophils yield predominantly LTB_4.

Subclasses of Cellular Receptors for Products of Mast Cell Activation

Specific high- and low-affinity LTB_4 receptors have been identified on neutrophils; since this leukotriene is the dominant product of the cells, these receptors produce an obvious mechanism for self-amplification. The reality of this phenomenon in humans has been demonstrated by the injection of purified LTB_4 into the skin of normal humans. In nanomolar amounts the leukotriene induces a local lesion that is palpable and painful; on biopsy the lesion reveals only neutrophils, confirming not only the potency of LTB_4 but also an in vivo activity completely consistent with its in vitro behavior.

Perhaps of greater interest in the context of human allergic disease is the evidence for subclass receptors for the three sulfidopeptide leukotrienes (C_4, D_4, and E_4). The possibility of such heterogeneity was first suggested by studies of the rank order of their spasmogenic potencies on three different tissue assay preparations, guinea pig ileum, guinea pig pulmonary parenchymal strips, and guinea pig tracheal rings. It was observed that the relative potencies of the three leukotrienes were completely different, with three contractile tissues in the same species. Most strikingly, it was found that with guinea pig lung parenchyma, LTC_4 and LTE_4 each gave a monophasic dose response, whereas LTD_4 elicited a biphasic dose response that began with concentrations as low as 10^{-13} M. As this concentration was increased, the contractile response plateaued, but then

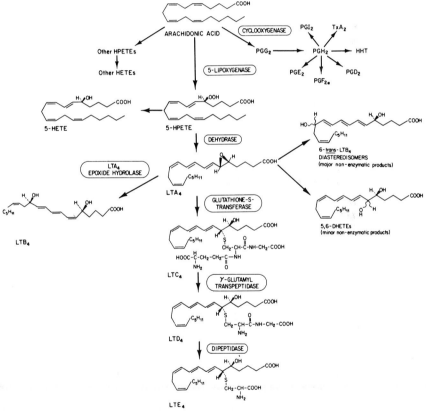

Figure 11–5. Biosynthetic pathways of leukotriene generation: enzymatic cascade for the oxidative metabolism of arachidonic acid. The enzymes of the 5-lipoxygenase pathway are specifically indicated. 5,6-DiHETE, 5,6-dihydroxy-eicosatetraenoic acid; 5-HETE, 5S-hydroxy-6-*trans*-8,11,14-*cis*-eicosatetraenoic acid; HHT, 12-hydroxy-heptadecatrienoic acid; PGD_2, PGE_2, $PGF_{2\alpha}$, PGG_2, PGH_2, and PGI_2, prostaglandins D_2, E_2, $F_{2\alpha}$, G_2, H_2, and I_2, respectively; TXA_2, thromboxane A_2. (Reproduced, with permission, from Lewis, R. A., and Austen, K. F.: The biologically active leukotrienes: biosynthesis, metabolism, receptors, functions, and pharmacology. J. Clin. Invest. 73:889, 1984.)

started to rise again at 10^{-10} M. Furthermore, a putative inhibitor of SRS-A, FPL55712, blocked the low-dose contraction to LTD_4, while leaving the high-dose response to LTD_4 and the entire response to LTC_4 unaffected. These physiologic and pharmacologic studies prompted the suggestion in 1980 that there were subclasses of receptors for the sulfidopeptide leukotrienes.

The presence of separate receptors for LTC_4 and LTD_4 has been confirmed by radioligand binding studies with nonvascular smooth muscle cells in culture, intact guinea pig ileal segments, and intact rat renal glomeruli as well as with subcellular fractions of guinea pig and rat lung. More recently, the physiologic evidence for a separate LTE_4 receptor, namely, its greater potency relative to LTC_4 and LTD_4 in contracting guinea pig tracheal spirals, has been extended by finding that this agonist, but not the others, induces hyperresponsiveness of this tissue to a subsequent contraction by histamine.

EFFECTS OF SRS-A (AND ITS CONSTITUENT LEUKO-TRIENES) ON PERIPHERAL AND CENTRAL AIRWAYS OF ASTHMATIC SUBJECTS

For more than a decade it has been recognized that SRS-A and its constituent sulfidopeptide leukotrienes have a preferential action on peripheral as compared with central airways in terms of elicited contraction or compromised pulmonary function in the guinea pig, and it can now be suggested that an additional function may be the elicitation of central airway hyperirritability. Furthermore, in normal human subjects, inhaled LTC_4 and LTD_4 were 4000 and 6000 times as potent as histamine in eliciting an impairment of pulmonary function by a measurement that emphasized peripheral airway effects. In contrast, by the same measurement, asthmatic subjects were only 200 times more reactive to LTD_4 than to histamine, and less than 10 times more responsive than normals. The failure of asthmatics to be substantially hyperresponsive to LTD_4 suggests that their lesions are in central, rather than peripheral, airways and that this distinction could be recognized only through the use of the sulfidopeptide leukotrienes because of their potency and marked preference for peripheral airways. Furthermore, based upon their potency at any airway level and the hyperreactivity of central airways in asthmatics to sulfidopeptide leukotrienes, it is also suggested that these substances are important contributors to the central lesion of bronchial asthma.

SUMMARY

To summarize with regard to immediate hypersensitivity reactions, the biologic response to which the mast cell is central, there is increasing evidence for diversity with the attendant clinical implications for a greater appreciation of the role of the mast cell in health and disease. At a minimum this diversity will involve the participation of mast cell subclasses, the elaboration of different mediators in quantitative and qualitative terms by these subclasses in response to IgE-Fc–dependent activation, and the action of these mediators through different subclass receptors distributed differently to specific target cells. Furthermore, while one mast cell subclass is held to be relatively stable in tissue concentration, the other appears to be expansile in concert with an immune response. The latter provides the biologic effector system for the trace antibody of the IgE class in helminthic infections.

Bibliography

Austen, K. F.: Histamine and other mediators of allergic reactions. *In* Samter, M. (ed.): Immunological Diseases. Boston, Little, Brown & Co., 1965, p. 211.

Austen, K. F.: Biologic implications of the structural and functional characteristics of the chemical mediators of immediate-type hypersensitivity. *In* The Harvey Lecture Series. New York, Academic Press, 73:93, 1979.

Austen, K. F., and Lewis, R. A.: Historical and continuing perspectives on the biology of the leukotrienes. *In* Chakrin, L. W., and Bailey, D. M. (eds.): The Chemistry and Biology of the Leukotrienes and Related Substances. New York, Academic Press, 1984, p. 1.

Creticos, P. S., Peters, S. P., Adkinson, N., Jr., et al.: Peptide leukotriene release after antigen challenge in patients sensitive to ragweed. N. Engl. J. Med. 310:1626, 1984.

Griffin, M., Weiss, J. W., Leitch, A. G., et al.: Effects of leukotriene D on the airways in asthma. N. Engl. J. Med. 308:436, 1983.

Krilis, S., Lewis, R. A., Corey, E. J., et al.: Specific receptors for leukotriene C_4 on a smooth muscle cell line. J. Clin. Invest. 72:1516, 1983.

Lewis, R. A., and Austen, K. F.: The biologically active leukotrienes: biosynthesis, metabolism, receptors, functions and pharmacology. J. Clin. Invest. (Perspectives) 73:889, 1984.

Lewis, R. A., Soter, N. A., Diamond, P. T., et al.: Prostaglandin D_2 generation after activation of rat and human mast cells with anti-IgE. J. Immunol. 129:1627, 1982.

Orange, R. P., Austen, W. G., and Austen, K. F.: Immunological release of histamine and slow reacting substance of anaphylaxis from human lung. I. Modulation by agents influencing cellular levels of cyclic 3′,5′-adenosine monophosphate. J. Exp. Med. 134:136s, 1971.

Razin, E., Mencia-Huerta, J.-M., Stevens, R. L., et al.: IgE-mediated release of leukotriene C_4, chondroitin sulfate E proteoglycan, β-hexosaminidase, and histamine from cultured bone marrow-derived mast cells. J. Exp. Med. 157:189, 1983.

Samuelsson, B.: Leukotrienes: mediators of immediate hypersensitivity reactions and inflammation. Science 220:568, 1983.

Soter, N. A., Lewis, R. A., Corey, E. J., et al.: Local effects of synthetic leukotrienes (LTC$_4$, LTD$_4$, LTE$_4$ and LTB$_4$) in human skin. J. Invest. Dermatol. 80:115, 1983.

Weiss, J. W., Drazen, J. M., Coles, N., et al.: Bronchoconstrictor effects of leukotriene C in humans. Science 216:196, 1982.

Weller, P. F., Lee, C. W., Foster, D. W., et al.: Generation and metabolism of 5-lipoxygenase pathway leukotrienes by human eosinophils: predominant production of leukotriene C$_4$. Proc. Natl. Acad. Sci. USA 80:7626, 1983.

Winslow, C. M., and Austen, K. F.: Role of cyclic nucleotides in the activation-secretion response. *In* Ishizaka, K., Kallos, P., Waksman, B. H., and deWeck, A. L. (eds.): Progress in Allergy. Basel, S. Karger, 34:236, 1984.

12

Mechanisms Involved in the Regulation of IgE Synthesis

KIMISHIGE ISHIZAKA, M.D.

INTRODUCTION

It is now established that IgE antibodies against allergens are responsible for hay fever and are probably involved in other allergic (reaginic) diseases. The crucial role of IgE antibodies in reaginic hypersensitivity suggests that partial or total suppression of IgE antibody responses to allergens may constitute a fundamental treatment for allergic diseases. During the past 15 years, mechanisms for the IgE antibody response were analyzed and several attempts made to regulate the IgE antibody response in animals. This chapter briefly summarizes attempts to suppress IgE antibody formation through antigen-specific mechanisms and

193

discusses current developments in isotype-specific regulation of the IgE response.

ANTIGEN-SPECIFIC REGULATION OF THE IgE RESPONSE

Regulation of the IgE antibody response by antigen-specific mechanisms has been attempted through either (a) tolerization of B cells or (b) manipulation of the population of antigen-specific T cells. Thus, Katz and coworkers induced B-cell tolerance by injecting hapten coupled to a nonimmunogenic carrier, D-glutamic acid D-lysine copolymer (DGL).

Lee and Sehon (1981) employed dinitrophenyl (DNP) conjugates of polyvinylalcohol (PVA) to terminate the anti-DNP IgE antibody response. Not only can DNP-PVA conjugates, like DNP-DGL, inactivate hapten-specific B cells but they can also induce DNP-specific suppressor T cells that regulate the antibody response of all isotypes.

An important practical problem involves regulation of the IgE antibody response to allergens and protein antigens. Because DNP-DGL conjugates are tolerizing, Liu and coworkers prepared DGL conjugates with ovalbumin or ragweed antigen E and studied the effect of these conjugates on the IgE response. Conjugates of ovalbumin suppressed, in mice, both the primary and secondary IgE antibody response to ovalbumin, by mechanisms entirely different from those obtained by DNP-DGL. Similar observations were made using ragweed antigen E, the major allergen in ragweed pollen.

IgE production to protein antigens may be regulated by inducing antigen-specific T cells, because antigenic determinants recognized by T cells may not be the same as the major antigenic determinants in such antigens as ragweed antigen E and ovalbumin. For example, the major antigenic determinants in these antigens are lost by denaturation in urea, and these antigens do not react with antibodies against native antigen or B cells specific for the major antigenic determinants. However, the modified antigens can stimulate T cells specific for the native antigen, and an injection of a large dose of urea-denatured antigen without adjuvant results in the induction of antigen-specific suppressor T cells. Lee and Sehon (1978) noted that ovalbumin–polyethylene glycol (PEG) conjugates have similar immunogenic properties, and injections of the conjugates, without adjuvant, induce suppressor T cells specific for native antigen.

An advantage of modified antigen over native antigen for

the treatment is that the modified antigen does not cause severe side effects, because the antigens do not react with the antibodies against native antigen. However, the antigens stimulate both helper and suppressor T cells. Animals already primed with antigen have a large population of antigen-specific helper T cells, and injected antigen expands the population of helper T cells rather than inducing suppressor T cells. The treatment may enhance rather than suppress the IgE antibody formation in certain circumstances.

ISOTYPE-SPECIFIC REGULATION OF THE IgE ANTIBODY RESPONSE

A unique feature of IgE antibody formation is that the antibody response is obtained under restricted conditions. A persistent formation of IgE antibody is obtained in the mouse only when genetically high responder strains are immunized with a minute dose of potent immunogen together with an appropriate adjuvant. Dissociation between the IgE antibody response and the IgG antibody response is frequently observed under a variety of conditions; some examples are as follows:

1. *Bordetella pertussis* vaccine (BP) and aluminum hydroxide gel are good adjuvants for the IgE antibody response, while complete Freund's adjuvant (CFA) is an excellent adjuvant for IgG antibodies but a poor adjuvant for the IgE isotype.

2. Some mouse strains, such as SJL, fail to form IgE antibodies but have a substantial IgG antibody response to the same antigen.

3. Repeated injections of CFA result in the suppression of IgE antibody response to an unrelated antigen.

4. Irradiation of mice with low-dose x-ray or an injection of cyclophosphamide prior to immunization selectively enhances the IgE response.

5. In both humans and rodents, infection with nematodes selectively enhances IgE synthesis. Infection of antigen-primed rats with the nematode *Nippostrongylus brasiliensis* (Nb) results in the enhancement of IgE antibody formation against the priming antigen. Augmentation of the antibody response after the nematode infection is restricted to the IgE isotype; the IgG_1 and IgG_2 antibody responses to the same antigen were not affected by the infection.

Dissociation between the IgE and IgG antibody responses suggests that the IgE response is regulated not only by antigen-specific helper and suppressor T cells but also by isotype-specific mechanisms. This possibility was studied using *Nippostrongylus* infection as an experimental model. T cells in the mesenteric lymph nodes (MLN) of Nb-infected rats released a soluble factor that has affinity for IgE and is capable of selectively enhancing the IgE response. The binding factor was spontaneously released from T cells that were obtained 14 days after the infection. However, MLN cells obtained 7 days after Nb infection and incubated with IgE released another IgE-binding factor that selectively suppressed the IgE response. Both the IgE-potentiating factor and the IgE-suppressive factor are derived from W-3/25$^+$ (Lyt-1$^+$) T cells and are of comparable molecular weight (13,000 to 15,000 daltons). As shown in Table 12–1, the major difference between the two factors is that the IgE-potentiating factor has affinity for lentil lectin and Con A while the IgE-suppressive factor does not, but does have affinity for peanut agglutinin. These findings show that both IgE-potentiating factor and IgE-suppressive factor are glycoproteins and indicate that the two factors contain different oligosaccharides.

The formation of IgE-binding factors is not restricted to Nb infection. After repeated injections of rats with CFA, their spleen cells released IgE-suppressive factor in vitro, and their serum contained IgE-suppressive factor. An injection of *Bordetella pertussis* (BP) vaccine, the best adjuvant for the IgE response in the rat, induced IgE-potentiating factor, and T cells in their peripheral blood spontaneously released potentiating factor. IgE-binding factors are also produced during an immune response. IgE antibodies are produced by Lewis rats injected with keyhole-limpet hemocyanin (KLH) absorbed to aluminum hydroxide gel. Spleen cells of these animals do not spontaneously secrete IgE-binding factor, but stimulation of the cells with KLH antigen yields IgE-potentiating factor. In contrast, immunization of rats with the same antigen in CFA, followed by the stimulation of

Table 12–1. Comparisons Between IgE-Potentiating Factor
and IgE-Suppressive Factor

Properties	IgE-Potentiating Factor	IgE-Suppressive Factor
Source	Fc$_\epsilon$R$^+$W 3/25$^+$ T cells	W 3/25$^+$ T cells
Molecular weight	13,000–15,000 daltons	13,000–15,000 daltons
Affinity for IgE	+	+
Affinity for:		
Lentil lectin	+	−
Concanavalin A	+	−
Peanut agglutinin	−	+

their spleen cells with the antigen, results in the formation of IgE-suppressive factor. Subsequent experiments provided evidence that genetic differences in the IgE antibody response may also be related to the nature of IgE-binding factors formed, i.e., high-IgE responder mice (BDF_1), and low-IgE responder mice (SJL) were immunized with alum-absorbed ovalbumin (OA) and their spleen cells were stimulated with OA. As expected, BDF_1 mice responded with persistent formation of IgE antibody, and their spleen cells formed IgE-potentiating factor. SJL mice, however, failed to form IgE antibody, and their spleen cells formed IgE-suppressive factor upon antigenic stimulation.

Apparently IgE-potentiating factor is detected whenever the IgE synthesis and/or IgE antibody response is enhanced. In contrast, IgE-suppressive factor is formed when IgE response is selectively suppressed. This strongly suggests that IgE-binding factors are involved in regulation of IgE antibody response in vivo.

RELATIONSHIP BETWEEN IgE-POTENTIATING FACTOR AND IgE-SUPPRESSIVE FACTOR

IgE-potentiating factor and IgE-suppressive factor are formed by Con A–activated T cells as well. T cells activated by 10 μg/ml Con A formed IgE-potentiating factor upon incubation with IgE, while those activated with 1 μg/ml Con A formed IgE-suppressive factor (Fig. 12–1). Since the major difference between IgE-potentiating factor and IgE-suppressive factor appears to reside in carbohydrate moieties of the molecules, T cells activated with 10 μg/ml Con A were incubated with IgE in the presence of tunicamycin, which inhibits the assembly of N-glycosidically linked oligosaccharide to peptide. Tunicamycin switched the Con A–activated cells from formation of IgE-potentiating factor to formation of IgE-suppressive factor, which suggests that N-linked, mannose-rich oligosaccharide in IgE-potentiating factor is essential for its biologic activity.

Switching of T cells from the formation of IgE-potentiating factor to the formation of IgE-suppressive factor was also achieved by pretreatment with glucocorticoid of cells activated by 10 μg/ml Con A or by adding lipomodulin (phospholipase inhibitory protein) during the synthesis of IgE-binding factor. In contrast, T cells activated with 1 μg/ml Con A, which form IgE-suppressive factor, could be made to switch to produce IgE-potentiating factor if the cells were incubated with IgE in the

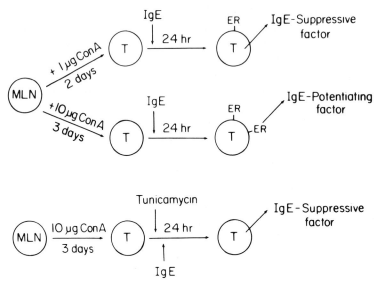

Figure 12–1. Schematic model of IgE-binding factor formation by Con A–activated lymphocytes. Lymphocytes from mesenteric lymph nodes (MLN) activated by 1 μg/ml of Con A formed IgE-suppressive factor upon incubation with 10 μg/ml IgE, whereas those activated by 10 μg/ml Con A formed IgE-potentiating factor. However, T cells activated with 10 μg/ml Con A formed "IgE-suppressive factors" if the cells were incubated with IgE together with 1 μg/ml tunicamycin (ER = $Fc_\epsilon R$).

presence of an activator of phospholipase, such as melittin or monoclonal antibody against lipomodulin. These findings imply that the same T cells can form both IgE-potentiating factor and IgE-suppressive factor, and that the nature of IgE-binding factors is determined by the environment of the cells. It is speculated that the IgE-potentiating factor and the IgE-suppressive factor share common precursors, and that the nature of IgE-binding factors is decided by a post-translational glycosylation process. Indeed, IgE-potentiating factor, IgE-suppressive factor, and Fc_ϵ receptor ($Fc_\epsilon R$) on both T and B cells share a common antigenic determinant.

Knowledge of the peptide portion of IgE-binding factors was quite limited until recent collaboration with Drs. Kevin Moore and Chris Martens, of the DNAX Institute of Molecular Biology, on gene cloning of rat IgE-binding factors succeeded in obtaining cDNA encoding the IgE-binding factor. Moore and Martens incubated 23B6 hybridoma cells with rat IgE, and messenger RNA was obtained from the cells. An injection of mRNA into *Xenopus* oocytes resulted in the formation of IgE-binding factors. Thus, cDNA libraries were constructed from the mRNA, and cDNA-encoding IgE-binding factors were selected. As the result of these experiments, four cDNA clones were obtained, the expression of which, in monkey kidney cells, resulted in the formation of IgE-binding factors. None of the IgE-binding factors so formed suppressed the IgE response, but the products of two cDNA clones selectively potentiated the IgE response. IgE-binding factors derived from one of the cDNA clones (clone 8.3) consisted of two species of IgE-binding factors, one with a molecular weight of about 60,000 and the other with a molecular weight of 11 to 12,000. Both species had affinity for lentil lectin and selectively potentiated the IgE response. These cDNA clones were prepared from messenger RNA of 23B6 cells, which forms IgE-suppressive factor, suggesting that IgE-potentiating factor and IgE-suppressive factor share a common structural gene, with the difference between the factors being decided by post-translational glycosylation processes.

The molecular weight of IgE-binding factor, calculated from the predicted amino-acid sequence, is about 62,000. Thus, the biologically active 11,000 IgE-potentiating factor must be a cleavage product of the 62,000 factor. Not yet known is which portion of the 62,000 peptide is responsible for binding to IgE; gene cloning of the IgE-binding factor may provide a structural basis for the function of IgE-binding factors.

MECHANISMS FOR THE SELECTIVE FORMATION OF IgE-POTENTIATING FACTOR OR IgE-SUPPRESSIVE FACTOR

An important question is why IgE-potentiating factor is formed under certain circumstances, such as 14 days after Nb infection and BP treatment, while IgE-suppressive factor is formed in such other conditions as after 7 days of Nb infection or after immunization with CFA. Analysis of various systems revealed that the nature of IgE-binding factors is determined by two T-cell factors that either enhance or inhibit the glycosylation of IgE-binding factors (Fig. 12–2). The cell sources of IgE-binding factors are always $Lyt-1^+$ T cells, which bear either $Fc_\epsilon R$ or $Fc_\gamma R$, or both, and which form IgE-binding factors when stimulated with IgE or an interferon-like substance ("inducer"). Interferon-like substance, which induces the formation of IgE-binding factors, is derived from $Lyt-1^+$ T cells, $Lyt-2^+$ T cells, or macrophages, depending on the system. For example, treatments with an adjuvant, such as CFA or BP, stimulate macrophages to form an interferon, while stimulation of antigen-primed $Lyt-1^+$ helper

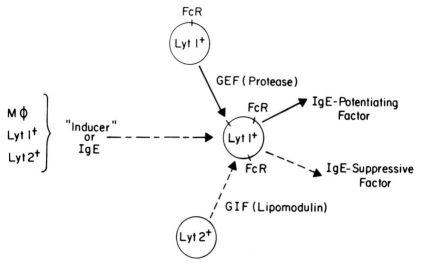

Figure 12–2. Schematic models for the selective formation of IgE-potentiating factor or IgE-suppressive factor. $Fc_\epsilon R^+$ Lyt-1$^+$ T cells form IgE-potentiating factor in the presence of GEF, but the same cells form IgE-suppressive factor in the presence of GIF. (GEF = glycosylation-enhancing factor; GIF = glycosylation-inhibiting factor; FcR = Fc receptor site; "inducer" = interferon-like substance.)

T cells with homologous antigen results in the release of "inducer" that, in turn, stimulates FcR$^+$ T cells to form IgE-binding factors (see Fig. 12–2). However, neither IgE nor "inducer" determines the nature of IgE-binding factors formed. For the selective formation of IgE-potentiating factor, another soluble factor is required (Fig. 12–2). One of them, called glycosylation enhancing factor (GEF), is derived from Lyt-1$^+$ T cells and enhances the N-glycosylation of IgE-binding factors during their biosynthesis. Subsequent studies showed that GEF is a kallikrein-like protease with lectin-like properties.

In contrast, FcR$^+$ T cells selectively form IgE-suppressive factor when the cells are stimulated with IgE or interferon-like substance ("inducer") in the presence of glycosylation inhibiting factor (GIF). This factor is formed by Lyt-2$^+$ T cells upon treatment of the donor of the cells with CFA. Antigen-specific suppressor T cells also release GIF, a fragment of phosphorylated lipomodulin that inhibits assembly of N-linked oligosaccharides to IgE-binding factors through inactivation of phospholipase. A series of experiments suggests that the nature and biologic activities of IgE-binding factors formed by FcR$^+$ T cells are decided by the balance between GEF and GIF in the environment. There is experimental evidence suggesting that the same principle may explain genetic differences between BDF_1 and SJL mice in the IgE response. Following immunization of both strains of mice with alum-absorbed ovalbumin, and stimulation of their spleen cells with the antigen, Lyt-1^+ T cells of BDF_1 mice form not only IgE-potentiating factor but also GEF, while Lyt-1^+ T cells of SJL mice form IgE-suppressive factor and GIF.

POSSIBLE APPROACHES FOR THE REGULATION OF IgE ANTIBODY RESPONSE

It is important to ascertain whether human lymphocytes produce T-cell factors similar to those detected in rodent systems. Peripheral blood lymphocytes of ragweed-sensitive patients produce IgE-binding factors when incubated with specific antigen and homologous IgE. Saryan and coworkers reported that IgE-specific potentiating factor, which has affinity for IgE and lentil lectin, was produced by peripheral blood T cells of patients with hyper-IgE syndrome (atopic dermatitis). They also detected, in the serum of normal individuals having extremely low IgE levels, an IgE suppressive factor that has affinity for IgE but which did not bind to lentil lectin. Among six human T-cell hybridomas that produce IgE-binding factors upon incubation with human IgE, one was obtained that formed 60K, 30K, and 15K species of IgE-binding factors upon incubation with human IgE. All three species have affinity for human IgE and Con A, and nearly one half of the factors bound to lentil lectin. The human IgE-binding factors have some affinity for rat IgE, and both the 60K and 15K IgE-binding factors selectively enhanced the IgE response of antigen-primed rat mesenteric lymph node cells to homologous antigen. Evidence was also obtained that the same cells produced IgE-suppressive factor under certain circumstances. An obvious approach for clinical application is to use human IgE-suppressive factors. Gene cloning of human IgE-binding factors is in progress, using cDNA libraries of 166A2 cells.

Another approach to consider is to regulate the nature of IgE-binding factors in vivo. If the nature of IgE-binding factors is determined by the balance between GEF and GIF (see Fig. 12–2), administration of GIF might suppress the IgE response. Experiments in the mouse showed that GIF is actually immunosuppressive. Repeated injections of mice with purified GIF during the primary antibody response did completely suppress both IgE and IgG antibody formation. GIF was also effective in suppressing the ongoing antibody formation. When BDF_1 mice were immunized with alum-absorbed antigen and then treated with GIF after the IgE antibody titer reached maximum, IgE antibody titer declined to one eighth, and IgG antibody titer to one half, of that present in control animals. It is hoped that the administration of either human IgE-suppressive factor or GIF may suppress the IgE antibody formation in atopic patients and provide clinical benefit to the patient with IgE-mediated disease.

Bibliography

Huff, T. F., and Ishizaka, K.: Formation of IgE-binding factors by human T cell hybridomas. Proc. Natl. Acad. Sci. USA 81:1514, 1984.

Huff, T. F., Yodoi, J., Uede, T., et al.: Presence of an antigenic determinant common to rat IgE-potentiating factor, IgE-suppressive factor and Fc_ϵ receptors on T and B lymphocytes. J. Immunol. 132:406, 1984.

Ishizaka, K.: Cellular events in the IgE antibody response. Adv. Immunol. 23:1, 1976.

Ishizaka, K.: Regulation of IgE synthesis. Ann. Rev. Immunol. 2:159, 1984.

Iwata, M., Munoz, J. J., and Ishizaka, K.: Modulation of the biologic activities of IgE-binding factor. IV. Identification of glycosylation enhancing factor as a kallikrein-like enzyme. J. Immunol. 131:1954, 1983.

Katz, D. H., Hamaoka, T., and Benacerraf, B.: Induction of immunological tolerance in bone-marrow-derived lymphocytes of the IgE antibody class. Proc. Natl. Acad. Sci. USA 7:2776, 1973.

Lee, W. Y., and Sehon, A. H.: Suppression of reaginic antibodies with modified allergens. II. Abrogation of reaginic antibodies with allergens conjugated to polyethylene glycol. Int. Arch. Allergy 56:193, 1978.

Lee, W. Y., and Sehon, A. H.: Suppression of the anti-DNP IgE response with tolerogenic conjugates of DNP with polyvinylalcohol. II. Induction of hapten-specific suppressor T cells. J. Immunol. 126:414, 1981.

Lee, W. Y., Sehon, A. H., and Akerblom, E.: Suppression of reaginic antibodies with allergens conjugated to polyethylene glycol (PEG) and monomethyl PEG with ovalbumin. Int. Arch. Allergy 64:100, 1981.

Liu, F. T., Bogowitz, C. A., Bargatze, R. F., et al.: Immunological tolerance to allergic protein determinants: properties of tolerance induced in mice treated with conjugates of protein and a synthetic copolymer of D-glutamic acid and D-lysine (D-GL). J. Immunol. 123:2456, 1979.

Martens, C. L., Huff, T. F., Jardieu, P., et al.: cDNA clones encoding IgE-binding factors from a rat-mouse T cell hybridoma. Proc. Natl. Acad. Sci. USA 82:2460, 1985.

Saryan, L. A., Leung, D. Y., and Geha, R. S.: Induction of human IgE synthesis by a factor from T cells of patients with hyper-IgE states. J. Immunol. 130:242, 1983.

Takatsu, K., and Ishizaka, K.: Reaginic antibody formation in the mouse. VII. Induction of suppressor T cells for IgE and IgG antibody responses. J. Immunol. 116:1257, 1976.

13

Anaphylaxis

MICHAEL A. KALINER, M.D.

INTRODUCTION

Portier and Richet used the word anaphylaxis to describe the fatal reaction induced by the introduction of minute amounts of antigen into dogs that had been previously sensitized to that antigen. The dramatic and unexpected fatal response was the opposite (*ana* = Greek: back, backwards) of protection (*phylax* = Greek: guard). Knowledge and comprehension of anaphylaxis have paralleled the understanding of the components of the immune system and, while there are still areas of uncertainty, our understanding of anaphylaxis is now rather complete.

Anaphylaxis is the syndrome elicited in a hypersensitive subject upon subsequent exposure to the sensitizing antigen. The spectrum of *anaphylactic responses* ranges from localized to systemic. Systemic anaphylaxis can cause *anaphylactic shock* and death. The necessary components of the anaphylactic response are (1) a sensitizing antigen, usually administered parenterally; (2) an IgE-class antibody response resulting in systemic sensitization of mast cells (and basophils); (3) reintroduction of the sensitizing antigen, usually systemically; (4) mast cell degranulation with mediator release and/or generation; and (5) production of a number of pathologic responses by the mast cell–derived mediators and manifested as anaphylaxis.

Because the mediators that are released or generated by mast cells cause anaphylaxis, any event associated with mast cell activation may produce the same clinical disease. Anaphylaxis usually refers to IgE-mediated, antigen-stimulated mast cell activation, while *anaphylactoid* reactions denote other, non-IgE mediated responses, such as may be produced by chemical agents capable of causing mast cell degranulation (e.g., opiates).

CLASSIFICATION OF CAUSES OF ANAPHYLAXIS (See Table 13–1)

IgE-Mediated Anaphylaxis

IgE-mediated anaphylaxis has been implicated in untoward reactions elicited by many drugs, chemicals, insect stings, foods, preservatives, and environmental factors. An agent capable of causing IgE antibody formation must be either an antigen or a hapten. For example, horse serum, formerly used as a source of antitoxin, contains many antigenic proteins. Subsequent reexposure to horse sera predictably caused anaphylaxis. Horse serum is now rarely used therapeutically, and more common sources of antigens include allergenic extracts, insulin, chymopapain (used to treat herniated vertebral discs), Hymenoptera venom, foods, and seminal plasma.

Haptens are molecules that are too small to elicit immune responses. However, haptens may bind to endogenous proteins such as serum globulins and become antigenic. The most important haptens are penicillin and related antibiotics. Penicillin is metabolized to a major determinant, benzylpenicilloyl, and a series of minor determinants including penicillin itself, penicilloate, penilloate, and penicilloyl-amine. These haptens circulate bound to serum proteins and produce IgE antibodies that can be

Table 13–1. Causes of Anaphylaxis/Anaphylactoid Reactions

IgE-Mediated Reactions
Antibiotics and other drugs
Foreign proteins (horse serum, chymopapain)
Foods
Immunotherapy
Hymenoptera stings
Seminal plasma

Complement-Mediated Reactions
Blood; blood products

Nonimmunologic Mast Cell Activators
Opiates (narcotics)
Muscle depolarizing agents
Radiocontrast media

Modulators of Arachidonic Acid Metabolism
Nonsteroidal anti-inflammatory agents
Tartrazine (possible)

Idiopathic Recurrent Anaphylaxis

Sulfiting Agents

Monosodium Glutamate

Exercise-Induced Anaphylaxis

detected in the positive skin test responses found in 4 to 10 percent of subjects who have completed a course of penicillin therapy. Thus, a sizeable portion of the population is at risk for penicillin reactions. One to 2 percent of the courses of penicillin therapy in the United States are complicated by systemic allergic reactions, and 10 percent of these reactions are serious or life-threatening. While serious reactions occur about twice as frequently after systemic administration, oral penicillin administration may also cause anaphylaxis and death. It is estimated that from 400 to 800 deaths per year in the United States are caused by penicillin reactions (Table 13–2).

Other beta-lactam antibiotics may act as haptens in their own right or may cross-react with penicillin. About 10 percent of penicillin-sensitive subjects will react to cephalosporins, and penicillin-sensitive subjects are 4 times more likely to have an allergic reaction to cephalosporins.

Table 13–2. Incidence of Reactions and Frequency of Anaphylactic Deaths

Agent	Mild	Severe	Deaths/Year (U.S.)
Penicillin	1:100–200	1:2500	400–800
Hymenoptera stings	1:200	1:2000	100 or more
Contrast media	1:20	1:1000	250–1000

Venoms of the Hymenoptera (bees, yellow jackets, hornets, and wasps) contain several protein antigens that are capable of eliciting an IgE antibody response. Between 0.5 and 4.0 percent of the population will experience a systemic reaction after being stung, and at least 100 subjects die per year as a consequence of such stings. Imported South American fire ants, *Solenopsis invicta* (Buren) and *Solenopsis richteri* (Forel), pose a similar risk. Imported fire ants were introduced into the United States in 1920 and now inhabit 13 southern states. The natural boundary for the fire ant is a minimal temperature of $-12°F$, and it is therefore likely that this insect will eventually spread more extensively. It is too early to know the frequency of systemic response to its sting, but anaphylaxis and death have occurred.

Ingestion of food-derived antigens provides a potentially huge antigen load and may cause anaphylaxis in a sensitive individual. Certain foods are more frequent offenders, including nuts, peanuts (which are actually legumes), fish, eggs, and seeds. Some subjects exhibit such extreme sensitivity that even exposure limited to the odor of cooked fish, for example, may cause a systemic response. Other, less frequently implicated, foods include milk, shellfish, chocolate, cola drinks, grains (particularly corn), fruits, and vegetables.

Immunotherapy for allergic diseases is among the most common triggers of mild anaphylaxis in that this treatment is based upon the progressively increasing dose of antigens to sensitive individuals (see Chapter 6 in *Principles of Immunology and Allergy*). However, immunotherapy rarely results in severe anaphylaxis or death because of the small incremental dose of the usual treatment plan and the expertise of the physicians who prescribe it.

Seminal fluid, but not sperm, has been implicated in anaphylaxis experienced after sexual intercourse in some women. The reactions reported range from pain and swelling restricted to the vaginal area to systemic anaphylaxis.

Complement-Mediated Reactions

Anaphylactic responses have been observed after the administration of whole blood or its products, including serum, plasma, fractionated serum products, and immunoglobulins. One of the mechanisms responsible for these reactions is the formation of immune complexes resulting in the activation of the complement cascade. Of the active by-products generated by complement activation, the anaphylatoxins, C3a, C4a, and C5a, are capable of causing mast cell (and basophil) degranulation, mediator release and generation, and consequent systemic reactions. In addition, the anaphylatoxins may directly induce vascular permeability and contract smooth muscles. This "aggregate-anaphylaxis" is thus immunologically mediated, but not through IgE. The immune complexes causing this reaction may involve aggregated IgG formed in vivo or in vitro, or IgG-IgA complexes. Indeed, individuals who are congenitally deficient for serum proteins may become sensitized to the missing factor. Patients with selective IgA deficiency (1:600 of the general population, 1:100 in the atopic population) have a greater chance of developing anaphylaxis when repeatedly given blood products, owing to the formation of anti-IgA antibodies (probably IgE–anti-IgA; see Chapter 6).

Cytotoxic (Type II) reactions can also cause anaphylaxis, via complement activation. Antibodies (IgG and IgM) against red blood cells, as occur in a mismatched blood transfusion reaction, activate complement. This reaction causes agglutination and lysis of red blood cells and perturbation of mast cells, which results in anaphylaxis.

Nonimmunologic Mast Cell Activators (Anaphylactoid Reactions)

Mast cells may degranulate when exposed to neuromuscular blocking agents, opiates and other narcotics, radiocontrast media, dextrans, and a myriad of low-molecular-weight chemicals. The clinically most important agents include radiocontrast media, narcotics, and depolarizing agents. These reactions are commonly referred to as anaphylactoid reactions.

Mild reactions are experienced by about 5 percent of subjects receiving radiocontrast dyes. Severe systemic reactions occur in 1:1000 exposures, with death in 1:10,000–40,000 exposures. In 1982, there were 10 million injections of contrast media in the United States, and it is estimated that from 250 to 1000 deaths resulted. Contrast media cause mast cell degranulation and may also lead to activation of complement. Documentation of elevated urine histamine levels in subjects experiencing adverse reactions lends additional support to the concept that this adverse reaction is an anaphylactoid response.

Narcotics and neuromuscular relaxing agents are recognized mast cell activators capable of causing elevated plasma histamine levels and anaphylactoid reactions, observed most commonly by anesthesiologists. No estimate of the frequency, morbidity, or mortality of these reactions is available.

Modulators of Arachidonic Acid Metabolism

About 5 percent of asthmatics react to nonsteroidal anti-inflammatory drugs (NSAID), such as aspirin and indomethacin, with rhinorrhea, bronchorrhea, bronchospasm, and, rarely, vasomotor collapse. Clinical indicators of the "aspirin triad" are chronic sinusitis, nasal polyposis, and asthma; eosinophilia may also be present. Nonasthmatics may react to NSAID with urticaria and angioedema, and, rarely, with vasomotor collapse. The mechanism underlying NSAID sensitivity is not known. No convincing evidence exists implicating IgE antibodies in this syndrome. While the clinical manifestations may resemble anaphylaxis, studies have failed to identify mast cell mediator release after aspirin challenge. The most likely cause is modulation of arachidonic acid metabolism by interference with cyclooxygenase enzyme pathways. There are two consequences of this action: reduction in the formation of prostaglandins, thromboxanes, and prostacyclin; and enhanced formation of lipoxygenase products. As subjects who are reactive to NSAID respond to each of the many drugs operative at the cyclooxygenase site, it is most reasonable to conclude that it is through modulation of arachidonic acid metabolism that the untoward response occurs.

This reaction is thus not anaphylaxis but closely resembles its clinical spectrum. NSAID-sensitive subjects may also react to tartrazine (F.D. and C.#5 yellow dye) as well as to benzoates and acetaminophen. The true incidence of these additional reactivities is unknown but is probably quite rare, and therefore does not warrant excluding these agents from the NSAID-sensitive subject.

Idiopathic Recurrent Anaphylaxis

A group of subjects who recurrently experience anaphylaxis due to no recognized cause has been identified. This group commonly experiences flushing (100%), tachycardia (100%), angioedema (96%), upper airway obstruction (76%), urticaria (72%), bronchospasm (48%), gastrointestinal complaints (32%), and syncope or hypotension (28%). The diagnosis is based upon the spectrum of clinical signs and symptoms, evidence of elevated urine histamine, and an exhaustive search for causative factors.

Sulfiting Agents

Sulfiting agents (sodium and potassium sulfites, bisulfites, metabisulfites, and gaseous sulfur dioxide) are added to foods as preservatives, to prevent discoloration. Foods to which these substances are added in the highest concentrations include leafy salad greens (particularly at salad-bar restaurants); light-colored fruits and vegetables (particularly dried fruits like apples or golden raisins, and instant potatoes); wine, beer, dehydrated soups, fish, and shellfish (particularly shrimp); and rapidly perishable foods such as avocados. Ingestion of sulfites may provoke asthma and anaphylaxis in susceptible persons. The magnitude of the problem is unclear, but provocation challenges indicate that less than 10 mg of potassium metabisulfite can cause asthma and anaphylaxis in a portion of the asthmatic population (<5%). Sulfite sensitivity should be suspected in subjects who relate symptoms to eating, particularly if restaurants or processed foods are implicated. Trials with oral sulfiting agents suggest that anaphylaxis is a very rare consequence.

Monosodium glutamate (MSG), a seasoning, is known to cause the "Chinese restaurant syndrome," which is usually manifested as flushing, lightheadedness, and tachycardia. MSG can rarely also cause asthma and/or anaphylaxis of a life-threatening nature.

Exercise-Induced Anaphylaxis

Strenuous exercise may lead to anaphylaxis in susceptible subjects. This reaction can be differentiated from exercise-induced asthma by the frequency with which the responses follow exercise. In the asthmatic, exercise (especially in the cold) regularly causes asthma, while individuals with exercise-related anaphylaxis experience the reaction only intermittently. The response resembles anaphylaxis in every respect, including elevated urine and plasma histamine levels. The syndrome sometimes requires both exercise and ingestion of particular foods for development. This reaction should be suspected in any subject who collapses after exercise, particularly if flushing, urticaria, and angioedema are evident.

CLINICAL FINDINGS IN ANAPHYLAXIS

The primary anaphylactic shock organs in humans are the cutaneous, gastrointestinal, respiratory, and cardiovascular systems (Table 13–3). Characteristically, patients describe an immediate sense of impending doom, coincident with flushing, tachycardia, and often pruritus (either diffuse, localized to the

Table 13–3. Clinical Findings in Anaphylaxis and Anaphylactoid Reactions

System	Signs	Symptoms
Cutaneous	Flushing, urticaria, angioedema	Flushing, pruritus
Cardiovascular	Tachycardia, hypotension, shock, syncope, arrhythmias	Faintness, palpitations, weakness
Gastrointestinal	Abdominal distension, vomiting, diarrhea	Bloating, nausea, cramps, pain
Respiratory	Rhinorrhea, laryngeal edema, wheezing, bronchorrhea, asphyxiation	Nasal congestion, shortness of breath, difficulty breathing, choking, cough, hoarseness, lump in throat
Others	Diaphoresis, fecal or urinary incontinence	Feeling of impending doom, conjunctival pruritus and edema, sneezing, disorientation, hallucinations, genital burning, headaches, metallic taste

palms and soles, and/or noted particularly in the genital and inner-thigh areas). These initial signs and symptoms rapidly evolve to urticaria, angioedema, rhinorrhea, bronchorrhea, nasal congestion, asthma, laryngeal edema, abdominal bloating, nausea, vomiting, cramps, arrhythmias, faintness, syncope, prostration, and death. The organ systems involved in these responses have two features in common: They are exposed to the external environment and they contain the largest number of mast cells. It is predictable that those organs richest in mast cells would be the "shock organs," since mast cell degranulation causes anaphylaxis.

Involvement of the cutaneous and cardiovascular systems is the most significant as regards mortality. The most common causes of death are cardiovascular collapse and asphyxiation secondary to laryngeal edema. In most cases, laryngeal edema is preceded by a sensation of "a lump in the throat," hoarseness, and difficulty in breathing. Hypotension due to anaphylactic shock is usually preceded by diffuse flushing, urticaria, light-headedness, faintness, and syncope.

The usual progression of symptoms begins within minutes of exposure to the inciting agent, peaks within 15 to 30 minutes, and is complete within hours. Some subjects have spontaneous recrudescence of anaphylaxis 8 to 24 hours later. Anaphylaxis may be complicated by myocardial infarction or stroke, and death may ensue from these complications.

PATHOGENESIS

When mast cells degranulate, preformed and rapidly generated mediators are released into the connective tissue along with the molecules that constitute the granular matrix (see Chapter 11). While many of these mediators induce dramatic local effects, few other than histamine are capable of entering the circulation in an active state. Thus, the symptoms of anaphylaxis can be attributed primarily to the local actions of the many mast cell mediators and the circulating effect of histamine. As summarized in Table 13–4, the majority of the changes occurring in anaphylaxis can be attributed to histamine (acting through H_1 and H_2 receptors), prostaglandins, and leukotrienes.

With the exception of the disease systemic mastocytosis, in which prostaglandin D_2 can be detected, the only mast cell mediator regularly observed in the circulation is histamine. Infusion of histamine into normal subjects causes the following signs and symptoms, which can be diminished by antagonists of specific histamine receptors (as noted in parentheses): flushing (H_1 plus H_2); hypotension (H_1 plus H_2); headache (H_1 plus H_2); tachycardia (H_1); pruritus (H_1); rhinorrhea (H_1); and bronchospasm (H_1).

The consequences of mast cell mediator release include *increased vascular permeability* due to the formation of intercellular gaps between endothelial cells in postcapillary venules. The increased vascular permeability causes tissue edema leading to urticaria (if the reaction is restricted to the epidermis); angioedema (if the reaction is in the dermis); laryngeal edema; nasal congestion; and gastrointestinal swelling, with abdominal bloating and cramps. *Contraction of smooth muscle* leads to bronchospasm and asthma as well as abdominal cramping and

Table 13–4. Processes Involved in the Symptoms of Anaphylaxis

Pathologic Process	Sign or Symptom	Putative Mediator Responsible
Vascular permeability	Urticaria, angioedema, laryngeal edema, abdominal swelling, cramps	Histamine (H_1), leukotrienes, prostaglandins
Vasodilation	Flushing, headache	Histamine (H_1 and H_2), leukotrienes, prostaglandins
Smooth muscle contraction	Wheezing (asthma), GI cramps, diarrhea	Histamine (H_1), leukotrienes, prostaglandins
Tachycardia	Palpitations	Histamine (H_1), leukotrienes
Reduced peripheral vascular resistance	Faintness, syncope	Histamine (H_1 and H_2)
Mucus secretion	Rhinorrhea, bronchorrhea	Histamine (H_2), prostaglandins, leukotrienes

diarrhea. *Vasodilation* leads to flushing, headaches, reduced peripheral vascular resistance, hypotension, and syncope. Other specific processes are stimulated as well: Sensory nerve endings in the skin are stimulated, leading to *pruritus,* and cardiac histamine receptor stimulation leads to *tachycardia* and possible *arrhythmias.*

DIFFERENTIAL DIAGNOSIS (Table 13–5)

The diagnosis of anaphylaxis is not difficult, given the constellation of an acute exposure to a provocative condition followed within minutes by the evolution of multisystem manifestations, including flushing, urtication, pruritus, and angioedema. Anaphylaxis is most easily confused with a vasovagal reaction. The clearest differential considerations in deciding between these two diagnoses are the presence in vasovagal reactions of pallor, extreme diaphoresis, and bradycardia or normal sinus rhythm, and the absence of flushing, urticaria, angioedema, pruritus, and asthma.

The correct diagnosis is much more difficult in a syncopal patient. The usual differential diagnoses include cardiac arrhythmias, myocardial infarction, pulmonary embolism, seizures, asphyxiation, hypoglycemia, and stroke. In analyzing the syncopal subject, anaphylaxis should be considered if urticaria, angioedema, or asthma are present or if the history suggests an acute exposure to conditions associated with anaphylaxis (e.g., Hymenoptera sting).

If laryngeal edema is the presenting problem, hereditary angioedema (HAE) must be considered (see Chapter 3; see also

Table 13–5. Differential Diagnosis of Anaphylaxis and Anaphylactoid Reactions

Anaphylaxis
  IgE mediated
  Complement mediated
  Nonimmunologic mast cell degranulation
  Idiopathic
  Exercise-related
  Sulfiting agents
Nonsteroidal anti-inflammatory drug reaction
Vasovagal collapse
Hereditary angioedema
Serum sickness
Systemic mastocytosis
Pheochromocytoma
Carcinoid syndrome

Chapter 12 in *Principles of Immunology and Allergy*). This disorder is usually inherited (although a smaller portion of the affected population may acquire the defect) and is accompanied by painless (and pruritus-free) angioedema, GI cramps and distension, recurrent attacks, and usually a family history of similar attacks and/or sudden death. HAE is not associated with flushing, asthma, or urticaria, is of slower onset, and, in the absence of severe airway obstruction, is not a cause of hypotension.

Serum sickness is characterized by fever, lymphadenopathy, maculopapular and urticarial rashes, arthralgias and arthritis, and, less frequently, nephritis and neuritis. Serum sickness generally develops 5 to 10 days after antigen exposure and may persist for 2 to 3 weeks.

Systemic mastocytosis is a generalized disease of mast cells, usually of a benign or very low-grade malignancy. Urticaria pigmentosa is a more frequently encountered benign growth of mast cells restricted to the skin. In either disease, it is possible for the mast cells to degranulate, generally producing local effects, or more rarely, causing systemic effects exactly like anaphylaxis. Degranulation of the mast cells can occur spontaneously and/or after exposure to NSAID, alcohol, narcotics, and other nonimmunologic mast cell degranulating agents. The diagnosis should be suggested by the recognition of the classic fawn-colored macular-to-low-papular skin lesions that urticate on trauma (Darier's sign), the history of flushing attacks, evidence of bone involvement (pain, abnormal bone scans, abnormal x-rays), GI pain and peptic ulcers, histaminuria, histaminemia, and increased urinary PGD_2 metabolites.

Other conditions that might also be considered include overdoses of medications, cold urticaria, cholinergic urticaria, pheochromocytoma, carcinoid tumors, and sulfite or monosodium glutamate ingestion in sensitive subjects.

TREATMENT OF ACUTE ANAPHYLAXIS

Anaphylaxis is an acute medical emergency requiring prompt and appropriate attention (Table 13–6). If possible, remove the source of antigen or retard its systemic circulation. If a bee sting is responsible, carefully remove the stinger, apply a venous tourniquet to the extremity, and inject aqueous epinephrine (0.1–0.2 ml, 1:1000) directly into the antigen source in order to reduce the local circulation. Aqueous epinephrine (1:1000, 0.3–0.5 ml SC) is the mainstay of the treatment plan. This drug

Table 13–6. Treatment of Acute Anaphylaxis (Adult)

1. When possible, apply a tourniquet to obstruct the draining blood flow from the source of the antigen or inciting medication. When possible, remove the stinger if an insect sting. Release the tourniquet every 15 minutes.
2. Place patient in recumbent position, elevate lower extremities, keep warm, provide O_2.
3. Epinephrine aqueous 1:1000, 0.3–0.5 ml SC; inject epinephrine 1:1000, 0.1–0.2 ml directly into source of antigen to reduce blood flow. Give 0.1 ml aqueous epinephrine 1:1000, mixed in 10 ml saline, slowly IV in cases of severe hypotension.
4. Diphenhydramine, 25–50 mg IM or IV.
5. Cimetidine, 300 mg IV over 3–5 minutes.
6. Establish and maintain airway; administer racemic epinephrine by metered dose inhaler to closed airway if laryngeal edema is present.
7. Maintain blood pressure with fluids, volume expanders, or pressors: dopamine hydrochloride, 2–10 µg/kg/min, or norepinephrine bitartrate, 2–4 µg/min.
8. If wheezing is a problem, administer aminophylline, 5.6 mg/kg over 20 minutes, with maintenance dose of 0.9 mg/kg/hr thereafter.
9. For prolonged reactions, repeat epinephrine every 20 minutes × 3; give hydrocortisone, 100 mg IV every 6 hours.

maintains the blood pressure, antagonizes many of the adverse actions of the mediators of anaphylaxis, and reduces the subsequent release of mediators through its action on mast cells and basophils.

In moderate to severe cases in which epinephrine alone is not adequate therapy, administer both H_1 and H_2 antihistamines, diphenhydramine, 25 to 50 mg IM, and cimetidine, 300 mg *slowly* IV (over 3 to 5 minutes). If upper airway obstruction is evident (lump in the throat, hoarseness, stridor), have the patient spray epinephrine from a metered-dose inhaler against a closed glottis in order to try to reduce the local swelling. If the obstruction is progressing, *immediately* place a nasopharyngeal airway or perform a tracheostomy. Once laryngeal edema has developed, it is impossible to place a nasopharyngeal tube! One of our subjects developed severe recurrent laryngeal edema during recurrent anaphylaxis and was effectively treated only after the opening of a tracheal fenestration.

Blood pressure should be maintained with fluid, plasma expanders, and pressors, as needed. Asthma that has not responded to diphenhydramine should be treated with aminophylline (loading dose = 5.6 mg/kg/20 min followed by 0.9–1.0 mg/kg/hr) and inhaled β_2-adrenergic agonists. Corticosteroids have no immediate effect but should be administered to prevent prolonged or recurrent sequelae. The usual dose is 100 mg hydrocortisone every 6 hours.

Treatment of anaphylaxis has been complicated by the increased use of β-adrenergic blocking agents in many subjects (e.g., for headaches, hypertension, heart arrythmias, and glaucoma). β-adrenergic receptor antagonists potentiate allergic reactions, possibly by reducing the normal homeostatic influences induced by circulating catecholamines. Treatment of anaphylaxis in the presence of β-adrenergic blockade should be essentially unchanged, recognizing the fact that agents such as epinephrine, which ordinarily stimulate both α- and β-adrenergic receptors, will act predominantly upon α-receptors under these circumstances.

PREVENTION AND PROPHYLAXIS OF ANAPHYLAXIS

Subjects with known sensitivity should avoid reexposure to causative agents, if possible. For instance, insect sting–sensitive individuals should (a) avoid areas in which there is an increased likelihood of insect encounters, (b) always wear shoes when outside, (c) avoid hair sprays, perfumes, after-shaving lotion, and flowered or brightly colored clothing, and (d) carry an anaphylaxis emergency treatment kit at all times. The "stinging insect emergency kit" contains epinephrine (in a spring-loaded injectable form that facilitates self-administration) and a rapidly absorbed antihistamine. Anyone given such a kit should be carefully instructed in its use. Appropriate immunotherapy should also be considered (see Chapters 6 and 8 in *Principles of Immunology and Allergy*).

A careful history of previous exposures and possible reactions to therapeutic and diagnostic materials is the best prophylaxis of adverse reactions. Even in the best circumstances, however, patients may experience profound anaphylaxis having had no recognizable previous adverse response. Only a few drugs are available for diagnostic skin testing. Penicillin and its major determinant, benzylpenicilloyl-polylysine, are used for diagnostic testing, and a mixed minor determinant preparation should soon be available for routine use.

While parenteral administration of drugs is more likely to cause anaphylaxis, oral dosing is also associated with the potential for profound reactions. Nonetheless, when in doubt, the oral route is preferred, because the antigen load is absorbed more slowly and anaphylaxis, if it occurs, is usually less severe.

When in doubt or when the medication is required despite likely reactivity, the subject should be treated with prophylactic H_1 and H_2 antihistamines: hydroxyzine, 25 mg qid, and cimetidine, 300 mg qid, for several doses before exposure. Subjects at increased risk, e.g., previous reactors to iodinated contrast media, should also be pretreated with prednisone, 50 mg q 6 h × 3, before reexposure. Agents such as penicillin can be administered in progressively larger doses given orally or parenterally in order to desensitize the patient (see Chapter 7 in *Principles of Immunology and Allergy*).

CONCLUSION

Anaphylaxis is a dramatic, major medical emergency. Comprehension of its pathogenesis, together with a thorough knowledge of the emergency treatment required and subsequent prophylactic measures to be taken, can reduce the morbidity and mortality. The most important component in the avoidance of anaphylaxis is a conscientious physician who carefully weighs each therapeutic decision and obtains a complete history of prior reactions. Prompt medical attention to individuals experiencing anaphylaxis should reduce mortality.

Bibliography

Austen, K. F.: The anaphylactic syndrome. *In* Samter, M. (ed.): Immunological Diseases. 3rd ed. Boston, Little, Brown & Co., 1978, p. 885.

Burks, A. W., Sampson, H. A., and Buckley, R. H.: Anaphylactic reactions after gammaglobulin administration in patients with hypogammaglobulinemia. N. Engl. J. Med. 314:560, 1986.

Kaliner, M., Shelhamer, J. H., and Ottesen, E. A.: Effects of infused histamine: correlation of plasma histamine levels and symptoms. J. Allergy Clin. Immunol. 69:283, 1982.

Metcalfe, D. D., Donlon, M. A., and Kaliner, M.: The mast cell. Crit. Rev. Immunol. 3:23, 1981.

Patterson, R., and Anderson, J.: Allergic reactions to drugs and biologic agents. JAMA, 248:2637, 1982.

Patterson, R., and Valentine, M.: Anaphylaxis and related emergencies including reactions to insect stings. JAMA 248:2632, 1982.

Sonin, L., Grammer, L. C., Greenberger, P. A., et al.: Idiopathic anaphylaxis: a clinical summary. Ann. Intern. Med. 99:634, 1983.

Summers, R. J., and Kaliner, M.: Current concepts of histamine actions through H1 and H2 receptors. Comprehensive Therapy 8:6, 1982.

Wasserman, S. I.: Anaphylaxis. *In* Middleton, E., Jr., Reed, C. E., and Ellis, E. F. (eds.): Allergy, Principles and Practices, 2nd ed. St. Louis, C. V. Mosby Co., 1983, p. 689.

14

Eosinophilia*

GERALD J. GLEICH, M.D.,
and JOSEPH H. BUTTERFIELD, M.D.

*From the Department of Immunology and the Division of Allergic Diseases and Internal Medicine, Mayo Clinic and Mayo Foundation, Rochester, Minnesota 55905. Supported by grants from the National Institutes of Health, AI 15231, AI 09728, AI 11483, AI 20416, and from the Mayo Foundation.

INTRODUCTION

The eosinophil was discovered by Paul Ehrlich in 1879 when he stained blood smears with aniline dyes. By the first decade of this century, the associations of eosinophilia with helminth infestation and with asthma had been made. Over the past decade, the eosinophil's likely roles in parasitic resistance and hypersensitivity have been elucidated. This chapter discusses certain basic information about the eosinophil, especially its production by the bone marrow, its distribution in tissue, the properties of its granule proteins, and its probable role in disease.

BIOLOGY

Eosinophil Production and Tissue Localization

Eosinophilopoiesis

Eosinophils are produced by the bone marrow and are briefly present in the blood before they enter tissues. Thus, the eosinophil is a tissue cell rather than a blood cell, because it resides chiefly in the tissues. Cells committed to eosinophil differentiation, eosinophil colony–forming cells, can be identified by their ability to form colonies (groups of 50 or more eosinophils) in soft agar or methylcellulose. The eosinophil colony–forming cell is a null lymphocyte bearing an Ia antigen marker. The growth of these colony-forming cells is influenced by factors that have not been thoroughly characterized. Eosinophil colonies are small (50–150 cells), mature slowly, and generally are compact. Mixed colonies of eosinophils and basophils are present, which suggests a common precursor cell for these leukocytes.

Eosinophils in the Peripheral Blood

Eosinophils are normally present in small numbers in peripheral blood, with a mean of 115 cells per mm^3 and a range of 11 to 678 cells per mm^3. The number of circulating eosinophils may be affected by their rate of release from the bone marrow, by changes in their circulation time, and by their margination in the circulation. Studies with radiolabeled cells have shown that eosinophils are present in the circulation for about 12 hours. Rare patients lacking peripheral blood eosinophils have been reported; such individuals may be clinically normal. Administration of glucocorticoids consistently lowers circulating eosinophils, and this decrease is associated with a corresponding increase in bone marrow eosinophils.

Peripheral blood eosinophilia in response to a stimulus has many of the characteristics of an immune response, including (1) a lag between the stimulus and the increase in eosinophils, (2) an anamnestic response following repeat antigen challenge, (3) a dependence on T lymphocytes, and (4) the ability to transfer eosinophilia adoptively with thoracic duct lymphocytes. Studies in thymectomized mice and nude mice showed that T cells are necessary for an eosinophilic response to infection with helminths.

Factors Determining Tissue Eosinophilia

Eosinophil chemotactic factors (ECF) have the ability to attract eosinophils across a concentration gradient and thereby increase the number of eosinophils in tissues. IgE-mediated (Type I) allergic reactions cause release of the eosinophil chemotactic factor of anaphylaxis (ECF-A) from human lung. ECF-A activity resides in two acidic tetrapeptides, Val-Gly-Ser-Glu and Ala-Gly-Ser-Glu, and with other low-molecular-weight substances. IgE-mediated reactions cause histamine release, and histamine has ECF activity. Eosinophils are also attracted by C5a, a potent chemotactic factor, or by a lymphocyte-derived ECF. The latter appears quite specific for eosinophils and does not cause neutrophil attraction. Several derivatives of arachidonic acid have ECF activity, including leukotriene B4, 12-L-hydroxy-5,8,10,14-eicosatetraenoic acid (HETE), and 12-L-hydroxy-5,8,10-heptadecatetraenoic (HHT). However, none of these are specific for eosinophils; they also attract neutrophils. Finally, various tumors produce substances with ECF activity.

Eosinophil-Associated Proteins

The eosinophil contains distinctive granules that stain avidly with acid dyes and have a characteristic fine structure. Primary granules are round, are uniformly electron dense, and are seen in eosinophilic promyelocytes. During differentiation, these granules develop electron-dense cores and an electron-radiolucent matrix, and are called secondary or specific granules (Fig. 14–1). The granule core shows a longitudinal and cross-sectional periodicity and is termed a crystalloid.

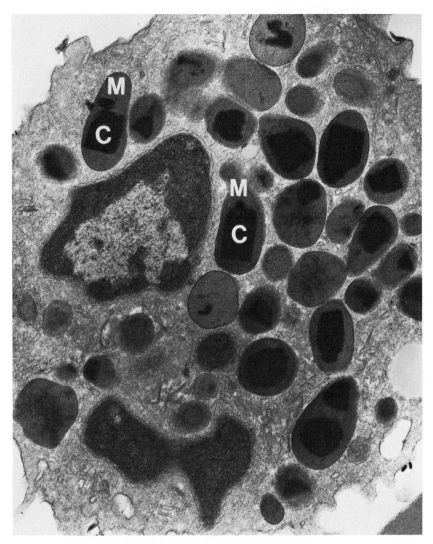

Figure 14–1. Electron photomicrograph of crystalloid-containing granules in a human eosinophil leukocyte showing dense cores (C) of various shapes embedded in a less dense matrix (M) (×15,000). (Photomicrograph generously provided by Dr. M. S. Peters.)

Membrane-Associated Proteins

Receptors. Eosinophils express receptors for IgG, IgE, and C3b. During the eosinophil's attack on schistosomula of *Schistosoma mansoni*, eosinophils are bound by their Fc receptors to IgG antibody to schistosomula. Similarly, eosinophils can bind by their C3b receptors to C3b on the schistosomula. Evidence for

IgE-dependent eosinophil cytotoxicity has been shown, and anti-sera have been developed that are preferentially reactive to eosinophils, which indicates that they possess unique markers.

Lysophospholipase. Degenerating eosinophils give rise to a characteristic crystalline structure, the Charcot-Leyden crystal (CLC) (Fig. 14–2), which possesses lysophospholipase activity.

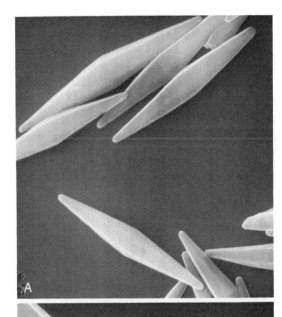

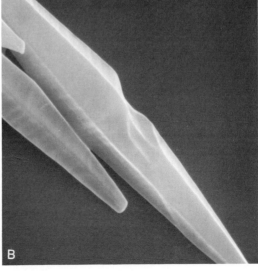

Figure 14–2. Scanning electron photomicrograph of human Charcot-Leyden crystal (CLC) (*A*, ×580; *B*, ×2800). Note the hexagonal bipyramidal structure of CLC. (Used with permission from Gleich, G. J.: The eosinophil: new aspects of structure and function. J. Allergy Clin. Immunol. 60:79, 1977.)

The CLC, which also forms from human basophils, may be seen in any organ heavily infiltrated with eosinophils and in secretions derived from these organs, such as stools of patients with helminth infestation or after allergic reactions to foods. CLCs derived from eosinophils in vitro yield a single protein with lysophospholipase activity. Conversely, purified lysophospholipase forms crystals with the morphology of the CLC. Lysophospholipase (CLC protein) appears to be localized in the plasma membrane of the eosinophil.

Granule-Associated Proteins

Major Basic Protein. Studies of isolated guinea pig eosinophil granules revealed the presence of a major basic protein (MBP), so named because (1) it accounted for over 50 percent of the granule protein, (2) its isoelectric point (pI) was too high to measure, and (3) it was a protein. Subsequently, an MBP-like molecule was found in human and rat eosinophils. Because MBP comprises essentially all of the protein in the crystalloid core of the granule, the core can be regarded as a crystal of MBP.

MBP is also present in human basophils, which contain about 3 percent of the MBP content of eosinophils. The presence of both MBP and CLC in basophils and eosinophils indicates biochemical similarities between these cell types. Furthermore, studies of granulocyte colonies from human peripheral blood indicate that "eosinophil-type" colonies may contain a mixture of eosinophils and basophils, suggesting a common precursor for eosinophils and basophils.

MBP is able to kill the following parasites in vitro: schistosomula of *S. mansoni,* newborn larvae of *Trichinella spiralis,* and the bloodstream trypomastigote stage of *Trypanosoma cruzi.* MBP, in vitro, also damages cells from organs known to be infiltrated with eosinophils in disease states, e.g., cells from tumors, skin, intestine, spleen, peripheral blood, and tracheal and bronchial epithelium. There is some evidence suggesting that the eosinophil causes tissue damage during hypersensitivity reactions (see below).

Eosinophil Peroxidase (EPO). EPO is localized in the granule matrix of numerous species. The intensity of peroxidase staining is so great that it can be used to enumerate eosinophils, as in the automated continuous-flow cytochemistry devices used to perform differential counts.

EPO catalyzes the oxidation of many substances by hydrogen

peroxide. Because eosinophils generate considerable H_2O_2, the activities of the EPO + H_2O_2 + halide system in the killing of microorganisms have been explored. EPO, in the presence of H_2O_2 and halide, kills bacteria, schistosomula, toxoplasma, trypanosoma, mast cells, and tumor cells.

EPO also binds to mast cells, and the EPO–mast cell complex catalyzes iodination of proteins and killing of microorganisms. Furthermore, EPO supplemented by H_2O_2 and halide induces mast cell degranulation and histamine release. Thus eosinophils, by releasing EPO in the presence of H_2O_2 (generated by eosinophils or other phagocytes in the area), chloride, or iodide, can induce mast cell secretion. These findings suggest that the EPO + H_2O_2 + halide system may play a role in the inflammatory response and in hypersensitivity reactions. This possibility is strengthened by reports showing leakage of EPO from granules into cytoplasm and apparent extracellular release following allergen provocation of human nasal mucous membranes. EPO binds to microbes such as *Staphylococcus aureus, Toxoplasma gondii,* and *T. cruzi* and markedly potentiates their killing by mononuclear phagocytes. Tumor cells also adsorb EPO, and this potentiates their lysis by H_2O_2 and by macrophages. These results point to a synergistic action in tumor cell destruction between the cytophilic cationic EPO and H_2O_2.

Eosinophil Cationic Proteins (ECP). Analyses of cationic proteins of human leukemic myeloid cells found seven cationic components. Components 5, 6, and 7 are from eosinophils, and they are termed eosinophil cationic proteins (ECP). ECPs are rich in arginine, and their isoelectric points are greater than pH 11. ECP differs from MBP in several respects, including its amino acid composition and its antigenicity.

ECP binds to heparin and neutralizes its anticoagulant activity. ECP also enhances hydrolysis of a plasmin-specific substrate by plasmin in a dose-related fashion. ECP produces the Gordon phenomenon (see below) at very low concentrations (0.1–0.3 micrograms), amounts about 10- to 100-fold less than those needed for the eosinophil-derived neurotoxin (see below). ECP is also a potent toxin for schistosomula of *S. mansoni* and, on a molar basis, is 8 to 10 times more potent than MBP.

Eosinophil-Derived Neurotoxin (EDN). Eosinophils contain a powerful neurotoxin that can severely damage myelinated neurons in experimental animals, causing symptoms of stiffness, progressive ataxia, weakness, and incoordination. M. H. Gordon first described this neurotoxic reaction in 1932; it is now known as the "Gordon phenomenon." Because patients with the hypereosinophilic syndrome or with cerebrospinal fluid eosinophilia exhibit varied neurologic abnormalities, EDN may play an important role in central nervous system disease in humans. The only function presently associated with EDN is its ability to provoke the Gordon phenomenon. Using the production of the Gordon phenomenon as an assay, EDN was purified from extracts of whole human eosinophils and eosinophil granules. Additional granule-derived proteins, ECP and eosinophil protein X (EPX), also produced the Gordon phenomenon. EPX may be identical to EDN, which raises the possibility that ECP accounts for the only neurotoxic activity, the activity reported for EPX and for EDN being due to contamination with ECP. CLC protein (lysophospholipase) and MBP do not produce the Gordon phenomenon. Clearly, further studies are needed to determine whether there is more than one granule molecule with neurotoxic activity.

Eosinophil-Associated Enzymes (see Weller et al., 1980). Enzymes associated with the eosinophil include: acid glycerophosphatase, adenosine triphosphatase, alpha-mannosidase, arylsulfatase, collagenase, beta-glucuronidase, ribonuclease, cathepsin, acid and alkaline phosphatase, histaminase, and phospholipase D. The subunit composition of the arylsulfatase from eosinophils has been determined. Collagenase activity for collagen Types I and III has also been associated with eosinophils.

Eosinophil Function in Helminth Infection

Evidence for Eosinophil Participation in Helminth Killing

The evidence for a role played by the eosinophil in parasite damage includes (1) reduction of immunity to helminths by antieosinophil serum (AES), (2) direct killing of helminths by eosinophils, and (3) demonstration of eosinophil degranulation and infiltration around the parasite.

1. The effect of AES has been tested on hosts infected with three helminths: *S. mansoni, T. spiralis, Trichostrongylus columbriformis,* and a tick, *Amblyomma americanum.* The ablation of eosinophils by AES caused a clear-cut reduction in immunity to the helminth. The immunity of guinea pigs infected with the tick *A. americanum* was completely abolished by antibasophil serum (ABS) and significantly reduced by AES. AES treatment reduced only the number of eosinophils in tissues from tick-

feeding sites, whereas ABS treatment reduced both basophils and eosinophils. These results point not only to a role for the basophil in tick immunity but also to its cooperation with the eosinophil in that immunity. Presumably basophils attract eosinophils to the tissue sites, and both participate in the attack on the tick.

2. Eosinophils attack schistosomula coated with IgG antibody, and their attack on the parasite is associated with degranulation and release of MBP. There is a synergy between eosinophils and mast cell–derived mediators in the damage to the schistosomula. In rats, C3 bound to schistosomula mediates eosinophil adherence, and classical pathway activation of the complement cascade enhances antibody-dependent eosinophil-mediated killing.

3. Eosinophils accumulate and degranulate around parasites in vivo. Microfilariae of *Onchocerca volvulus* and eosinophils are found in the skin of humans with onchocerciasis. Treatment with diethylcarbamazine exacerbates chronic onchocercal dermatitis, resulting in intense pruritus, edema, erythema, and urticaria (Mazzotti reaction). Immunofluorescent staining for MBP in skin biopsy specimens from patients with the Mazzotti reaction shows marked extracellular MBP deposition around degenerating microfilariae. Thus, a toxic granule protein is present on damaged helminths in vivo.

Mechanisms of Eosinophil Damage to Parasites

The eosinophil granule is a rich source of toxic cationic proteins, and three of these, MBP, ECP, and EPO, damage helminths directly. MBP and EPO are released during the assault on the schistosomulum's membrane. EPO may kill schistosomula directly or together with H_2O_2 + halide. Eosinophils generate H_2O_2 on stimulation by a parasite, and therefore H_2O_2 should be available for reaction with EPO and halide.

Enhancement of Eosinophil Damage to Parasites

The numerous factors that increase the eosinophil's capacity to damage parasites include the T-cell–derived eosinophil stimulation promoter ECF-A, eosinophil colony stimulating factor, and factors derived from monocytes. ECF-A, a product of mast cells, increases the number of complement receptors on eosinophils, which then show an enhanced ability to kill schistosomula. Partially purified eosinophil colony stimulating factor both enhances eosinophil cytotoxicity to parasites and promotes eosinophil colony growth. Factors derived from monocytes also enhance eosinophil killing of schistosomula, but the mechanism of their action is unknown.

Hypersensitivity Reactions

The above results indicate that the eosinophil destroys multicellular parasites. These findings are in keeping with an inimical role for the eosinophil in hypersensitivity reactions. The eosinophil, however, also possesses enzymes able to degrade mediators of anaphylaxis and had been regarded as a modulator cell for control of immediate hypersensitivity reactions. This view must now be modified to include a role for the eosinophil as an effector of injury in hypersensitivity reactions.

Eosinophil Modulation of Immediate Hypersensitivity Reactions

Eosinophils are attracted to sites of IgE-mediated reactions, and they possess certain enzymes that neutralize mediators of anaphylaxis. Therefore, it was suggested that one function of the eosinophil was containment of the inflammation following immediate-type hypersensitivity reactions. Stimulation of human eosinophils by allergens or anti-IgE was also found to liberate prostaglandins E_1 and E_2, which inhibit leukocyte histamine release. MBP binds heparin, neutralizing its anticoagulant activity. EPO + H_2O_2 + halide degrades leukotrienes, which are important mediators of hypersensitivity and chemotaxis.

Experiments do not support the hypothesis that the eosinophil down-regulates immediate hypersensitivity reactions. For example, leukotrienes (LT) C4, D4, and E4 are now recognized as accounting for the activity of the slow-reacting substance of anaphylaxis. LT-C4 is an acidic lipid substituted at the 6-position with the tripeptide glutathione through a thio-ether linkage. The absence of a sulfate ester suggests that LT-C4 is not susceptible to the hydrolytic action of arylsulfatase. Also, purified eosinophil arylsulfatase does not inactivate contraction of the guinea pig ileum by synthetic LT-C4 and LT-D4. Furthermore, there is evidence to suggest that eosinophil phospholipase D degrades a factor having platelet lytic activity but not the platelet activating factor. Lastly, a test of the hypothesis that eosinophils inactivate mediators was conducted using methylprednisolone and to abolish eosinophils from passively sensitized guinea pigs. Administration of neither AES nor methylprednisolone altered passive or systemic anaphylactic reactions, and there was a decreased release of histamine from the passively sensitized peritoneal cavity of the guinea pig. This test study concluded that the presence of eosinophils might actually contribute to histamine release.

Effector Function in Hypersensitivity Reactions

Asthma

In Vitro Studies. Because certain hypersensitivity diseases are associated with eosinophilia and because there is a positive association between eosinophilia and lung dysfunction in bronchial asthma, the possibility that the eosinophil mediates damage to the bronchi was tested.

Studies of respiratory epithelium in vitro showed that MBP produced exfoliation of epithelial cells and impairment of ciliary beating. The exfoliated cells were disrupted and their cell contents were liberated. These MBP effects on bronchial epithelium were similar to the pathologic changes in human bronchial asthma. In bronchial asthma, excessive shedding of cells and desquamation of the bronchial epithelium are reported as constant findings. The superficial columnar cells undergo detachment, leaving behind them a layer of basal cells from which regeneration of the mucosa takes place.

Clinical Studies. The in vitro studies suggested that eosinophils, a hallmark of bronchial asthma, damage human bronchial epithelium in asthma. If so, MBP should be present in the sputum of patients with asthma in concentrations approximating those in the toxic range. Therefore, MBP was measured in the sputa of 100 patients with various respiratory diseases. The sputa of 13 patients contained elevated MBP levels, and 11 of these 13 had asthma. The sputa of 15 additional patients hospitalized for asthma showed that all had elevated MBP levels; the peak level was approximately tenfold greater than the lowest concentration causing damage in vitro. These results indicate that elevated sputum MBP is a marker for bronchial asthma, and that high concentrations of MBP are present in the sputa of some patients with asthma.

If eosinophils damage bronchial tissues, MBP might be localized at the damaged site. Therefore, lung tissues from autopsies of patients who died of asthma were examined for MBP by immunofluorescence. Examination of sections stained with hematoxylin and eosin (H&E) showed that those from patients with severe asthma stained positively for MBP that was inside the eosinophil (cellular staining) as well as outside the eosinophil (extracellular staining). Striking epithelial damage and extracellular staining by MBP were observed in patients who died of asthma, while patients with asthma but dying of other causes showed lesser changes. Patients with a history of asthma, but whose deaths were not due to asthma, showed no damage or extracellular MBP. One pattern of MBP immunofluorescence (Fig. 14–3) was diffuse staining of mucous plugs with brilliant

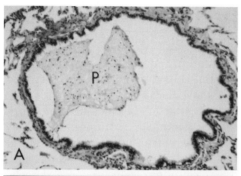

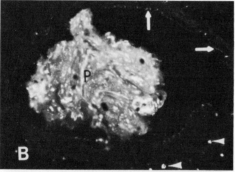

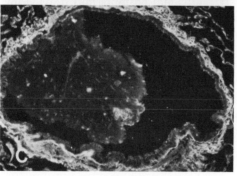

Figure 14–3. Serial sections of a bronchiole with mucous plug (P). Sections stained with (A) H & E, (B) anti-MBP serum, and (C) normal rabbit serum. Note diffuse fluorescence of the plug (P) and patchy staining of the luminal surface of the respiratory epithelium (arrows). There are also discrete eosinophils in the peribronchiolar area (arrowheads) (×100). (Used with permission from Filley, W. V., et al.: Identification by immunofluorescence of eosinophil granule major basic protein in lung tissues of patients with bronchial asthma. Lancet 2:13, 1982.)

streaks and whirls, and patchy staining of the epithelial surface of the bronchiole. Other patterns included (1) diffuse extracellular MBP immunofluorescence in the lamina propria, corresponding to the presence of necrotic, amorphous, eosinophilic material on the H&E stained section, and (2) intense extracellular MBP staining of damaged epithelium associated with eosinophil infiltration in the lamina propria and frank destruction of the basement membrane zone.

Leukotrienes, Mast Cells, and Basophils. These observations indicate that eosinophils degranulate in tissues and that MBP, a toxic granule constituent, is present at sites of tissue damage in asthma. Other studies found that both human and horse eosinophils produce leukotrienes, including both LT-C4 and D4. Purified normal human neutrophils produce 7.5 ± 4 ng of LT-$C4/10^6$ cells, whereas eosinophils produce 38 ± 3 ng/10^6 cells. These results indicate that local eosinophils might, in the asthmatic, secrete these potent smooth muscle contractants around bronchial smooth muscle, thus inducing bronchospasm. Eosinophils may also induce inflammation by stimulating mast cells via the $EPO + H_2O_2 +$ halide system. Furthermore, MBP activates purified human basophils and rat mast cells to release histamine in an energy-, temperature-, and calcium-dependent manner, and it stimulates wheal-and-flare skin reactions in a dose-related manner. Thus, eosinophils possess the ability to cause inflammation, bronchospasm, and tissue damage in bronchial asthma through a variety of mechanisms (summarized in Fig. 14–4).

Skin Disorders

Inflammatory Skin Diseases. The eosinophil may also participate in inflammatory skin diseases. Peripheral blood eosinophilia is, in general, associated with increased levels of serum MBP. In chronic urticaria serum MBP was elevated in 38 percent of patients, even in the absence of peripheral blood eosinophilia. Immunofluorescence localization of MBP in skin from patients with chronic urticaria showed that extracellular MBP was present in 12 of 28 biopsies (43 percent); in contrast, skin from patients with a variety of other skin diseases did not show extracellular MBP. Because eosinophils can stimulate mediator release from mast cells, it is possible that they act upon the mast cell in certain cases of chronic urticaria. ECP was also found outside eosinophils in chronic urticaria.

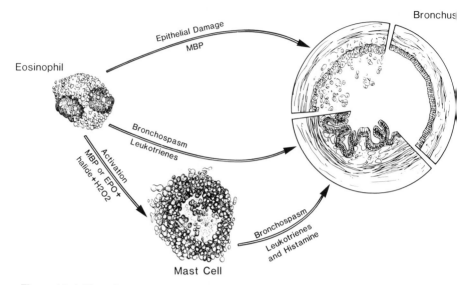

Figure 14–4. The role of eosinophils in airway obstruction in bronchial asthma. The effects on the bronchus are shown by comparing a section of normal bronchus (upper right) with a section damaged by MBP (upper left) that shows epithelial desquamation and with a section (bottom) that shows smooth muscle hypertrophy, constriction, and edema of the lamina propria, resulting in a reduction in the caliber of the airway (MBP, eosinophil granule major basic protein; EPO, eosinophil peroxidase; H_2O_2, hydrogen peroxide). (Used with permission from Gleich, G. J., et al.: Eosinophils and bronchial inflammation. *In* Kay, A. B., Austen, K. F., and Lichtenstein, L. M. (eds.): Asthma: Physiology, Immunopharmacology and Treatment. New York, Academic Press, 1984, p. 204.)

Episodic Angioedema with Eosinophilia. Another syndrome in which eosinophils may play a pathogenetic role is episodic angioedema associated with eosinophilia. Four patients with this syndrome presented with recurrent attacks of angioedema, urticaria, fever, and weight gain of up to 18 percent. During attacks, leukocyte counts were as high as $108,000/mm^3$, with up to 88 percent eosinophils. The disease waxed and waned in concert with the number of eosinophils in the peripheral blood. By electron microscopy, dermal eosinophils showed a spectrum of abnormalities, including frank destruction and loss of their contents into the dermis. Immunofluorescence showed extracellular MBP around blood vessels and collagen bundles. Mast cells showed evidence of degranulation by electron microscopy. These observations suggest that activated eosinophils localize in the skin, release their granule constituents, and cause mast cell degranulation with resultant edema.

Cardiac Disease

Peripheral blood eosinophilia is associated with the development of cardiac disease, especially in the hypereosinophilic syndrome. Because ECP damages myocardial cells in vitro, eosinophil degranulation onto myocardium could be important in the pathogenesis of the disease. Immunofluorescent localization of MBP in cardiac tissue from patients with the hypereosinophilic syndrome shows diffuse extracellular staining of subendomyocardium and of the basement membrane. In contrast, during the fibrotic stage of the disease, no extracellular MBP was present, and eosinophils themselves were scanty.

Activated eosinophils have been demonstrated in granulomas and necrotic lesions from patients with allergic granulomatosis (the Churg-Strauss syndrome), in keeping with the concept that the eosinophil may be an important effector cell in this disease.

DISEASES ASSOCIATED WITH EOSINOPHILIA

Eosinophils are produced in the bone marrow and travel to various tissues through the circulation. A high proportion of eosinophils is in the bone marrow, and a much smaller proportion is in the peripheral blood (Table 14–1). Of interest are the large

Table 14–1. Distribution of Eosinophils in the Organs of the Rat*

Organs	Mean per 100 g Body Weight
Bone Marrow	430,000,000
Skin (Dermis)	93,000,000
Gastrointestinal Tract	52,000,000
Stomach	2,000,000
Ileum	37,000,000
Colon	12,000,000
Lungs	14,000,000
Uterus	
Diestrus	70,000
Estrus	3,500,000
Blood	1,400,000
Spleen	470,000
Liver	470,000

*The total number of eosinophils in an adult rat is between 1,500,000,000 and 1,800,000,000. The ratio of eosinophils between the bone marrow and the blood is about 300:1 and between the tissue and the blood is about 200–300:1.

Table reprinted with permission from Rytomaa T: Organ distribution and histochemical properties of eosinophil granulocytes in rat. Acta Path et Microbiol Scand Suppl 140 (Vol. 50):73–76, 1960.

numbers of eosinophils in the skin, gastrointestinal tract, and lungs; these associations are valuable to keep in mind, because diseases of these organs are also associated with eosinophilia.

In the past, association of a given disease and the eosinophil has been made on the basis of an elevation of the number of eosinophils in the peripheral blood or in tissues from the diseased organ. Using granule proteins as probes, tissue deposition of MBP in the absence of eosinophilia has been found. For example, the granule MBP is elevated in the serum of about 40 percent of patients with chronic urticaria, even though peripheral blood eosinophils are not elevated. Similarly, immunofluorescence of granule proteins in analyses of skin from patients with chronic urticaria, atopic dermatitis, and episodic angioedema has shown marked deposition of the granule MBP in the virtual absence of eosinophils. These findings suggest that eosinophils, at least in certain situations, lose their morphologic integrity after tissue infiltration. Presumably eosinophils are activated by various factors that then cause degranulation. Finally, the released eosinophil granule proteins, such as MBP and ECP, may be toxic to cells and may stimulate mediator release from mast cells and basophils.

Helminth Infections

A number of diseases have been associated with peripheral blood eosinophilia (see Beeson and Bass, 1977; Cohen and Ottesen, 1984). Probably the most common association, when considered from a global viewpoint, is between eosinophilia and helminth infection. There are hundreds of millions of patients with helminthiasis, including schistosomiasis and filariasis. These helminths have a tissue invasive stage; intestinal parasites without a tissue invasive stage are associated with slight eosinophilia.

Allergic Diseases

Allergic diseases, especially allergic bronchial asthma, may be accompanied by peripheral blood eosinophilia. When asthma is associated with marked eosinophilia, such complications as allergic bronchopulmonary aspergillosis (ABPA), eosinophilic pneumonitis, and the Churg-Strauss syndrome should be kept in mind. Ordinarily, allergic rhinitis is not associated with marked eosinophilia, although there may be an increased number of eosinophils following the peak of the pollination season. Drug allergy may be accompanied by striking eosinophilia.

Skin Diseases

Skin diseases, especially bullous pemphigoid and atopic dermatitis, may be associated with eosinophilia. Eosinophilic cellulitis (Wells' syndrome) is associated with peripheral blood eosinophilia, tissue eosinophilia, and deposition of the granule MBP in the pathognomonic "flame figures" (brightly eosinophilic areas usually surrounded by eosinophils early in formation and later by mononuclear cells).

Lung Diseases

Lung diseases often coincide with peripheral blood eosinophilia. The syndromes of pulmonary infiltration with tissue eosinophilia, including Loeffler's syndrome, lung infiltration associated with allergic bronchopulmonary aspergillosis, tropical pulmonary eosinophilia with filarial infection, eosinophilic pneumonitis, and bronchiocentric granulomatosis, may be associated with striking blood eosinophilia.

GI Diseases

Gastrointestinal diseases, especially allergic gastroenteropathy and eosinophilic gastroenteritis, may be accompanied by marked eosinophilia. Allergic gastroenteropathy occurs in patients with atopic diseases, such as asthma and allergic rhinitis, and is often associated with dramatic increases in serum IgE levels and with allergic reactions to foods.

Neoplastic Diseases

Neoplastic disease, especially lymphomas and Hodgkin's disease, may be associated with marked eosinophilia, but this is not common. Nonetheless, one should bear these possibilities in mind when investigating patients with marked eosinophilia.

Hypereosinophilic Syndrome

Finally, the hypereosinophilic syndrome is seen in patients with a spectrum of diseases ranging from pulmonary infiltration with eosinophilia to Loeffler's endomyocarditis, eosinophilic leukemia, and eosinophilic collagen vascular disease. Diagnostic criteria for the hypereosinophilic syndrome include (1) persistent eosinophilia of 1500 cells/mm^3 for 6 months or longer, (2) lack of evidence of other known causes of eosinophilia, and (3) signs and symptoms of organ involvement. The heart is the organ most commonly affected in this disease. The prognosis of the hypereosinophilic syndrome is grave, even after optimal therapy; in one series there was a 30 percent mortality during 7 years of follow-up.

Table 14–2. Syndromes Associated with Eosinophilia*

Gastro*i*ntestinal diseases† (I)
Arteritis (A)
Malignancy (M)
Skin diseases (S)
Allergy (A)
Drug reaction (D)
Heart diseases (H)
Hypereosinophilic syndrome (E)
Lung diseases (L)
Parasites (P)

*These letters form a useful mnemonic: I AM SAD, HELP.
†The *i* in gastrointestinal and *e* in hypereosinophilic syndrome are used in the mnemonic and are italicized for emphasis.

Episodic Angioedema Associated with Eosinophilia

Another group of patients with marked eosinophilia are those with episodic angioedema (see above). At the peak of an attack of angioedema one patient had a total leukocyte count of 108,000 cells/mm³ and 88 percent eosinophils. Although these patients satisfy the criteria of the hypereosinophilic syndrome, we believe their condition constitutes a separate entity. In contrast to patients with the hypereosinophilic syndrome, the patients with episodic angioedema have a good prognosis, have not developed cardiac disease, and have a distinctive clinical syndrome.

Table 14–2 summarizes certain of the syndromes associated with eosinophilia and proposes a mnemonic for ease in remembering them.

Bibliography

Beeson, P. B., and Bass, D. A.: The eosinophil. *In* Smith, L. H., Jr.: Major Problems in Internal Medicine. Philadelphia, W.B. Saunders Co., 1977, pp. 1–269.

Butterfield, J. H., Maddox, D. E., and Gleich, G. J.: The eosinophil leukocyte: maturation and function. Clin. Immunol. Rev. 2:187, 1984.

Cohen, S. G., and Ottesen, E. A.: The eosinophil, eosinophilia and eosinophil-related disorders. *In* Middleton, E., Jr., Reed, C. E., and Ellis, E. F. (eds.): Allergy: Principles and Practice, Vol. 2. St. Louis, C. V. Mosby Co., 1984, pp. 701–769.

Gleich, G. J., and Loegering, D. A.: Immunobiology of eosinophils. Ann. Rev. Immunol. 2:429, 1984.

Gleich, G. J., Schroeter, A. L., Marcoux, J. P., et al.: Episodic angioedema associated with eosinophilia. N. Engl. J. Med. 310:1621, 1984.

Weller, P. F., Wasserman, S. I., and Austen, K. F.: Selected enzymes preferentially present in the eosinophil. *In* Mahmoud, A. A. F., and Austen, K. F.: The Eosinophil in Health and Disease. New York, Grune & Stratton, 1980, pp. 1–364.

Yoshida, T., and Torisu, M.: Immunobiology of the Eosinophil. New York, Elsevier Biomedical, 1983, pp. 1–399.

15

Hypersensitivity in Infectious Diseases

MICHAEL H. GRIECO, M.D.

Introduction	**Viral Infections**
Streptococcus Pyogenes	Urticaria and Vasculitis
Acute Rheumatic Fever (ARF)	Heart Disease, Myocarditis,
Poststreptococcal Acute Glo-	and Valvulitis
merulonephritis (AGN)	Renal Disease
Other Sequelae	**Fungal Infections**
Mycobacterial Infections	**Parasitic Infections**

INTRODUCTION

Immune responses to infectious agents usually protect the host, but in some instances they may induce hypersensitivity diseases. This chapter reviews examples of immune hypersensitivity to bacterial, viral, fungal, and parasitic infectious agents (Table 15–1).

STREPTOCOCCUS PYOGENES

Group A streptococci are important human bacterial pathogens. This bacterium is the most frequent cause of pharyngitis

Table 15–1. Examples of Probable or Possible
Hypersensitivity Reactions to Infectious Organisms

Organism/Infection	Manifestation	Type of Immunologic Mechanism Implicated*
A. *Streptococcus pyogenes*	Acute rheumatic fever	II, IV
	Acute glomerulonephritis	II, III
	Acute urticaria	I, III
	Erythema multiforme	I, III
	Venulitis	III
	Arteritis	III
	Erythema nodosum	III
B. *Mycobacterium tuberculosis*	Tuberculin test	IV
C. Viral Infections	Urticaria, vasculitis	I, III
	Myocarditis, valvulitis	IV
	Renal disease	III, IV
D. Fungal Infections	Acute histoplasmosis	III
	Acute coccidioidomycosis	III
E. Parasitic Infections	Urticaria, anaphylaxis	I

*Gell and Coombs (G.C.) classification.

and may cause erysipelas and pyoderma. However, it may also induce such nonsuppurative sequelae as acute rheumatic fever and poststreptococcal acute glomerulonephritis.

The somatic constituents of these coccal organisms include the capsule (hyaluronic acid); cell wall (proteins M, T, and R; group-specific carbohydrates N-acetyl-glucosamine and rhamnose; and peptidoglycan-mucopeptides N-acetyl-glucosamine and N-acetyl-muramic acid); and cytoplasmic membrane (phospholipids and proteins). The hyaluronic acid capsule retards phagocytosis by host neutrophils and macrophages. The group-specific carbohydrate in the cell walls of group A strains is a dimer of N-acetyl-glucosamine and rhamnose, and the mucopeptide layer of the cell wall is composed of polymers of N-acetyl-glucosamine and N-acetyl-muramic acid connected by amino acid side chains.

M-protein in the cell wall is the major virulence antigen affecting resistance to phagocytosis. There are more than 60 serotypes of Group A streptococci, based on antigenic differences in M-protein molecules. Immune protection is type specific and dependent on development of opsonizing antibodies.

Acute Rheumatic Fever (ARF)

ARF is a nonsuppurative complication of Group A streptococcal pharyngitis. Cutaneous streptococcal infections do not cause cardiac sequelae. Either the pharyngeal site is essential to initiate this reaction, or pyodermal strains lack rheumatogenicity.

The exact mechanism by which this organism induces the disease is unclear, but a Type II hypersensitivity autoimmune mechanism is suspected (Fig. 15–1). Direct immunofluorescence studies reveal that rabbit antibodies against Group A streptococci bind to sarcolemma and subsarcolemmal sarcoplasm in myofibers of human heart and to smooth muscle of vessel walls. Antigens, cross-reactive with human heart myofibers, have been localized to the cell wall and cell membrane of Group A streptococci. Cross-reactions have also been described between protein in the hyaluronate capsule and human synovial tissue. These cross-reacting antigens may explain autoimmunity due to exogenous Group A streptococcus, but direct evidence to confirm these mechanisms is lacking. Delayed hypersensitivity (Type IV) to streptococcal antigens is being examined. HLA-A5 has a high statistical association with lymphoproliferative responses to streptococcal extracellular products, suggesting selective genetic control.

The revised Jones criteria are useful to diagnose ARF. The presence of two major criteria or of one major and two minor criteria indicates a high probability of rheumatic fever, if supported by evidence of a preceding streptococcal infection. This includes a history of documented streptococcal pharyngitis or scarlet fever, a positive throat culture, or demonstration of elevated serum titer of antistreptococcal antibodies. A battery of three streptococcal antibody tests (antistreptolysin-O [ASO], anti-DNAse B, antihyaluronidase) would yield 95 percent positive reactions with serum obtained after onset. Failure to demonstrate recent streptococcal infection makes the diagnosis of ARF doubtful, except in the case of chorea.

Poststreptococcal Acute Glomerulonephritis (AGN)

AGN usually results from pharyngeal and/or cutaneous infections with Group A organisms. An exception has been described in Romania, where nephritis has been encountered complicating Group C streptococcal pharyngitis. In contrast to ARF, the serotypes involved are limited. Type M-12 serotype is most frequent following pharyngitis, and M-49 is most commonly associated with pyoderma-associated nephritis. There are no reliable biologic markers to distinguish nephritogenic from nonnephritogenic strains, even within specific serotypes.

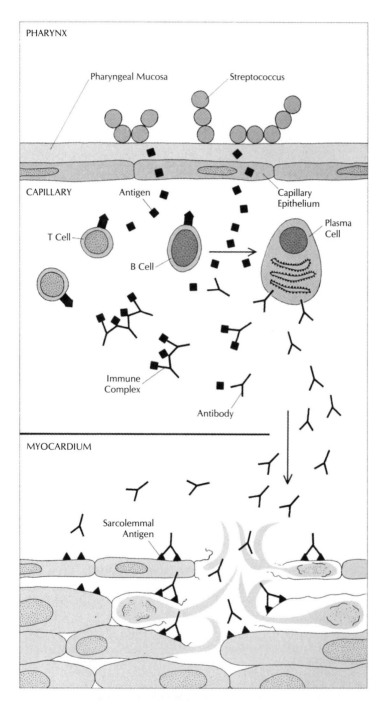

Figure 15–1. *See legend on opposite page*

Antibody-mediated immunity is probably involved, and both Type II and Type III mechanisms have been implicated. Cross-antigenicity of streptococcal cell membrane and glomerular antigen has been described, which may indicate that these are exogenously induced autoimmune antibodies. Subepithelial nodular deposits favor immune complex deposition, and circulating immune complexes are detectable early in the illness. There are antigenic determinants present in glomeruli that are identical to constituents in the streptococcal plasma membrane.

As with ARF, the diagnosis of AGN depends on confirmatory evidence of antecedent streptococcal infection. Usually streptococcal antibodies are elevated in serum. ASO responses are frequently poor, and it may be necessary to perform assays for anti-DNAse B, antihyaluronidase, or antistreptozyme.

Other Sequelae

Thus, Type II and Type IV hypersensitivity states in ARF, and Types II and III in AGN, have been linked to Group A streptococcal antigens. Group A infections have also been associated with acute urticaria, erythema multiforme, allergic venulitis and arteritis, and erythema nodosum, but the pathogenesis of these diseases remains unknown.

MYCOBACTERIAL INFECTIONS

Cell-mediated immune responses to microbial agents usually protect the host. However, this response may contribute to the clinical manifestations of disease by augmenting inflammation and cytotoxicity. Type IV hypersensitivity includes both delayed-type cell-mediated reactions and direct T-cell cytotoxicity. The tuberculin skin test is an example of the former mechanism in which T-helper lymphocytes recognize intracutaneous tuberculoprotein. They react to the tuberculin antigen and release lymphokines that activate and recruit inflammatory cells, particularly macrophages, which make up the majority of the cells recruited to the tuberculin test site.

Figure 15–1. In generalized scheme for immunopathogenesis of rheumatic fever and rheumatic carditis, one starts with colonization of pharynx by group A streptococci. A systemic immune response ensues, with sensitization of B lymphocytes (and possibly also of T cells) by streptococcal antigens, elaboration of antistreptococcal antibody, formation of immune complexes and cross-reaction with cardiac sarcolemmal antigens, and myocardial inflammatory response involving valvular and perivalvular structures. (Reprinted, with permission, from Williams, R. C., Jr.: Host factors in rheumatic fever and heart disease. Hosp. Pract. 16(8):127, 1982. Drawing by Alan D. Iselin.)

A positive Mantoux skin test using 5 tuberculin units of polysorbate-80–stabilized purified protein derivative (PPD) identifies past or present infection with *Mycobacterium tuberculosis* but does not necessarily signify clinical disease. Most infected persons will respond to a 5-TU PPD test with ≥10 mm of induration in 48 to 72 hours. False-positive reactions result from sensitization to nontuberculous *Mycobacteria*, while false-negative responses reflect immunologic nonresponsiveness or anergy.

Type IV hypersensitivity is of major importance in host protective mechanisms against a wide variety of intracellular infecting organisms, including *Salmonella*, *Listeria*, *Nocardia*, *Histoplasma*, *Cryptococcus*, *Candida*, herpesviruses, *Pneumocystis*, and *Toxoplasma*.

VIRAL INFECTIONS

Urticaria and Vasculitis

The several viral infections that have been associated with exanthems include measles, rubella, varicella zoster, enteroviruses such as ECHO Types 16 and 9, Coxsackie Group A, Types 16 and 9, and Coxsackie Group B, Type 5. Urticarial pruritic lesions are associated with Coxsackie Group A, Type 16 infections, but the mechanism has not been studied. Immune complex or Type III hypersensitivity has been implicated in hepatitis B infections and is associated with maculopapular and urticarial eruptions, palpable purpura, polyarteritis nodosa, glomerulonephritis, and cryoglobulinemia. Gianotti-Crosti syndrome, or papular acrodermatitis, is an infectious disease that primarily affects children. A cell-mediated immune response to hepatitis B surface antigen may be responsible for this nonrelapsing erythematopapular dermatitis of the face and limbs.

Heart Disease, Myocarditis, and Valvulitis

Coxsackie B viruses are the most commonly identified causative agents of viral heart disease in man. Viral replication in the heart results in necrosis of myofibers and accumulation of mononuclear inflammatory cells in the pericardium, myocardium, and endocardium. Chronic experiments in cynomolgus monkeys have established long-term effects of Coxsackie B4 disease. Since replicating virus is not detected in the heart beyond the first week of infection, it has been suggested that immunologic reactions implicating T lymphocytes play a role in cardiac damage. Coxsackie viral antigen has been detected in 31 percent of routine autopsies at the Charity Hospital in New

Orleans. Viral agents and concomitant immunologic responses are also being investigated for their possible relationship to arteriosclerosis.

Renal Disease

Coxsackie B antigen was found in renal tissue in 11 percent of 104 patients routinely autopsied at Charity Hospital in New Orleans. Glomerulonephritis and/or pyelonephritis has been associated with the following viruses: Coxsackie Group B, coronavirus (Balkan nephropathy), hemorrhagic fever viruses, influenza, mumps, rubella, cytomegalovirus (especially following allogeneic transplantation), and varicella. In some instances the histologic picture is identical to that described for poststreptococcal disease.

Type III and Type IV hypersensitivity mechanisms may play important roles in the pathogenesis of acute and chronic cardiac and renal diseases.

FUNGAL INFECTIONS

Cell-mediated immune responses are believed to play important protective roles in defense against several geographic and opportunistic fungal infections. The best example of a likely hypersensitivity manifestation is in acute histoplasmosis. About 90 percent of cases described in epidemics are probably primary infections. The symptoms are influenza-like except that myalgia is less prominent. In some epidemics, erythema nodosum and erythema multiforme have been described, more frequently in young women. It is estimated that the overall incidence of these cutaneous manifestations of hypersensitivity is 1 in 200 cases, but they have been observed more frequently in certain outbreaks. Acute polyarthritis has been noted on occasion.

Primary infection with *Coccidioides immitis* is associated with a rash in 50 percent of the cases. The rash appears at the onset of disease and is often generalized, pruritic, maculopapular, and sometimes exfoliating without weeping. Some lesions are urticarial. Erythema nodosum, 2 to 10 times more common in women, or an erythema multiforme involving the upper trunk and extremities, may occur. These patients are sometimes incorrectly diagnosed as having contact dermatitis.

PARASITIC INFECTIONS

A number of host defenses provide variable resistance against parasites. From the biologic point of view, invading parasites must not eliminate the susceptible host population. Effector mechanisms include T lymphocytes, antibodies, and nonspecific cytotoxic and serum factors.

Type I hypersensitivity is important in the pathogenesis of urticaria, angioedema, and even anaphylaxis with some protozoal, nematode, and trematode infections. Characteristically these infections are associated with invasive stages in which there are elevated levels of both total IgE and specific IgE antibodies. The hypersensitivity is detectable with protozoa such as *Amoeba* and *Giardia* and with invasive nematodes such as *Ascaris*, hookworm, *Strongyloides*, human filariasis, animal filariasis (tropical pulmonary eosinophilia from *Brugia* sensitivity), *Capillaria philippinensis*, visceral larva migrans, cutaneous larva migrans, *Trichinella spiralis*, and echinococcosis.

High IgE levels are present in most patients with hydatid disease. The majority of infections with *Echinococcus granulosus* are asymptomatic. Patients with symptomatic infections usually present with the features of space-occupying lesion. The most important complications of hydatid cysts are rupture or infection. A leaking cyst may give rise to urticaria or precipitate an anaphylactic reaction. On occasion surgical rupture and spillage of an *Echinococcus* cyst is associated with fatal anaphylaxis.

Bibliography

Daniel, T. M.: The immunology of tuberculosis. Clin. Chest Med. 1:189, 1980.

Gocke, D. J.: Extrahepatic manifestations of viral hepatitis. Am. J. Med. Sci. 270:49, 1975.

Goodwin, R. A., Jr., and Des Prez, R. M.: Histoplasmosis. Am. Rev. Resp. Dis. 117:929, 1978.

Greenberg, L. J., Gray, E. D., and Yunis, E.: Association of HLA-A5 and immune responsiveness in vitro to streptococcal antigens. J. Exp. Med. 141:934, 1975.

Kaplan, M. H., and Meyeserian, M.: An immunological cross-reaction between group A streptococcal cells and human heart tissue. Lancet 1:706, 1962.

Lange, C. F.: Chemistry of cross reactive fragments of streptococcal cell membrane and human glomerular basement membrane. Transplant Proc. 1:959, 1969.

Lawley, T. J., Bielory, G. P., Yancey, K. B., et al.: A prospective clinical and immunologic analysis of patients with serum sickness. N. Engl. J. Med. 311:1407, 1984.

Lerner, A. M., Klein, J. O., Cherry, J. D., et al.: New viral exanthems. N. Engl. J. Med. 269:678, 1963.

Popp, J. W., Jr., Harrist, T. J., Dienstag, J. L., et al.: Cutaneous vasculitis associated with acute and chronic hepatitis. Arch. Intern. Med. 141:623, 1981.

Schiller, C. F.: Complications of *Echinococcus* cyst rupture. JAMA 195:158, 1966.

Shusterman, N., and London, W. T.: Hepatitis B and immune-complex disease. N. Engl. J. Med. 310:43, 1984.

Woodruff, J. F., and Woodruff, J. J.: Involvement of T lymphocytes in the pathogenesis of Coxsackie virus B3 heart disease. J. Immunol. 113:1776, 1974.

Zabriskie, J. B., and Freimer, E. H.: An immunological relationship between group A streptococcus and mammalian muscle. J. Exp. Med. 124:661, 1966.

16

Active and Passive Immunization

RAMA GANGULY, M.D.,
and ROBERT H. WALDMAN, M.D.

Introduction	Comments About Certain
Passive Immunization	Vaccines
Active Immunization	Hazards of Immunization
The Decision to Immunize	Conclusions

INTRODUCTION

It has long been recognized that most individuals become immune, often permanently, to an infectious disease after having had the disease. From this observation, methods were developed to induce this immune state without causing illness. This prevention of infectious diseases by immunization is one of the outstanding achievements of medical science (Fig. 16–1).

Immunization procedures can be divided into two forms, passive and active. Each, in turn, can be thought of as mediated by either humoral or cell-mediated mechanisms. Active immunization usually stimulates both parts of the immune system, whereas passive subcutaneous or intravenous administration of

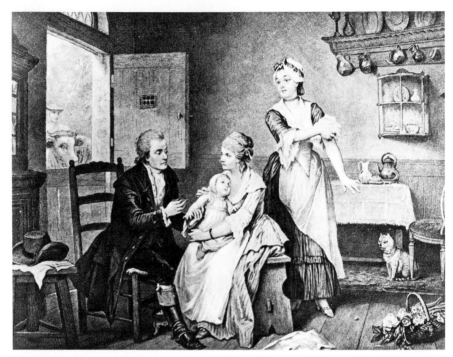

Figure 16–1. Scene of Jenner administering live smallpox vaccine to a child. (Photograph of engraving by C. Manigaud after E. Hamman. Reprinted courtesy of the Fisher Collection of Alchemical and Historical Pictures, Pittsburgh, PA.)

antibody, transfer factor, or lymphocytes obtained from another human or from an animal results in passive immunity, which is short-lived and transient.

PASSIVE IMMUNIZATION (Table 16–1)

The antibody content of human immune serum globulin (HISG) is predominantly IgG and is obtained by fractionating pooled human sera. The fractionation procedure not only concentrates IgG but also removes hepatitis viruses. Gamma globulin is usually administered for postexposure prophylaxis when there is insufficient time for active immunization, e.g., in cases of tetanus and diphtheria. Passive immunization is also required when a vaccine is not available for active immunization, e.g., in hepatitis A exposure and botulism poisoning.

HISG is usually not effective if given after onset of the disease. Immune globulin preparations, i.e., stabilized sterile solutions of human plasma proteins, are also used intravenously to confer passive immunity, primarily in patients with acquired or congenital agammaglobulinemia (Chapters 6 and 9). Special preparations of HISG derived from persons known to have high titers of antibodies against specific infectious agents are also available for immunoprophylaxis against hepatitis B (HISG), rabies (HRIG), tetanus (TIG), vaccinia (VIG), and varicella zoster (VZIG). HISG also is effective against Rh disease.

Horse antitetanus antiserum, which was used for many years to treat tetanus, frequently caused serum sickness. It has been replaced with human tetanus antitoxin. Human immunoglobulins are also immunogenic, but this is rarely clinically significant. Horse-derived gamma globulin is still used to treat snake and other animal envenomation, since human gamma globulin is not available for these diseases.

The disadvantages of passive immunization are as follows: (1) the protection conferred is short-lived; (2) the immunoglobulins are themselves immunogenic, especially when obtained from other species; (3) intramuscular gamma globulin injections are painful; and (4) these biologic products are usually expensive.

ACTIVE IMMUNIZATION (Tables 16–2 to 16–5)

Active immunization stimulates the individual's own protective mechanisms. The most important aspect of a vaccine's development is assessing its efficacy. This can be determined by measuring immune responses in appropriate subjects. Unfortunately, there are only a few infectious diseases, e.g., tetanus, in which protective mechanisms have been elucidated where the degree of protection correlates with serum antibody titers to toxin. Circulating antibody is easily measured; however, since serum titers do not always correlate with immunity, other parameters are needed. Measurements of secretory antibody and of cell-mediated immunity have been even less useful than serum antibody titers in assessing vaccine efficacy. Field trials to determine vaccine efficacy are both expensive and time consuming. Furthermore, direct challenge studies do not always reflect natural infectious disease situations, and they involve artificial infection of volunteers, which raises serious ethical questions because this may cause morbidity and mortality.

Table 16–1. Passive Immunization*

Disease	Preparation	Indication	Dose and Route	Comments[a]
Botulism	Trivalent (A,B,E) horse antibotulism serum	Therapeutic	8–32 ml, half IM and half IV, depending on severity, period of incubation, and amount of contaminated food ingested Per 8 ml: A, 7500 U; B, 5500 U; E, 8500 U	Effects definite Effectiveness not certain in botulism in infants
Snake bite[b] (pit viper)	Horse antivenom serum	Therapeutic	IV, 1:1 to 1:10 dilution of reconstituted antivenin in normal saline; dose given ranges from 20 to 150 ml, depending on the best estimate of the severity of envenomation at the time treatment is begun	Effects definite
Diphtheria	Horse antidiphtheria serum	Therapeutic	30,000–80,000 U, depending upon extent of disease (IV preferred, but IM acceptable)	Effects definite Active immunization preferred for nonimmune contacts
Gas gangrene[c]	Pentavalent anticlostridial horse serum	Therapeutic	26,000–104,000 U, IV	Clinically ineffective
Hepatitis A	Human immune serum globulin	Prophylactic	0.02–0.06 ml/kg, IM	Effects definite Given as soon as possible after exposure
Hepatitis B	Human hyperimmune serum globulin (HBIG)	Prophylactic	0.05–0.07 ml/kg, IM; repeat in 4 weeks	Definitely effective
	Human immune serum globulin	Prophylactic	5–10 ml, IM; repeat in 4 weeks	Efficacy unknown Use when hepatitis B hyperimmune serum globulin is not available
Measles	Human immune serum globulin	Prophylactic	Preventive dose: 0.25 ml/kg, IM Modifying dose: 0.04 ml/kg, IM	Effects definite Rarely indicated; give immediately after exposure

Mumps	Human hyperimmune serum globulin	Prophylactic	5–10 ml, IM	Questionable efficacy in preventing orchitis in postpubertal males
Pertussis	Human hyperimmune serum globulin	Prophylactic	2.5 ml, IM	Efficacy unproved
Poliomyelitis	Human immune serum globulin	Prophylactic	0.35 ml/kg, IM	Efficacy proved
Rabies	Human immune serum globulin (preferred agent)	Prophylactic	20 U/kg, half IM, half into wound	Effects definite. If human rabies immunoglobulin not available, equine rabies immune serum should be used
	Horse antirabies serum	Prophylactic	40 U/kg, IM (part infiltrated into wound)	
Rubella	Human immune serum globulin	Prophylactic	20–50 ml, IM	Doubtful efficacy
Tetanus	Human hyperimmune serum globulin (TIG)	Prophylactic	250–500 U, half IM and half locally	If TIG unavailable, tetanus antisera from equine sources (TAT) may be used. Prophylactic effects: definite. Therapeutic effects: probable
	Horse antitetanus serum (TAT) available but not recommended	Therapeutic	3000–6000 U, half IM and half locally. Used at 10 times the dose of tetanus immune globulin	
Smallpox and vaccinia	Human hyperimmune serum globulin (VIG)	Prophylactic	0.3 ml/kg, IM	Effects definite
		Therapeutic (for vaccinia)	0.6 ml/kg, IM	Effects probable
Varicella	Human hyperimmune serum globulin	Prophylactic	1.25–5.00 ml, IM	When given within 24 hours after exposure, effects definite. Not indicated with active infection

*Modified from Pichon, H. E.: Vaccination and immunotherapy. In Yoshikawa, T. T., Chow, A. W., and Guze, L. B. (eds.): Infectious Diseases: Diagnosis and Management. Boston, Houghton Mifflin Professional Publishers, 1980.

[a] Administration of horse sera may involve side effects, e.g., hypersensitivity, serum sickness, and anaphylaxis; human sera may cause pain and tenderness at site of injection.

[b] Different snake bites require specific antisera—see package insert.

[c] C. perfringens is cultured from 60 to 90 percent of cases of clostridial myonecrosis. There are five types of C. perfringens, A to E, separated according to their production of four major lethal toxins.

Note: For all products used, consult manufacturer's brochure for instructions for storage, handling, and administration. Biologicals prepared by different manufacturers may vary, and those of the same manufacturer may change from time to time. The package insert should be consulted for a specific product.

Table 16–2. Recommended Schedule for Active Immunization of Normal Infants and Children*

Recommended Age	Vaccine[a]	Adverse Effects	Comments
2 mo	DTP[b], OPV[c]	DTP can cause fever, local induration, and pain	Can be initiated earlier in areas of high endemicity
4 mo	DTP, OPV		2 mo interval desired for OPV, to avoid interference
6 mo	DTP, OPV		OPV optional for areas where polio might be imported (e.g., some areas of southwest United States)
12 mo	Tuberculin test[d]		May be given simultaneously with MMR at 15 mo
15 mo	Measles, mumps, rubella (MMR)[e]	Fever, rash, local pain, and arthralgia in older patients	MMR preferred; one dose, subcutaneously
18 mo	DTP, OPV		Consider as part of primary series; DTP essential
24 months to 6 years	Hib vaccine (Haemophilus b polysaccharide vaccine)	Minor erythema and induration at injection site and fever lasting 24 hr	Immunization of children 18 to 23 mo of age in known high risk groups Seroconversion is not as high as with older children Vaccination for infants younger than 18 mo of age is not recommended
4–6 yr[f] 14–16 yr	DTP, OPV Td[g]	Local induration and pain and rare allergic reactions	Repeat every 10 years of lifetime

*Modified from Heggie, A. D.: Immunization against infectious diseases. Med. Clin. North Am. 67:17, 1983.
[a]DPT, Td, OPV, and MMR give ≥ 90 to 95 percent protection.
[b]DTP contains diphtheria toxoid, 33 flocculating units (Lf) U/ml; tetanus toxoid, 10 Lf U/ml; heat-killed *Bordetella pertussis*. Adult booster not recommended.
[c]OPV = oral, attenuated poliovirus vaccine; contains poliovirus Types 1, 2, and 3.
[d]Tuberculin test = Mantoux (intradermal PPD) preferred. Frequency of test depends on local epidemiology. Annual or biennial testing unless local circumstances dictate less frequent or no testing.
[e]MMR = live measles, mumps, and rubella viruses in a combined vaccine. No childhood or adult booster recommended.
[f]Up to the seventh birthday.
[g]Td = adult tetanus toxoid (full dose) and diphtheria toxoid (4 Lf U/ml) in combination. Usually 0.5 ml IM at 10-year intervals.
Note: For all products used, consult manufacturer's brochure for instructions for storage, handling and administration. Biologicals prepared by different manufacturers may vary, and those of the same manufacturer may change from time to time. The package insert should be consulted for a specific product.

Vaccines are most often administered by the parenteral route, although other methods have been used. The route of immunization should depend upon identification of the immune host defense mechanisms responsible for protection. Application of the antigen by nose drops, eye drops, intranasal inhaled aerosols, or oral ingestion is most effective if stimulation of secretory antibody or cellular immunity on secretory surfaces is of primary importance. Polio vaccine is an excellent example of a successfully used oral vaccine. Duration of protection is an important consideration in active immunization, and immunity can often be prolonged by periodic reimmunization and by use of adjuvants or attenuated live vaccines. Live organisms may multiply at the site of deposition, and the resultant increase of antigenic mass results in superior protection. Live vaccines require cautious handling and refrigeration, which is not always available in underdeveloped countries. Moisture may ruin lyophilized (freeze-dried) vaccines. Live vaccines are more likely to contain adventitious agents. This is especially true of viral vaccines, since viruses require cultivation in a living cellular milieu from which it is impossible to exclude the presence of other agents.

There is little data on time intervals and number of booster immunizations needed to confer proper immunity or extend the immune process. Two doses of a particular vaccine decreases the number of persons susceptible to a disease from 10 percent to 1 percent, and a third booster lowers it to below 1 percent. Boosters stimulate an anamnestic response (memory response) and result in a faster and greater antibody production. Immunologic memory prolongs immunity and mobilizes host defense mechanisms rapidly upon reexposure to the offending organism. For example, with tetanus toxoid, a booster immunization every 10 years results in virtually 100 percent immunity.

THE DECISION TO IMMUNIZE

The decision to immunize an individual is a complex one in which the physician must weigh the risks and the consequences of the patient's acquiring a natural, unmodified illness, the availability of a safe and effective immunogen, and the duration of its effects. Diphtheria and tetanus (Fig. 16–2) can be prevented by highly effective vaccines that are associated with few side effects. The causative agents for these diseases are ubiquitous, and only immunized individuals are protected. Therefore, im-

Table 16–3. Components and Routes of Administration of Vaccines in Use*

Vaccine	Components	Route of Administration
Frequently Used		
DPT[a]: Diphtheria	Diphtheria toxoid (formalin-inactivated *Corynebacterium diphtheriae* toxin) adsorbed to aluminum phosphate[b]	Intramuscular
Pertussis	Whole killed pertussis bacteria (*Bordetella pertussis*)	Intramuscular
Tetanus	Tetanus toxoid (formalin-inactivated toxin of *Clostridium tetani*) adsorbed to aluminum phosphate	Intramuscular
OPV (oral poliomyelitis vaccine)	Live attenuated polioviruses Types I, II, and III grown in African green monkey kidney cell cultures	Oral
MMR[c]: Measles	Live attenuated measles virus grown in chick embryo cell cultures	Subcutaneous
Rubella	Live attenuated rubella virus grown in human embryonic lung cell cultures	Subcutaneous
Mumps	Live attenuated mumps virus grown in chick embryo cell cultures	Subcutaneous
IPV (inactivated poliomyelitis vaccine)	Virulent polioviruses Types I, II, and III grown in monkey kidney cell cultures and inactivated with formalin	Subcutaneous
Influenza vaccine	Recently prevalent influenza viruses, strains A and B, grown in embryonated eggs, inactivated with formalin, and purified by zonal centrifugation to reduce amount of egg protein. Whole virus vaccine contains intact virus particles. Split product vaccine contains antigenic fragments of the virus	Subcutaneous
Hepatitis B vaccine	Surface antigen of hepatitis B virus, obtained from human plasma, purified, and inactivated by treatment with urea, pepsin, and formalin. Alum adsorbed	Intramuscular (in buttock)
Pneumococcal vaccine	Capsular polysaccharide antigens from the 14 serotypes of pneumococci most frequently involved in bacteremic pneumococcal infections. Contains no live organisms	Subcutaneous or intramuscular

	capsular polysaccharides antigens of groups A or C, or A and C meningococci. Contain no live organisms	Subcutaneous
Rabies vaccine	Rabies virus grown in human embryonic lung fibroblast cultures and inactivated with beta-propiolactone	Intramuscular
Yellow fever vaccine	Live attenuated yellow fever virus grown in embryonated eggs	Subcutaneous
Less Frequently Used		
Anthrax	Cell-free alum-concentrated inactivated protein antigen of *Bacillus anthracis*	Subcutaneous
Cholera	Phenol-inactivated *Vibrio cholerae* of Ogawa and Inaba serotypes	Subcutaneous or intramuscular
Plague	Formaldehyde-inactivated *Yersinia pestis*	Intramuscular
Tuberculosis	BCG (an attenuated strain of *Mycobacterium bovis*)	Subcutaneous or multiple percutaneous
Typhoid	Acetone-killed *Salmonella typhi*	Subcutaneous
Rickettsia typhi	Formaldehyde-inactivated *Rickettsia prowazekii* grown in chick embryos	Subcutaneous
Smallpox	Live attenuated vaccinia virus in lyophilized or glycerinated vaccine	Multiple puncture jet injection
Recently Approved for Usage		
Haemophilus b polysaccharide vaccine	Haemophilus b capsular polysaccharide (polymer of ribose, ribitol phosphate)	Subcutaneous

*Modified from Heggie, A. D.: Immunization against infectious diseases. Med. Clin. North Am. 67:17, 1983.

[a]DPT can be administered as the combination, or if a child has an adverse reaction to the combination, diphtheria and tetanus can be given together without pertussis (DT or TD), or tetanus can be given alone.

[b]Aluminum phosphate acts as an adjuvant. Immunization with absorbed toxoids results in higher antibody titers and more prolonged immunity than when unadsorbed (fluid) toxoids are used.

[c]MMR can be administered as the combination, or each of the components can be given alone.

Note: For all products used, consult manufacturer's brochure for instructions for storage, handling, and administration. Biologicals prepared by different manufacturers may vary, and those of the same manufacturer may change from time to time. The package insert should be consulted for a specific product.

Table 16–4. Bacterial and Viral Vaccines Currently
Under Laboratory and Clinical Investigation*

Bacterial Vaccines	Type of Product(s)
A. *Bacterial components or products*	
Meningococcal group B	Serotype protein isolated from outer membrane protein
	O-acetylated K, polysaccharide
Meningococcal groups Y, 29E, and WI-35	Isolated capsular polysaccharide
Gonococci	Pili (attachment protein)
	Outer membrane proteins
	IgA proteinase
Typhoid vaccine	Isolated capsular polysaccharide (Vi antigen)
Group B streptococci	Type IIIa, isolated capsular polysaccharide
Enteropathogenic *E. coli*	Pili (attachment protein)—enterotoxin
Dental "caries vaccine"	Extracellular dextran-synthesizing enzymes
B. *Live*	Live bacteria
Cross-reacting nonpathogenic enteric bacteria (*H. influenzae* type b and perhaps others)	

Viral Vaccines	Live	Inactivated
C. *Respiratory viruses*		
Influenza	Temperature-sensitive mutants, cold-adapted recombinant viruses (embryonated chicken egg)	Subunit hemagglutinin and neuraminidase vaccines (embryonated chicken egg)
Respiratory syncytial	Temperature-sensitive mutants (primary bovine embryonic kidney cell culture)	
	Serially passaged viruses (WI-38 cell culture)	
Adenoviruses	Types 4, 7, 21 virus administered in enteric-coated capsules (WI-38 cell culture)	Subunit vaccines (cell cultures)
D. *Herpesviruses*		
Herpes simplex Type I		Subunit vaccines (cell cultures)
Herpes simplex Type II		
Varicella	High-passage virus (WI-38 cell cultures)	
Cytomegalovirus	High-passage virus (WI-38 cell culture)	
E. *Togaviruses*		
Dengue	High-passage virus (guinea pig heart cell culture; DBS-FRhL-2 continuous fetal rhesus lung cell culture)	
Venezuelan equine encephalomyelitis	High-passage virus (chick embryo cell culture)	(Chick embryo cell culture)

*Modified from Parkman, P. D., Hopps, H. E., and Meyer, H. M.: Immunoprevention of infectious diseases. *In* Nahmias, A. J., and O'Reilly, R. J. (eds.): Comprehensive Immunology. New York, Plenum Medical Book Co., 1982, pp. 561–583.

Table 16–5. Trade Names and Manufacturers of Currently Available Vaccines*

Name of Vaccine	Trade Name	Manufacturer
Diphtheria toxoid, tetanus toxoid, and pertussis vaccine absorbed (DPT)	Same as name of vaccine Tri-Immunol	Connaught, Wyeth, Lederle
Diphtheria toxoid and tetanus toxoid absorbed for pediatric use (DT)	Same as name of vaccine	Lederle, Sclavo, Wyeth
Diphtheria toxoid and tetanus toxoid absorbed for adult use (TD)	Same as name of vaccine	Wyeth
Diphtheria toxoid absorbed for pediatric use	Same as name of vaccine	Sclavo
Tetanus toxoid absorbed	Same as name of vaccine	Connaught, Lederle, Sclavo, Wyeth
Live attenuated poliomyelitis vaccine (OPV)	Orimune Poliovirus Vaccine	Lederle
Inactivated poliomyelitis vaccine (IVP)	Poliomyelitis Vaccine	Connaught
Measles, mumps, and rubella vaccine	M-M-R	Merck Sharp & Dohme
Measles and rubella vaccine	M-R-VAX	Merck Sharp & Dohme
Rubella and mumps vaccine	Biavax	Merck Sharp & Dohme
Measles vaccine	Attenuvax	Merck Sharp & Dohme
Rubella vaccine	Meruvax II	Merck Sharp & Dohme
Mumps vaccine	Mumpsvax	Merck Sharp & Dohme
Haemophilus b polysaccharide	b-CAPSA I vaccine	Praxis Biologics; distributed by Mead Johnson
Influenza vaccine	Fluzone	Connaught
	Fluogen	Parke-Davis
	Influenza Virus (Vaccine Subvirion Type)	Wyeth
Rabies vaccine (human diploid cell vaccine)	Rabies vaccine, Human Wyvac	Merieux Wyeth
Hepatitis B vaccine	Heptavax-B	Merck Sharp & Dohme
Pneumococcal vaccine	Pneumovax	Merck Sharp & Dohme
	Pnu-Imune	Lederle
Meningococcal vaccine	Menomune A,C, and A/C	Connaught
	Meningovax-AC	Merck Sharp & Dohme
Yellow fever vaccine	YF-VAX	Connaught
Typhoid vaccine	Typhoid Vaccine	Wyeth
Cholera vaccine	Cholera Vaccine	Sclavo, Wyeth
	Cholera Vaccine (India strains)	Lederle
Smallpox vaccine	Dryvax	Wyeth
Plague vaccine	Plague Vaccine	Cutter Biological

*Modified from Heggie, H. D.: Immunization against infectious diseases. Med. Clin. North Am. 67:17, 1983.

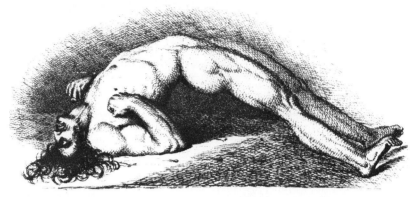

Figure 16–2. Sir Charles Bell's drawing (1832) of a British soldier suffering from tetanus (lockjaw) as a result of wounds received at the Battle of Corunna. Note the spastic paralysis resulting from opposing muscles pulling against each other, owing to tetanus toxin blocking synaptic inhibition. This man will certainly die. (From Braude, A. I. (ed.): Medical Microbiology and Infectious Diseases, Vol. II. Philadelphia, W. B. Saunders Co., 1981.)

munization is universally advised. Pertussis (whooping cough) attack rates correlate inversely with use of the vaccine. The available vaccine has significant side effects such as encephalopathy, convulsions, and other CNS complications. However, the benefits of pertussis immunization with the currently available vaccine still outweigh its risks. Smallpox vaccine is effective and usually safe. The last naturally acquired known case of smallpox was reported in Somalia in October, 1977, and it is now thought that smallpox has been eradicated from the earth. Even though there is a low complication rate from smallpox vaccine, the risks of vaccination now outweigh the benefits, and it is no longer recommended. There are vaccines that may be reserved for special situations, e.g., occupational exposure to rabid animals. Because the risk of human rabies is low in the United States, pre-exposure immunization is used only for travelers to hyperendemic areas or for persons with an occupational hazard.

Cholera vaccines offer low-grade protection for a short period of time, and the risk of exposure to the disease in developed countries is minimal. It is of little use to travelers and is used only if the risk of exposure to the vibrio bacterium is high or if the traveler is going to an area where regulations require its use. Immunity to Type A influenza virus is transient, because there are antigenic "shifts" and "drifts" in surface chemistry of the Type A influenza virus every few years. This usually renders previously developed vaccines obsolete. Rapid mobilization of resources is needed for sufficient production, distribution, and utilization of new antigenic flu vaccines to prevent an epidemic spread of an altered strain. Influenza vaccine should be given routinely to high-risk groups (see remarks under Comments About Certain Vaccines, below).

The age of the host is an important consideration for administration of a vaccine. Whooping cough, poliomyelitis, and diphtheria usually are childhood diseases, and therefore immunization against these diseases begins during infancy. Immunization for rubella is recommended for females prior to puberty or for seronegative nonpregnant females in childbearing ages. The purpose of rubella immunization is not to protect the vaccinee, but to prevent fetal infection, which may result in congenital abnormalities. Many vaccines contain multiple antigens, e.g., DPT (diphtheria, pertussis, and tetanus [nonliving antigens]) or MMR (measles, mumps, and rubella [live attenuated viruses]). Simultaneous immune responses are elicited against each component of the vaccine.

Adjuvants enhance the immunogenic potency of soluble proteins. Accordingly, inorganic gels (e.g., alum, aluminum hydroxide, or aluminum phosphate) with absorbed immunogens are used, which permits antigen to be released slowly over a period of time. Many adjuvants include dead bacteria and/or their products. The killed *Bordetella pertussis* vaccine itself acts as an adjuvant, providing a superior immune response against the added antigens. Endotoxins from gram-negative organisms also have immunoenhancing effects. The mycobacteria are powerful adjuvants. The attenuated bovine strain of *Mycobacterium tuberculosis*—the bacillus Calmette-Guérin (BCG)—has been used to augment immunologic responses against cancer. Freund's adjuvant (tubercle bacilli in water-in-oil emulsion) is employed to augment immunologic responses to protein in experimental work. The intense chronic inflammatory responses around the deposits of these emulsions precludes their use in man in routine immunization procedures. These adjuvants probably act by increasing macrophage and T-cell helper functions, but their complete mode of action is not understood.

COMMENTS ABOUT CERTAIN VACCINES (Table 16–6)

Influenza usually does not cause life-threatening disease in healthy young and middle-aged adults and children. However, influenza immunization is recommended for persons over age 65

Table 16–6. Recommended Vaccine Schedule for Heptavax-B[*a]

Vaccine Group	Immunization (Volume, ml)		
	First	*Second*[b]	*Third*[c]
Young children (3 mo–10 yr)	0.5	0.5	0.5
Adults and children (>10 yr)	1.0	1.0	1.0
Dialysis and immunocompromised patients	2.0	2.0	2.0[d]

[*]Modified from Gregory, D. H., II: Hepatitis B vaccine. Postgrad. Med. 75:199, 1984.
[a]Hepatitis B vaccine administered intramuscularly in buttock.
[b]One month after initial dose.
[c]Six months after initial immunization.
[d]Two 1-ml doses given intramuscularly in two different sites.

and for patients with cardiopulmonary disorders or other chronic diseases that make them at risk for serious illness from these viruses. Protection ranges from 75 to 90 percent, although the immunity conferred lasts several months. Influenza vaccines are grown in embryonated chicken eggs, and the virus is then inactivated by formaldehyde and concentrated by ultracentrifugation. The vaccines contain either whole viruses or subunit (split) viruses, the latter made by breaking the viral cell with organic solvents or detergents. Although split vaccines usually provoke fewer systemic side effects, they are less immunogenic. They are considered safer for use in children, since children below 13 years tend to have more side effects from influenza vaccines. Swine influenza vaccine (A/New Jersey/76) was associated with Guillain-Barré syndrome. However, other components of influenza vaccines, including all of the current constituents, have not been shown to have a statistically significant association with the Guillain-Barré syndrome.

Pneumococcal vaccines contain capsular polysaccharide antigens from the serotypes of pneumococci most frequently involved in bacteremic pneumococcal infections. A 14-valent vaccine was developed and was shown to confer protection to 75.9 percent of healthy adults of a selected group, i.e., South African gold miners who frequently acquire the infection. This vaccine, licensed in 1977, was recommended for patients over 2 years of age with sickle-cell disease, splenic dysfunction, anatomic asplenia, nephrotic syndrome, and other chronic illness, and for persons 50 years or older. Duration of the serum antibody response is at least 5 years, and the need for booster immunization is unknown. A newer preparation of pneumococcal vaccine, licensed in the United States in 1983, consists of a mixture of purified capsular polysaccharide from 23 pneumococcal types and has replaced the 14-valent polysaccharide vaccine. The 23 bacterial types represented in the current vaccine are responsible for 87 percent of bacteremic pneumococcal disease in the United States as reported to the CDC in 1983. This compares with 71 percent for the previous 14-valent formulation. Although the new polysaccharide vaccine contains only 25 μg of each antigen, in contrast to the 50 μg of antigen in the 14-valent vaccine, a study of 53 adults reveals comparable levels of immunogenicity of the two vaccines.

Although rabies rarely affects humans in the United States, every year thousands of persons receive rabies prophylaxis as a result of possible exposure, usually from animal bites. The currently available vaccine against rabies in the United States is made from virus grown in human diploid cells (embryonic lung, WI-38) and is inactivated with tri-N-butyl phosphate. It elicits a 10- to 20-fold higher level of protective antibodies than the previously used duck embryo vaccine. The recommended procedure for postexposure prophylaxis for rabies is to administer human rabies immunoglobulin (HRIG) and the 5-injection human diploid cell rabies vaccine.

Hepatitis B virus (HBV) vaccine is recommended for high-risk individuals (Table 16–6). These include health care workers, employees of institutions for the mentally retarded, hemodialysis patients, homosexually active males, intravenous-drug users, recipients of certain blood products, sexual and other contacts of HBV carriers, and inmates of long-term correctional facilities. The vaccine is a suspension of inactivated alum-adsorbed 22-nm surface antigen particles (20 μg/ml protein) separated from human plasma by a combination of biophysical and biochemical procedures. Inactivation of the virus is achieved by a threefold process using 8 M urea, pepsin at pH 2, and formalin (1:4000). This vaccine induces protective antibody titers in 90 percent of healthy individuals and in all infants and children (3 months to 9 years of age). Three intramuscular doses in the buttock are needed to achieve maximum protection; the second and third doses are given 1 and 6 months respectively after the primary dose. Immunity lasts for at least 3 years, and the need for boosters is unknown.

Hepatitis B immune globulin (HBIG) is recommended for postexposure prophylaxis. Infants born to a mother whose serum is positive for hepatitis B antigen are at high risk and should receive HBIG immediately after birth. The optimal age for active immunization in infancy with hepatitis B vaccine is not yet determined. The first dose of vaccine should be given to the high-risk infants 3 months after the HBIG infusion.

HAZARDS OF IMMUNIZATION

Vaccine recipients and contacts may be at risk when live attenuated organisms are used. For example, a pregnant mother can contract attenuated rubella virus from an immunized child and consequently infect her fetus, with a theoretical danger of developing fetal abnormalities. Parenteral active immunization may be associated with fever, malaise, and myalgia. Arthritis and arthralgia may follow rubella vaccination, and seizures have occurred following pertussis immunization.

The large-scale immunization program in 1976 against swine influenza A (Hsw1N1) was associated with a fivefold increase in Guillain-Barré syndrome in vaccinated persons. Traces of egg proteins and/or antibiotics in cell-cultured viral vaccines can provoke allergic reactions in hypersensitive individuals. Killed respiratory syncytial virus (RSV) vaccine used in an experimental field trial was associated with an increased severity of illness compared with the control group. The cause has not been determined, but it has been postulated as being an "imbalance" in the systemic and secretory antibody responses, i.e., serum antibody alone is stimulated by injection of the vaccine without stimulation of secretory antibody. Such an individual when exposed to the wild virus could conceivably develop an Arthus-like or Type III reaction, resulting in increased tissue damage. The killed measles vaccine has caused somewhat similar reactions when the immunized individuals were exposed to wild measles virus.

CONCLUSIONS

Disease often becomes less prevalent following the widespread use of a vaccine. The incidence of poliomyelitis and its paralytic sequelae decreased following the widespread use of Salk inactivated polio vaccine (IPV) in 1955 and Sabin's oral polio vaccine (OPV) in 1964. Such success has fostered some complacency about the need for immunization and may result in a large at-risk population. For example, the potential for polio in unimmunized persons remains, as illustrated by an outbreak in a religious community in which the members refused immunization. Immunization of the population remains one of the most objective and useful means of preventive medicine.

Bibliography

Edelman, P.: Vaccine adjuvants. Rev. Infect. Dis. 2:370, 1980.

Fulginiti, V.A.: A new pertusssis vaccine: hope for the future? J. Inf. Dis. 148:146, 1983.

Fedson, D. S.: Adult immunization: protocols and problems. Hosp. Pract. 21:143, 1986.

Ganguly, R., Stablein, J., Lockey, R. F., et al.: Defective antimicrobial functions of oral secretions in the elderly. J. Infect. Dis. 153:163, 1986.

Ganguly, R., and Waldman, R.H.: Local immunity and local immune responses. Prog. Aller. 22:1, 1980.

Heggie, A.D.: Immunization against infectious diseases. Practice and problems. Med. Clin. North Am. 67:17, 1983.

Hilleman, M.R.: New developments with new vaccines. Prog. Clin. Biol. Res. 47:21, 1980.

Hilleman, M.R.: Vaccines for the decade of the 1980's and beyond. S. Afr. Med. J. 61:691, 1982.

Krugman, S.: Hepatitis virus vaccines: present status. Yale J. Biol. Med. 55:375, 1982.

Lloyds, S.: Progress in immunization against parasitic helminths. Parasitology 83:225, 1981.

Morbidity and Mortality Weekly Report. Update: Pneumococcal Polysaccaride Vaccine usage—United States. 33:272, 1984.

Plotkin, S.A.: Rabies vaccine prepared in human cell cultures. Progress and Perspectives. Rev. Infect. Dis. 2:433, 1980.

Ponka, A., and Leinonen, M.: Adverse reactions to polyvalent pneumococcal vaccine. Scand. J. Infect. Dis. 14:67, 1982.

Sabin, A.B., Arechiga, A.F., de Castro, J.F., et al.: Successful immunization of infants with and without maternal antibody by aerosolized measles vaccine. JAMA 251:2363, 1984.

Schiff, G.M.: Active immunizations for adults. Ann. Rev. Med. 31:441, 1980.

Stuart-Harris, C. (from the National Institute of Allergy and Infectious Diseases): The present status of live influenza virus vaccine. J. Infect. Dis. 142:784, 1980.

Waldman, R.H., and Ganguly, R.: Immunization against viral infections. Postgrad. Med. 75:170, 1984.

17

Tumor Antigens

RALPH A. REISFELD, Ph.D.

INTRODUCTION

It has been apparent for some time that cancer is not a single disease but rather a variety of diseases that are most often expressed as the abnormal and continuous growth of cells of certain tissues. The events that lead to the development of cancer and the factors controlling it either at one site or at multiple metastatic sites are at best only partially understood at this time. Comprehensive studies of antigenic changes on cell surfaces accompanying malignant transformation were the most promising among many efforts made during the last 25 years to gain a better understanding of the complex phenomena involved in the neoplastic process. These cell surface changes were often found to be characterized by either the loss or the appearance of cell surface markers designated as tumor antigens. It is not at all the aim of this brief chapter to recount the extensive literature dealing with either classic concepts of tumor immunology or those leading to the development of different categories of tumor antigens, i.e., tumor-specific transplantation antigens (TSTA), antigens of either chemically or virally induced tumors, or in fact the much described oncodevelopmental tumor antigens, e.g., α-fetoprotein (AFP) or carcinoembryonic antigen (CEA). To gain an understanding of these tumor antigens, the reader is directed to some of the excellent reviews that have appeared in the literature, including, for TSTA, a review of Koldovsky (1969); for chemically induced tumors, a review of Heidelberger (1975); for virally induced tumors, a review by Klein (1975); for α-fetoprotein, a review by Sell (1980); and for CEA, reviews by Gold et al. (1979) and Kirkpatrick et al. (1982).

It is, however, the aim of this chapter to focus the reader on a few selected reports in the very recent literature that have led to new and exciting concepts, largely because of the development of monoclonal antibodies. These reagents, particularly when directed to human melanoma-associated antigens, have served as specific molecular probes for basic tumor biology and biochemistry and may ultimately pave the way for new and effective approaches to aid in the diagnosis and therapy of cancer.

MONOCLONAL ANTIBODIES AS PROBES

Delineation of Molecular Profiles of Tumor Antigens by Monoclonal Antibodies

Glycoproteins

A particularly good example of the use of monoclonal antibodies to thoroughly characterize a human tumor antigen is provided by a family of antigens designated p97 and preferentially expressed by human melanoma cells and tissues. A comprehensive structural characterization of p97 demonstrated, by sequential immunoprecipitation and SDS-PAGE (sodium dodecyl sulfate–polyacrylamide gel electrophoresis), that four different monoclonal antibodies recognized the same p97 molecule. Six additional monoclonal antibodies, reported earlier to be specific for a melanoma cell surface protein of M_r 95,000 (gp95), are also bound to the p97 antigen by sequential immunoprecipitation, indicating that p97 and gp95 are identical. Quantitation of the expression of p97 on SK-MEL 28 melanoma cells revealed at least 400,000 molecules of p97 per cell based on antibody binding data, which is roughly equal to HLA-A,B,C determinants identified by binding of anti-HLA monoclonal antibody W6/32 to these same cells. Regarding the expression of three different epitopes of p97, i.e., p97 a,b,c, types, it could be demonstrated that a melanoma, a lung carcinoma, and a B and T lymphoid cell line all bound each antibody defining these epitopes but in vastly different amounts. The melanoma line bound 300,000 to 380,000 molecules of each antibody per cell; the lung carcinoma line bound 4000 to 6200 molecules per cell; and the B and T cell lines bound only 250 to 1400 molecules per cell.

Concerning the chemical characerization of p97, it was found to be glycosylated and sialylated and to consist of a single polypeptide chain, most likely with some intrachain disulfide bridges. Partial digestion, with either papain or trypsin, of detergent solubilized p97 produced seemingly identical fragments of M_r 40,000, which are glycosylated and contain the p97 a,b,c, epitopes but lack the p97 d,e epitopes.

The human melanoma–associated antigen p97 was reported to be functionally related to transferrin, and it was proposed that the two proteins evolved from a common ancestral gene (Brown et al., 1982). This conclusion was based on the amino-terminal amino acid sequence homology between these two molecules, i.e., 7 from a total of 12 residues determined were found to be identical. This includes two of the least common amino acids, i.e., tryptophan and cystine. These conclusions were further supported by the finding that antiserum to denatured p97 cross-reacted with denatured transferrin and lactotransferrin and by the finding that p97 binds iron. Although p97 and transferrin receptors have a smiliar molecular weight, this same report also showed conclusively that these two molecules are not identical. Thus, following SDS-PAGE under nonreducing conditions, transferrin receptor forms a dimer of M_r 200,000, whereas p97 migrates slightly faster than the reduced protein. In addition, the tissue distribution of the two molecules differs considerably, and monoclonal antibody OKT9, which is specific for transferrin receptor, does not immunoprecipitate p97 from radioiodinated melanoma cells. The immunologic difference of these two molecules was also demonstrated by sequential immunoprecipitation experiments. Finally, p97 also failed to bind to a transferrin-Sepharose column. However, although p97 and transferrin receptor are structurally distinct, it was suggested that they may share some of their proposed biologic functions, e.g., mediation of cellular uptake of transferrin-bound iron, a proposal that was not possible to prove experimentally. Since trace amounts of p97 are present in normal adult tissue, it appears more likely that this function is carried out by transferrin receptor rather than by the p97 molecule. The fact that distribution of p97 is more or less limited to melanoma cells, nevi, and fetal intestine argues for a more specialized functional role of this molecule, which may be restricted to these tissues, a contention that requires experimental substantiation.

Another study produced a monoclonal antibody (mAb) (mAb 9.2.27) directed to a melanoma-associated antigen that later was identified as a glycoprotein–chondroitin sulfate–proteoglycan complex (Bumol and Reisfeld, 1982). One of the key features of the production of mAb 9.2.27 was that the immunogen, derived from a 4M urea extract of M14 melanoma cells, was partially purified by affinity chromatography on lentil lectin Sepharose and by removal, on gelatin Sepharose, of fibronectin, a competing immunogen. Another important feature of this approach was the use of a radioimmunometric antibody binding assay with a chemically defined spent medium of melanoma cells as a solid phase target to screen for suitable antibody-secreting hybridomas. The melanoma-associated antigen was used as an immunogenic vehicle devoid of competing antigens such as HLA-A,B,C, HLA-DR and fibronectin. This resulted in the production of 59 antibody-secreting hybridomas (3.7 percent of 1590 positive wells) that bound preferentially to melanoma targets. The antigen defined by mAb 9.2.27 appeared as two components by indirect immunoprecipitation and SDS-PAGE, one of very high molecular weight ($>780,000$) and the other with an M_r of 250,000 (Bumol and Reisfeld, 1982; Bumol et al., 1982). The latter component is highly sensitive to treatment with trypsin, and, although it appears to be part of the extracellular matrix, the 250K component is distinctly different from fibronectin by numerous biochemical criteria.

An mAb 155.8 produced against purified membranes of human melanoma cells was reported to react with a chondroitin sulfate proteoglycan (CSP) preferentially expressed on such cells. Binding inhibition studies indicated that mAb 155.8 reacts with an epitope different from that recognized by mAb 9.2.27 on the same proteoglycan molecule. The mAb 155.8 binds melanoma cells to a more limited extent than does mAb 9.2.27, suggesting that either the antibody recognizes determinant(s) found in smaller numbers on the cell surface or that the affinity constants of the two antibodies are different. The difference in reactivities of these two monoclonal antibodies with chondroitin sulfate proteoglycan is also revealed by immunodepletion analysis, which showed that mAb 155.8 determinants are present on only a subgroup of those molecules bearing the 9.2.27 epitope (Harper et al., 1984; Cheresh et al., 1984).

The proteoglycan nature of the molecules defined by mAb 155.8 was clearly evident from data of ^{3}H-leucine incorporation into the high-molecular-weight component (M_r >780,000) and analysis of $^{35}SO_4^=$-labeled material by cellulose acetate electrophoresis following β-elimination of O-linked glycosaminoglycans by alkaline-borohydride treatment. Data from this analysis along with chondroitinase ABC sensitivity confirmed that the sulfated glycosaminoglycans associated with antigen(s) identified by mAb 155.8 indeed contain chondroitin sulfate Type A and/or C. Similar to mAb 9.2.27, mAb 155.8 also recognizes determinants on the 250K core glycoprotein and the intact CSP. The disappearance of the CSP and concomitant intensification of the 250K component following chondroitinase digestion of immunoprecipitated proteoglycans proves that the 250K glycoprotein is included in the CSP and is, in fact, its core protein. Clear and direct evidence indicates that mAb 9.2.27 and mAb 155.8 recognize the proteoglycan in the absence of 250K, thus ruling out the possibility that the proteoglycan does not contain antigenic determinants but is only complexed with the 250K molecule and thus is merely a "passenger" in immunoprecipitates. Specifically, after resolving antigens extracted from human melanoma cells by $CsCl_2$ density centrifugation in the presence of detergent and high salt, it became possible to immunoprecipitate high-density proteoglycans alone as well as the free 250K component from lower density fractions of the gradient.

The topographic distribution of mAb 155.8–defined proteoglycans on the surface of paraformaldehyde-fixed human melanoma cells when examined by indirect immunofluorescence shows filamentous structures that sometimes connect cells with the underlying substratum. These molecules were not found distributed as substrate-attached material left behind when cells were removed. This raises interesting questions as to the involvement of CSP in melanoma cell adhesion and spreading on various substrata. In this regard, there is already some evidence that mAb 9.2.27 and mAb 155.8 inhibit adhesion and, to a greater extent, cytoplasmic spreading of human melanoma cells on plastic and collagen-fibronectin complex substrata. The finding of an mAb 155.8–defined CSP on freshly explanted melanoma tissues by indirect immunoperoxidase techniques, underlines its functional relevance. In fact, the distribution of the proteoglycans defined by mAb 9.2.27 and mAb 155.8 throughout normal fetal and adult tissues, as well as other tumor types, suggests that determinants recognized by these antibodies are not found in normal tissues known to be rich in CSP, e.g., cartilage. Consequently, from a strictly functional point of view, CSPs on melanoma cells may play more than simply a structural role proposed for such molecules in normal cartilage and other connective tissues (Harper et al., 1984).

Glycolipids

Dippold and coworkers (1980) were among the first to study monoclonal antibodies to cell surface antigens of melanoma cells that appeared to be directed against glycolipids. Thus, antigens defined within the R_{24} system by four monoclonal antibodies appeared to be glycolipids—i.e., they were found to be heat stable, and antibody binding could be inhibited with glycolipid fractions of reactive cells. It was shown that mAb R_{24}, of IgG3 isotype, was indeed directed to the disialoganglioside GD_3 that was isolated from melanoma cells. This finding was confirmed by compositional and partial structural analysis and by comparison with authentic GD_3 ganglioside by thin-layer chromatography (TLC). The mAb R_{24} reacted specifically with authentic GD_3 and a newly developed glycolipid-mediated immune adherence assay (GMIA) established that melanoma cells and tissues contained GD_3 and GM_3 as major gangliosides, whereas a series of other cells and tissues, including other tumor lines, contained these molecules in smaller amounts. The characteristic accumulation of GD_3 in melanoma cells is considered to be caused by either (1) low levels of N-acetyl-galactosaminyl transferase in the Golgi apparatus, where this well-known biosynthetic precursor of gangliosides would likely be concentrated, or (2) elevated levels of certain sialyltransferases promoting an overabundance of GD_3.

An mAb designated mAb 4.2 was found to react with a surface antigen expressed on most human melanomas (Nudelman et al., 1982). This antigen turned out to be a ganglioside with the carbohydrate structure (Neu Acα2 $\rightarrow$ 8 Neu Acα2 $\rightarrow$ 3 Galβ1 $\rightarrow$ 4 Glcβ1 $\rightarrow$ 1 Cer) that was established by enzymatic degradation and methylation analysis by mass spectrometry. Structurally, this antigen is identical with brain GD_3 ganglioside, although this melanoma-associated antigen has a ceramide characterized by a predominance of longer chain fatty acids. This is in contrast to brain GD_3, which has mainly C18:10 fatty acid. Interestingly enough, mAb 4.2 failed to react with gangliosides GT1a and GQ1b, which have a terminal sugar sequence identical to GD_3, i.e., the Neu Aca2 → 8 Neu Aca2 → 3 Galβ1 → 4 Glc → Cer sequence, including the innermost sugar, Glc residue. The mAb 4.2, which reacted with ~ 80 percent of human melanoma cell lines tested also reacted, although somewhat more weakly, with a variety of non-melanoma tumor cell lines. However, it is clear that mAb 4.2 does react with a GD_3 molecule that differs from ordinary GD_3 in its ceramide composition found in brain, a difference postulated by Nudelman and coworkers (1982) to possibly define the antigenic expression of GD_3 in melanoma.

Most recently, monoclonal antibody D1.1 was reported to be specifically reactive with human melanoma tumors and with a majority of melanoma cell lines tested (Cheresh et al., 1984). This particular antibody, prepared against the rat B49 cell line, was found to recognize a ganglioside on developing rat neuroectoderm. Interestingly enough, this particular antibody was found to be highly specific for human melanoma. In fact, the antigen recognized by mAb D1.1 is not detected on a variety of fresh frozen human fetal tissues and does not react by immunoperoxidase assays with any normal human tissues tested, including brain. This antibody also fails to react by immunoperoxidase tests with a wide variety of fresh frozen human tumor tissue sections and does not react in the enzyme-linked immunosorbent assay (ELISA) with a large variety of human tumor cell lines and lymphoblastoid lines. However, the antibody does react very well with a variety of human melanoma cell lines and fresh frozen melanoma tumor tissues. These findings set this particular antibody apart from the mouse monoclonal antibodies described above, i.e., mAb 4.2 and mAb R24. Results from analyses by one- and two-dimensional TLCs indicated that mAb D1.1 reacts with a ganglioside. Moreover, intermediate ammonia treatment of this ganglioside showed that it contains one or more base-labile O-acyl esters. Mild base hydrolysis of the ganglioside substrate, under conditions known to remove O-acyl esters, resulted in complete loss of reactivity with mAb D1.1, indicating that the alkali-labile moiety is a critical component of the epitope recognized by this monoclonal antibody. Analysis of the sialic acids of the total gangliosides from 6-[^{3}H] glucosamine-labeled melanoma cells showed that 10 percent of these molecules were O-acylated. A similar analysis of purified gangliosides indicated that 30 percent of the sialic acids migrated with authentic 9-O-acetyl-N-acetyl-neuraminic acid. This observation led to a follow-up study that demonstrated that the antigen specifically detected by mAb D1.1 was indeed a GD_3 disialoganglioside that was O-acetylated. The importance of the O-acetyl sialic acid moiety as an antigenic epitope specifically recognized by mAb D1.1 was further defined. Chemical acetylation of purified GD_3 with N-acetyl-imidazole made this molecule reactive with mAb D1.1, which otherwise does not react with nonacetylated GD_3, as clearly indicated by de-O-acetylation of GD_3 by treatment with ammonia. These results strongly suggest that the ganglioside recognized by mAb D1.1 differs from GD_3 only by a single O-acetyl ester on a sialic acid residue. The data also suggest that GD_3 may serve as a substrate for a specific O-acetyl-transferase responsible for aberrant O-acetylation in human malignant melanoma cells.

Biosynthesis and Structure of Tumor Antigens Defined by Monoclonal Antibodies

A follow-up study intended to define, chemically and immunochemically, the antigen recognized by mAb 9.2.27 found the antigen to be a unique glycoprotein-proteoglycan complex preferentially expressed by human melanoma cells (Bumol and Reisfeld, 1982; Bumol et al., 1982). A combination of biosynthetic and enzymatic studies of the antigenic determinant recognized by mAb 9.2.27 made it possible to identify this rather unique antigen on human melanoma cells. Specifically, mAb 9.2.27 recognizes an N-linked, sialylated glycoprotein of M_r 250,000 that is associated with a component of $M_4 > 780,000$, expressing all the characteristics of a chondroitin sulfate proteoglycan (CSP). The mAb 9.2.27 was also found to recognize both the free pool of core protein and the CSP monomer. While generally reacting preferentially with melanoma cell lines and freshly explanted surgical melanoma specimens, mAb 9.2.27 also binds to a neuroblastoma cell line. Finally, data obtained by tryptic peptide map analysis and chondroitinase lyase AC and ABC digestions suggest that the 250K molecule is contained within the CSP and possibly represents a "core" protein onto which CSP side chains are added.

In additional studies, the cationic ionophore monensin was found to block effectively the appearance of CSP monomers and polymers in immunoprecipitates obtained with mAb 9.2.27 from detergent extracts of intrinsically radiolabeled melanoma cells that had been previously exposed for 18 hours to $10^{-7}M$ monensin. These findings suggest that monensin can effect the biosynthesis of proteoglycans in melanoma cells. Pulse-chase analyses of the endoglycosidase H-treated antigen complex also suggested that the appearance of CSP is kinetically linked to biosynthetic functions of the Golgi apparatus, the site proposed for biosynthesis of proteoglycans involving glycosyltransferases. There is unique specificity of the mAb 9.2.27 for an M_r 250,000, N-linked, sialylated core glycoprotein associated with a common CSP. This suggests that the human melanoma cell may actually express modified or even unique gene products capable of serving as acceptors or core glycoproteins for common proteoglycan oligosaccharide side chains. Indeed, this type of alteration may account for the known changes in proteoglycans of the membranes and extracellular matrix of some tumor cells.

Biologic Function of Melanoma Antigens Defined by Monoclonal Antibodies

In Vitro Studies

Proteoglycans had been implicated in growth control, cell-substratum interaction, and other functional properties of potential relevance to tumor interaction and tumor metastasis. Therefore, mAb 9.2.27 was used as a specific probe to delineate the possible role of this extracellular matrix component in cell-to-cell interactions and growth control of human melanoma cells (Harper and Reisfeld, 1983). In this regard, mAb 9.2.27 inhibited anchorage-independent growth of human melanoma cells in soft agar, an event that had been shown to correlate with in vivo tumorigenicity. Data obtained from the double agar clonogenic assay indicated that the growth inhibitory effect by mAb 9.2.27 in this in vitro system was indeed specific. Thus, monoclonal anti–HLA-A,B,C antibodies that bind to human melanoma cells had no significant effect on the plating efficiencies of two mAb 9.2.27 antigen–negative cell lines.

The precise mechanism underlying this phenomenon is not entirely clear at this time. It is postulated that it relates to the physicochemical nature and location of the proteoglycan antigen recognized by mAb 9.2.27 on the surface of human melanoma cells. In this regard, it is known that human tumor cells maintained on the extracellular matrix exhibit higher growth rates and have lower serum requirements than do human tumor cells grown on plastic. It is believed that the major components of the extracellular matrix—i.e., collagens, laminin, fibronectin, and proteoglycans—work in concert to produce this effect. Although human melanoma cells were shown to lack an organized extracellular matrix, immunoperoxidase analysis of freshly explanted melanoma tumor tissue showed that melanoma cells in vivo synthesize and deposit CSPs pericellularly among other matrix components. Thus, when melanoma cells are grown in soft agar containing mAb 9.2.27, cell-to-cell interactions may actually be disrupted by interference of this antibody with the normal pericellular disposition and organization of the proteoglycans; consequently, mAb 9.2.27 may be involved in interactions important for the inhibition of growth of melanoma cells in an anchorage-independent fashion.

There are apparently no metabolic constraints on melanoma cells that are attached to and spread on a solid substratum, since it was observed that binding of mAb 9.2.27 to melanoma cells grown in liquid culture does not affect either DNA or protein synthesis, even after 3 days. When taken together, the data of Harper and Reisfeld strongly suggest that CSPs are among those molecules on the surface of human melanoma cells that are involved in cell-to-cell interactions important to anchorage-independent growth regulation. Studies of human tumor metastasis such as these using specific monoclonal antibody probes may provide a better understanding of the molecules involved in tumor growth and may eventually lead to a more effective treatment and ultimately to prevention of metastasis.

In studies of the functional role of CSPs in human tumor systems, mAb 9.2.27 was found to block early events of melanoma cell spreading on endothelial basement membranes while only slightly inhibiting cell adhesion. These data suggest that CSPs may play a part in stabilizing cell-substratum interactions in this in vitro model of metastatic invasion. Thus, CSPs commonly found in the extracellular matrices of normal cells may have different functional roles in tumor cells lacking a formal structural matrix, while maintaining an active biosynthesis of these molecules. This apparently is the case for those melanoma systems that actively synthesize CSPs but lack any organized fibronectin matrix.

Leukocytes possessing Fc receptors are known to lyse cells coated with specific antibody. Such antibody-dependent cell-mediated cytolysis (ADCC) is illustrated by the lysis of antibody-coated tumor cells by lymphocytes. This classic ADCC reaction has been extensively studied by measuring the lysis of antibody-coated target cells by nonimmune effector cells that were not previously exposed to antibody. Interactions of the Fc portion of the antibody molecule with Fc receptors on effector cells are a prerequisite for this in vitro reaction; however, this type of reaction is known to be easily inhibited by even low levels of aggregated IgG that competes with target-bound antibody for Fc receptors on effector cells. It is thus quite obvious that "ADCC-like reactions" in vivo would certainly be much impaired by circulating immune complexes that are often prevalent in the circulation of cancer patients. One way to avoid inhibition of ADCC by immune complexes is to attach specific antibody to effector cells. This in vitro reaction, i.e., "antibody-directed ADCC," proved more effective and less sensitive to inhibition by immune complexes and aggregates of nonimmune IgG than did the classic ADCC reaction.

In another study, Schulz and coworkers (1983) observed that murine effector cells armed with an IgG2a monoclonal antibody highly specific for melanoma (mAb 9.2.27) could specifically kill these cells in vitro by a "directed ADCC" reaction. In this case, polyethylene glycol 20,000 (8 percent) was used to enhance binding of the antibody IgG nonspecifically to effector cells and thus to "arm" the effector cells. Data from ^{51}Cr release assays indicated that the directed ADCC was at least twice as effective as the classic ADCC reaction in inducing specific tumor cell killing. In fact, only the directed ADCC reaction clearly exceeded background, as it showed a statistically significant reactivity (p <0.001) compared with that of natural killer (NK) cells.

The role of macrophages and monocytes as effector cells involved in tumor killing has not yet been critically evaluated in the human melanoma system. However, macrophages and monocytes have been implicated as effector cells in the killing of colorectal cancer cells. Fc receptors present in both of these cell types were found to strongly cross-react only with immuno-globulins of IgG2a isotype. Moreover, macrophages, in the presence of murine monoclonal antibody of IgG2a isotype, specifically mediated the killing of colorectal tumor cells in vitro. Taken together, all these data from experiments conducted in several laboratories strongly support the hypothesis that murine IgG2a monoclonal antibodies directed against human tumor-associated antigens may prove effective in aiding the therapy of human neoplasms.

In Vivo Studies

Initial experiments performed by Koprowski and colleagues (1978) demonstrated that monoclonal antibodies to melanoma were able to suppress the growth of human melanoma tumors in athymic (nu/nu) mice. These mice, which received 2×10^6 hybridoma cells secreting monoclonal antibody 2 days prior to receiving a challenge of 10^7 melanoma cells failed to establish tumors that grew rapidly in control animals that expired after 36 days. In another experiment, Bumol and coworkers (1983) also could suppress melanoma tumor growth in athymic (nu/nu) mice that received multiple doses (40 µg/each) of mAb 9.2.27 two to three days after the injection of tumor cells. While it was possible to suppress tumor growth by 60 percent in these experiments, it should be emphasized that residual melanoma cells formed tumors again, which ultimately killed the nude mice. Taken together, these data demonstrate that under ideal conditions, administration of monoclonal antibody per se may prevent a tumor from establishing itself, but that this regimen will not be useful to effectively inhibit the growth of well-established tumors.

It was against this background of events, and because of the encouraging results obtained in vitro with murine effector cell–antibody conjugates in the directed ADCC, that experiments were initiated to test this entire concept in vivo (Schulz et al., 1983). Some encouraging observations were made initially when nude mice implanted subcutaneously with human melanoma cells (7.5×10^6) received, 1 day later, several intravenous injections of 2×10^6 effector cells—i.e., mononuclear cells from normal BALB/c mice, "armed" with 40 µg of mAb 9.2.27 IgG. It was only in this group of animals that the tumors remained very small and necrotic and were "biologically dead" once the injection of conjugates was stopped after 12 days. Another group of animals that received an equal number of injections of 40 µg mAb 9.2.27 IgG per se showed ~ 60 percent suppression of tumor growth; however, the effect was transient. This was also true when effector cells, either alone or treated with 8 percent polyethylene glycol, were administered to several groups of animals. In other words, at day 32, when the experiments were terminated, tumors were growing rapidly in all treatment groups, with the notable exception of those animals that received the effector cells "armed" with mAb 9.2.27.

The results from these experiments, however, did not establish that effector cells "armed" with a specific antitumor monoclonal antibody could effectively inhibit the growth of established tumors. This concept was tested, and it was discovered that a single intravenous injection of 2×10^7 effector cells plus 400 µg mAb 9.2.27 IgG completely eliminated relatively large (mean volume = 90 mm^3) melanoma tumors that had been established in nude mice for 14 days prior to any injection of effector cell–antibody conjugates.

PERSPECTIVES

It was the purpose of this selective review to document the decisive impact made by monoclonal antibodies on structural and functional studies dealing with human tumor antigens. Indeed, these highly specific reagents have served as excellent molecular probes and have contributed considerably to recent progress made not only in melanoma antigens (used here as only one example) but in the entire field of tumor biology. This brief review also attempted to point to some of the limitations of monoclonal antibodies, especially when dealing with highly complex and heterogeneous populations of tumor cells. It is hoped that the reader realizes that the application of monoclonal antibodies to the diagnosis and therapy of human cancer is still very much at the beginning. It is obvious that new and imaginative ways will have to be explored to produce and apply monoclonal antibodies in such a way that they will effectively contribute toward the elimination of cancer.

ACKNOWLEDGMENTS

The author's research has been supported in part by NIH grant CA 28420. The author also would like to acknowledge that his colleagues, Drs. J. R. Harper, G. Schulz, and D. A. Cheresh, kindly made some of their data available that are either currently in press or submitted for publication. The author wishes to thank Ms. Bonnie Filiault for her excellent assistance in the typing of this manuscript.

Bibliography

Brown, J. P., Nishiyama, K., Hellstrom, I., et al.: Structural characterization of human melanoma–associated antigen p97 with monoclonal antibodies. J. Immunol. 127:539, 1981.

Brown, J. P., Hewick, R. M., Hellstrom, I., et al.: Human melanoma–associated antigen p97 is structurally and functionally related to transferrin. Nature 296:171, 1982.

Bumol, T. F., and Reisfeld, R. A.: Unique glycoprotein-proteoglycan complex defined by monoclonal antibody in human melanoma cells. Proc. Natl. Acad. Sci. USA 79:1245, 1982.

Bumol, T. F., Chee, D. O., and Reisfeld, R. A.: Immunochemical and biosynthetic analysis of monoclonal antibody–defined melanoma-associated antigens. Hybridoma 1:2;83, 1982.

Bumol, T. F., Wang, O. C., Reisfeld, R. A., et al.: Monoclonal antibody and antibody-toxin conjugate to a cell surface proteoglycan of melanoma cells suppress *in vivo* tumor growth. Proc. Natl. Acad. Sci. USA 80:529, 1983.

Cheresh, D. A., Varki, A. P., Varki, N. M., et al.: A monoclonal antibody recognizes an O-acylated sialic acid in human melanoma–associated ganglioside. J. Biol. Chem. 259:7453, 1984.

Dippold, W. G., Lloyd, K. O., Li, T. L., et al.: Cell surface antigens of human melanoma cells: definition of six antigenic systems with monoclonal antibodies. Proc. Natl. Acad. Sci. USA 77:6114, 1980.

Gold, P., Freedman, S. O., and Shuster, J.: Carcinoembryonic antigen. In Herberman, R. B., and McIntyre, K. R. (eds.): Immunodiagnosis of Cancer, Vol. 1. New York, Marcel Dekker, 1979, pp. 147–168.

Harper, J. R., and Reisfeld, R. A.: Inhibition of anchorage-independent growth of human melanoma cells by a monoclonal antibody to a chondroitin sulfate proteoglycan. J. Natl. Canc. Inst. 71:259, 1983.

Harper, J. R., Bumol, T. F., and Reisfeld, R. A.: Characterization of monoclonal antibody 155.8 and partial characterization of its proteoglycan antigen on human melanoma cells. J. Immunol. 132:2096, 1984.

Heidelberger, C.: Chemical carcinogenesis. Ann. Rev. Biochem. 44:79, 1975.

Kirkpatrick, C. H., and Fahey, J. H.: Tumor immunology: clinical aspects. JAMA 248:2722, 1982.

Klein, G.: The Epstein-Barr virus and neoplasia. N. Engl. J. Med. 293:1353, 1975.

Koldovsky, P.: Tumor specific transplantation antigens. In Rentchnik, P. (ed.): Recent Results in Cancer Research, Vol. 22. New York, Springer Verlag, 1969, pp. 113–133.

Koprowski, H., Steplewski, Z., Herlyn, D., et al.: Study of antibodies against human melanoma produced by somatic cell hybrids. Proc. Natl. Acad. Sci. USA 75:3405, 1978.

Nudelman, E. S., Hakomori, S., Kannagi, R., et al.: Characterization of a human melanoma–associated ganglioside antigen defined by a monoclonal antibody. J. Biol. Chem. 257:12752, 1982.

Schulz, G., Bumol, T. F., and Reisfeld, R. A.: Melanoma antibody–directed effector cells selectively lyse human melanoma cells in vitro and in vivo. Proc. Natl. Acad. Sci. USA 80:5407, 1983.

Schulz, G., Staffileno, C. U., Reisfeld, R. A., et al.: Eradication of established human melanoma tumors in nude mice by antibody directed effector cells. J. Exp. Med. 161:1315, 1985.

Sell, S.: Alpha-fetoprotein. In Sell, S. (ed.): Cancer Markers, Vol. 1. Clifton, NJ, The Humana Press, 1980, pp. 249–284.

18

Immunopharmacology: Immunosuppression and Immunopotentiation

JOHN W. HADDEN, M.D.,
and LYNNE MERRIAM, R.N.

INTRODUCTION

Immunopharmacology, a new field of study, is concerned with regulation of the immune system and its selective modification during treatment of human disease. Since the function of the immunoglobulins was first defined in the 1950s, they have been used for the treatment of agammaglobulinemia, prophylaxis of hepatitis, and in conjunction with live attenuated vaccines. Elucidation of severe combined immunodeficiency disease (SCID) by 1960 brought treatment by bone marrow transplantation, now a successful and currently accepted therapy. In recent years bone marrow transplantation has been done experimentally to treat marrow aplasia and certain leukemias, with encouraging results (see Chapter 9). Delineation of cellular immune functions and mechanisms of allograft rejection has led to immunosuppressive therapy for renal transplantation and for selected use in autoimmune disease. During the past 20 years, demonstration of the prevalence of cellular immune defects in cancer, aging, autoimmunity, and infectious diseases has generated interest in the development of immunotherapeutic agents, sometimes called "biologic response modifiers." Though currently largely experimental, work in this field to date indicates that a variety of biologicals and drugs will shortly be used in the therapy of a number of human diseases. This chapter summarizes salient features of this new field.

IMMUNOSUPPRESSIVE THERAPY (Table 18–1)

A great deal has been learned from experiences with kidney transplants, of which more than 76,000 had been completed by 1984, 5600 per year at the end of that period. Hepatic and cardiac transplants continue with increasing frequency. Although the goal of tolerance induction to alloantigens has not been achieved, high graft acceptance rates have been accomplished with intense initial immunosuppressive therapy and relatively nominal maintenance immunosuppression. The problem of secondary infections, particularly with certain viruses (CMV, Epstein-Barr, and Herpes), and a high, but acceptable, rate of cancer in these transplant patients may be overcome by more selective future therapies. The agents currently in use for renal transplants are azathioprine, glucocorticoids, antilymphocyte globulins (ALG), and cyclosporin A.

Renal Transplantation

Azathioprine (Imuran)

This nitroimidazole derivative of 6-mercaptopurine (6-MP) is thought to act as a specific antagonist of DNA synthesis and

Table 18–1. Immunosuppressive Agents

Immunosuppressive Agent	Source	Dose/Route	Mode of Action	Side Effects	Use
Azathioprine (Imuran)	Synthetic imidazolyl derivative of 6-MP	Initial: 3–5 mg/kg/day Maintenance: 1–3 mg/kg/day Oral	Interferes with nucleic acid metabolism — preferentially suppressive for T cells	Leukopenia Secondary cancer	Renal transplantation
Glucocorticosteroids (Prednisone, etc.)	Synthetic steroid hormones from adrenal gland	1–50 mg/day Oral	Impairs T-lymphocyte and macrophage function	Cushing's syndrome Peptic ulcer	Transplantation Autoimmunity Allergic disorders
Antilymphocyte globulin (ATGAM)	Antibody from heterologous species	For acute rejection: 10 mg/kg/day IV	Masks T-lymphocyte surface and lyses B and T cells	Serum sickness reactions	Transplantation
Cyclosporin A	Cyclic polypeptide derived from a strain of fungi imperfectii	10–25 mg/kg/day Oral	Preferentially suppressive for T cells	Hepatic and renal toxicity Secondary cancer	Transplantation GVH disease
Cyclophosphamide (Cytoxan)	Synthetic	Loading dose: 40–50 mg/kg IV	Destroys proliferating lymphoid cells and alkylates resting cells	Cystitis and pancytopenia, anemia GI toxicity Secondary cancer	Bone marrow transplantation Autoimmunity Cancer

cellular replication by inhibiting de novo purine synthesis, principally mediated by the intracellular metabolite thioinosinic acid. This drug is only moderately suppressive of the hematopoietic system, and at doses of 3 to 5 mg/kg/day initially (maintenance is 1–3 mg/kg/day) its major side effects are neutropenia and monocytopenia. Hair loss, GI toxicity, and lymphopenia are minimal, and lymphocyte function is readily restored by discontinuance of therapy. The effects of azathioprine and 6-MP are thought to be selective for T-cell–mediated responses. With usual clinical doses, immunoglobulin levels fall slightly and return to normal levels, and antibody-mediated responses remain intact. Secondary infections with high-grade pyogenic pathogens are not a significant problem. The effect of azathioprine on T cells includes inhibition of proliferation, lymphokine production, and cytotoxicity. Cytotoxic responses by NK cells and macrophages are also thought to be impaired, in part through inhibition of lymphokine production (interferon, interleukin 2, and migration inhibition factor [MIF]). The effects on T cells are manifested by allograft acceptance, anergy, and increased susceptibility to infection, particularly with fungi, mycobacteria, and viruses like CMV, as well as an increased incidence of cancer, especially lymphoblastic lymphoma and Kaposi's sarcoma (CMV-linked).

There is an alternative explanation for the reversible effects of azathioprine at clinically used doses. Lymphocytes preferentially reutilize rather than synthesize purines de novo and are exquisitely sensitive to enzymatic defects in the purine salvage pathway. Inhibition of RNA synthesis through action on enzymes of this pathway seems likely. Additionally, the capacity of murine T cells to bind to sheep erythrocytes is sensitive to low doses of azathioprine. A purine receptor has been postulated that regulates T-lymphocyte differentiation and function to account for the immunostimulating actions of certain purines and of transfer factor; it may be that azathioprine and 6-MP are antagonists of this receptor. Such a mechanism would explain the observed selectivity of azathioprine and 6-MP for T cells.

The potent anti-inflammatory activity mediated by these two drugs is partly due to their actions on macrophages and granule-containing cells, including polymorphonuclear leukocytes (PMNs) and mast cells. Azathioprine is generally used clinically in combination with glucocorticosteroids in the management of allograft transplantation and also in SLE (particularly when complicated by vasculitis and nephritis), autoimmune blood dyscrasias (anemia, neutropenia, and thrombocytopenia), Wegener's granulomatosis, chronic active hepatitis, and severe rheumatoid arthritis.

Glucocorticosteroids

These have been extensively used in the treatment of aberrent immune responses such as allergy and autoimmunity, as well as in organ allograft rejection, graft-versus-host (GVH) disease, and certain leukemias. The many steroid preparations available for local, oral, and parenteral administration vary in potency and side effects. Prednisone (5–100 mg/day) is most often used. It converts in vivo to its active metabolite, prednisolone. All preparations may induce side effects, among which are fluid accumulation, euphoria, hirsutism, "buffalo hump," moon facies, striae, and suppression of the pituitary-adrenal axis. These effects may be diminished or avoided by administering the drug on alternate days.

Glucocorticosteroids act by binding to a receptor protein and subsequently to nuclear receptor sites that regulate the synthesis of specific proteins. They induce specific responses, inhibit others, influence membrane enzyme activation, and modulate the sensitivity of the adenylate cyclase/cyclic AMP system.

The mechanisms by which corticosteroids influence the immune system are not entirely clear and vary in different species, e.g., glucocorticoids lyse immature T cells in the steroid-sensitive species mouse and rat, an effect not observed in man. In man, the traffic of lymphocytes is affected, and an intravenous injection of a short-acting steroid will induce an absolute lymphopenia of both T and B cells ($<1000/mm^3$), with a nadir at 4 to 8 hours followed by a return to normal levels by 24 hours. Lymphopenia results from altered recirculation and transient sequestration of lymphocytes, principally in bone marrow. Circulation of granulocytes is also affected, and injection of steroids causes neutrophilia, monocytopenia, and eosinopenia as the result of both altered release from the bone marrow and exodus from the circulation. Functions of the cells are also impaired; e.g., there is impaired macrophage proliferation and activation as well as impaired response to lymphokines. Mediator release is also impaired. These suppressive effects on mediator release probably account for the anti-inflammatory actions of steroids. Phagocytosis and bactericidal properties are relatively spared.

Effects on B-cell function in vitro are relatively minimal, and in vivo suppression of immunoglobulin and antibody production is mild and transient.

The T-cell effects are greater and are modulated by macrophages, which make a steroid binding and inactivating factor. All functions of mature T cells are affected, including proliferation, lymphokine production, cytotoxicity, and helper and suppressor activity. There is close correlation between serum prednisolone levels during therapy and suppression of lymphocyte proliferation and interleukin 2 production in mixed leukocyte cultures. The major mechanism of immunosuppression is thought to be on T-cell and macrophage function and on their collaboration through cytokine release. The clinical manifestations of these effects are anti-inflammatory and antiallergic at relatively low doses, and anergy with depression of cellular immune responses at higher doses. Immunosuppressive side effects generally involve infection with viruses (herpes zoster and simplex), fungi (*Candida albicans*), and intracellular pathogens (*Mycobacterium tuberculosis*).

Antilymphocyte Globulin (ALG)

Antilymphocyte antibody has been produced by horses, goats, and rabbits; partially purified globulins have been prepared from their sera, and one is now commecially available as ATGAM (horse gamma globulin—Upjohn). The antibody masks the lymphocyte surface, and in the presence of complement both T and B cells are lysed, resulting in lymphocytopenia that is reversible on discontinuance of therapy. Side effects are those of other immunosuppressives inhibiting both T and B cells. General use of this antibody was limited by unavailability and induction of allergic reactions to the heterologous proteins. Its use is adjunctive in allograft recipients who are steroid intolerant and in some autoimmune disorders. Monoclonal antibodies selective for T cells will in the future provide more specific therapy.

Cyclosporin A

Derived from the fungus *Tolypocladium inflatum gams*, this hexadecapeptide selectively inhibits T-cell proliferation, cytotoxicity, and lymphokine production, without destroying cells. At clinical doses (5–10 mg/kg/day) there are no antiproliferative effects on other organ systems. Although the mechanism of its action is not known, it has been shown to impair renal allograft rejection and, both alone and in combination with glucocorticoids, to inhibit GVH disease after bone marrow transplantation. Side effects of cyclosporin A include hepatic and renal toxicity, but to a tolerable degree because its steroid-sparing effect allows use of less toxic doses of those agents. Secondary malignancies occur with a significant incidence, comparable to that following azathioprine and steroids.

Cyclophosphamide

The most frequent uses for this drug are as an immunosuppressive and, with glucocorticosteroids, in severe rheumatoid arthritis and systemic lupus erythematosus. This alkylating agent specifically inhibits cell replication, preferentially of B lymphocytes, and therefore impairs both immunoglobulin and antibody production. At clinical doses (2–3 mg/kg), proliferating lymphoid cells are destroyed; side effects include depressed erythro- and myelopoiesis, hemorrhagic cystitis, alopecia, sterility, GI disturbances, secondary infection, and malignancy following long-term use. High doses destroy both B and T cells, and the drug may augment cellular immune responses, perhaps by a selective effect on T suppressor cells.

Other Immunosuppressive Therapies

Although total body or regional irradiation, methotrexate, thoracic duct drainage, surgical removal of lymphoid tissue, and high-dose interferon are known immunosuppressives, none are accepted for clinical use. Future prospects for drugs in this category include prostaglandin analogs, cyclomunine, procarbazine, oxisuran, niridazole, genetically engineered lymphoid specific chalones, and immunosuppressive alpha$_2$-macroglobulin.

IMMUNOTOXIC CHEMICAL AGENTS (Anticancer Drugs)

Anticancer drugs inhibit marrow and lymphoid proliferation, effects that define limiting toxicities. Granulocytopenia with secondary infection is the single most common effect, but anemia and thrombocytopenia are also common. Profound immunosuppression is a general feature of cancer chemotherapy, particularly with multiple agents. Infections with common pathogens as well as with opportunistic organisms are frequent in treated cancer patients, and infections are the most frequent cause of death. While anticancer agents differ in their immunosuppressive effects, intensive radiotherapy and such drugs as steroids, chlorambucil, busulfan, thioguanine, cyclophosphamide, hydroxyurea, daunorubicin, carmustine (BCNU), cytosine arabinoside, methotrexate, adriamycin, bleomycin, and L-asparaginase are potently immunosuppressive when used in combined protocols. These drugs singly, and others such as 5-fluorouracil and actinomycin-D, are less immunosuppressive.

These agents have different effects on the immune system, sometimes stimulating certain cells and functions. Actinomycin D, for example, restores immune response in mice by impairing tumor-induced immunosuppression. The successes of cancer immunotherapy have principally derived from combined chemoimmunotherapy protocols. Immunotherapy will be more specifically designed as the actions of the chemotherapeutic agents become better understood.

ENVIRONMENTAL CHEMICALS

These are included not as therapeutic agents but because modification of them may yield useful anticancer drugs, and prolonged exposure to them may induce cancer.

Benzene exposure, particularly when extreme, is associated with marrow and lymphoid suppression, and chronic exposure in man has been associated with suppression of complement and immunoglobulins.

Polychlorinated biphenyls (PCBs) are widespread environmental contaminants that, in high doses, induce immunosuppression in animals and decreased resistance to microbes.

Polybrominated biphenyls (PBBs), used as flame retardants, were introduced into a local food chain in Michigan in 1973 when they were accidentally mixed with livestock feed. Affected animals died of thymic atrophy, immune deficiency, and infection; local farmers, who ingested the meat and dairy products, manifested depressed T-cell numbers and augmented immunoglobulin levels and dermal reactivity.

Polycyclic aromatic hydrocarbons are products of combustion of fossil fuels; high doses are immunosuppressive for both T- and B-cell–mediated immunity and are carcinogenic.

Tetrachlorodibenzodioxin (dioxin), a contaminant of defoliants, is immunosuppressive in animals. Accidental exposure, including use in Vietnam, has been studied but has not been demonstrated to be immunosuppressive in man.

Asbestos, as asbestos fiber, is carcinogenic and has recently been linked to immune defects; asbestosis patients have been demonstrated to have impaired T-cell function, and some patients also have had increased serum immunoglobulin levels.

Insecticides—organophosphates, carbonates, and organochlorines—produce immunotoxic effects at high, near lethal, doses; low-level exposure is generally considered safe.

Metals, specifically industrial exposure to metals such as lead, mercury, nickel, and cadmium, have been associated with increased susceptibility to infection.

Abused drugs such as ethanol, cannabinoids, and opiates have been implicated, both directly and indirectly (i.e., through associated abnormal lifestyles and malnutrition), as contributors to impaired immune response and resistance.

Certain prescribed drugs, e.g., nonsteroidal anti-inflammatory drugs, dilantin, anesthetics, diethylstilbestrol, beta-lactam antibiotics, and cimetidine, have been demonstrated to modulate immune response.

IMMUNOSTIMULATION (Table 18–2)

Immunostimulatory agents were first used in a few primary and secondary cellular immune deficiency diseases. After the

Table 18–2. Immunostimulatory Agents

Immuno-stimulant	Mode of Action	Experimental and Clinical Uses				
		Immuno-deficiency	Vaccine	Cancer	Infection	Auto-immunity
Thymic hormone	T-cell differentiation / modulation	+	NT*	+	+	+
Lymphokine	Effector cell activation	NT	NT	+	NT	NT
Interferon	Antiviral	–	–	+ +	+	–
Drugs						
Levamisole	Potentiator	+	+	+	+	+ +
Isoprinosine	Thymomimetic	+	+	NT	+ +	+
MDP*	MØ activator*	NT	+ +	NT	NT	NT

*MDP = muramyl dipeptide; MØ = macrophage; NT = not tested.

association of cellular immunodeficiency with cancer was noted, the development of biologicals and drugs was expanded, and they were used experimentally to treat cancer. A number of these agents have produced a small increase in survival of patients who are potentially curable by primary cytoreductive therapy, i.e., chemotherapy, surgery, or irradiation. This is "remission stabilization," and such therapy is ineffective as a single therapy in active, progressive cancer. Some of the drugs in this class have been effective in the treatment of immunodeficiency associated with infection and autoimmunity, but their effect on the incidence of infection in treated cancer patients has not been adequately assessed. All of these agents are classed as experimental in the United States, and none have been approved by the FDA; a number have been licensed in Europe and Japan, where wide use appears to have supported their safety and efficacy.

Biologicals

Thymic Hormones

The epithelial cells of the thymus produce a number of hormones that collectively induce the maturation of immature T cells and modulate functionally mature T cells. The levels of those hormones that appear in the circulation decline rapidly after thymectomy, and slowly as the thymus involutes with age. Thymosin fraction 5 and thymostimulin are two partially purified thymic extracts in widespread use. Four other hormones, extracted from these preparations or from serum, include:

a. *Thymosin alpha 1*, which has been produced by genetic engineering.

b. *Thymulin,* which has been synthesized chemically, requires zinc for its activity.

c. *Thymopoietin,* which, along with its active site, thymopentin (TP5), has been synthesized.

d. *Thymic humoral factor,* which has not yet been sequenced.

Each of the purified hormones is chemically distinct, yet all function to modulate T-cell function and cell-mediated immunity in vivo and to mature and modulate the function of thymocytes. Expected differences in their activities remain to be clearly identified.

The extracts are derived from bovine sources and therefore are capable of inducing local or systemic allergic reactions. The purified preparations are all of low molecular weight (<4000) and are poorly or not at all immunogenic. Animal studies reveal that one or another of these hormone preparations will partially restore immune defects associated with aging, cancer, and autoimmunity, or following immunosuppressive therapy, and will increase survival after various pathogen and tumor challenges.

Administration of these preparations has, under a variety of circumstances, increased T-cell numbers and receptor display, reactivity to alloantigens and mitogens, and certain parameters of depressed cell-mediated immunity. Thymosin, thymopoietin, and thymulin have increased T-cell number and function in congenital immunodeficiency, particularly in the DiGeorge syndrome and SCID with B cells. Thymosin fraction 5 and/or thymosin alpha 1 have been active in lung, head and neck, and renal cell cancer. In patients with rheumatoid arthritis, thymulin and thymopoietin have both shown activity to reduce signs and symptoms and help to correct immunologic abnormalities as measured by laboratory tests. Thymic humoral factor has been reported to be effective in viral infections.

Lymphokines

These products of activated lymphocytes play a central role in regulating the cellular immune response. Examples are MIF, T-cell growth factor (TCGF, or interleukin 2), colony stimulating factor (CSF), and gamma interferon. Therapeutic potentials are under exploration. Crude preparations, which are devoid of interferon, are active in tumor-bearing mice and in human breast cancer. Several have been purified to homogeneity, and interleukin 2 and gamma interferon have been produced by gene cloning of bacteria. Defects of interleukin 2 have been described in cancer, AIDS, aging, and autoimmunity, and therapy trials in these conditions can be expected.* Interleukin 1 (produced by macrophages) and interleukin 2 promote maturation as well as function of the T-cell system, so their use in conjunction with thymic hormones can be envisioned.

Interferons

These are produced by several cell types on stimulation by viruses or other stimuli. Alpha interferon is produced by leukocytes of various types, and more than 16 distinct genetic types have been identified with some heterogeneity of action. Gamma, or immune, interferon is produced by antigen- or mitogen-activated T cells. All interferons share the capacity to inhibit replication of DNA and RNA viruses and of normal and malignant cells, as well as the ability to modulate the immune system. Interferons activate microbicidal function and, at lower doses, stimulate the immune system, principally by increasing cytocidal activity of natural killer (NK) cells, macrophages, and T cells. High doses inhibit both T- and B-cell proliferation and decrease humoral and, especially, cellular immune responses.

Interferons, given prophylactically, nasally or parenterally, can prevent certain virus infections but are therapeutically less active. They have been effective in virus infections such as chronic active hepatitis (HB+) and in herpes zoster and in virus-related disorders such as laryngeal polyposis and venereal warts. Given in high doses in treatment of various cancers they have had varied results:

a. Significant palliation has occurred in hairy cell leukemia, non-Hodgkin's lymphoma, and multiple myeloma; in nasopharyngeal, renal cell, and bladder carcinoma; in osteogenic sarcoma (following surgery) and Kaposi's sarcoma; and in malignant melanoma, when given in combination with cimetidine.

b. Complete regression has been observed occasionally in renal cell carcinoma and Kaposi's sarcoma.

c. Little or no effect has been observed with carcinoma of the lung or pancreas.

The antitumor effect of interferons results from immune modulation in part, and their efficacy will probably improve when combined with cytoreductive and other forms of therapy.

---

*A successful trial of interleukin 2 in therapy of advanced cancer has already been reported by Rosenberg.

Leukocyte Extracts

Leukocyte extracts that have been studied clinically have been identified as immunogenic RNA, dialyzed leukocyte extract (DLE), and transfer factor (TF). Their chemical structures have not been completely worked out, but both nonspecific immunoenhancement and specific transfer of delayed-type hypersensitivity have been demonstrated with them. TF contains inosine and may share activities identified with inosine-like compounds discussed in the next section. The preparations have been used with encouraging results in mucocutaneous candidiasis, leprosy, and Wiskott-Aldrich syndrome. Encouraging results have also been obtained in acute and chronic infections such as disseminated vaccinia, measles pneumonia, and congenital herpes simplex, herpes zoster, and CMV infection. A few reports of benefit of immunogenic RNA and TF in cancer are also encouraging. Improved in vitro assays and better chemical definition to assess cell targets and reveal mechanisms of action should provide the basis for improved clinical results.

Bacterial Products

BCG (bacille Calmette Guérin) and *Corynebacterium parvum* heralded the last decade of immunotherapeutic efforts, when encouraging results in treating antigenic animal tumors led to widespread clinical trials. However, it developed that the favorable responses with BCG (in cutaneous melanoma, bladder cancer and osteogenic sarcoma) were so rare and its toxicity so great that a general moratorium was called on the use of these agents, and emphasis shifted to the biologicals derived from the immune system and to chemically defined drugs. There are still some bacterial preparations under study, e.g., *Klebsiella, Brucella,* and mixed bacterial vaccines, but they are likely to share the same fate. Endotoxins or lipopolysaccharides (LPS) are immunologically active components of gram-negative organisms and have been recently detoxified by chemical modification without loss of immunologic activity, stimulating a resurgence of interest in them. Anti-infectious and antitumor activity have been reported when animals were treated with LPS in combination with BCG or *C. parvum* (which yields tumor necrosis factor [TNF]).

Fungal Products

A number of fungi have yielded β-1,3-polyglycans (glucans), which are high-molecular-weight compounds that activate macrophages and expand the reticuloendothelial (RE) system. Two preparations, krestin and lentinan, are licensed in Japan and have been used extensively in the treatment of cancer. A 20 to 40 percent increase in survival of gastric cancer patients treated with glucans in combination with other means of therapy has been reported. A few studies have been performed in the United States.

Chemically Defined Immunostimulating Agents

Levamisole

The discovery that this phenylimidothiazole antihelminthic reversed anergy in some cancer patients led to extensive evaluation of its effectiveness in treating cancer and other diseases and of its immunopharmacology. The compound potentiates the stimulating effects of antigen, mitogen, lymphokine, and chemotactic factors on lymphocytes, granulocytes, and macrophages, and therefore modifies proliferation, secretion, and motility. The effects, which are small and inconsistent, are mediated by changes in cellular levels of cyclic GMP and, via its sulfur moiety, by induction of a thymic hormone–like factor in blood. The effects in man are weak, and a considerable time span is often required before they occur. Enhancement of cell-mediated immunity is greater than that of humoral immunity. Clinical trials have shown small but consistent effects to increase survival by 15 percent in patients with head and neck, breast, lung, and gastrointestinal cancers. Benefits have been reported in rheumatoid arthritis (equivalent to penicillamine), aphthous stomatitis, recurrent herpes simplex, leprosy, erythema multiforme, and SLE. Side effects include nausea and vomiting, skin rash, a "flu-like" syndrome, and reversible agranulocytosis. Low efficacy and significant side effects have prompted a search for more active agents. Since the sulfur moiety of the compound is immunologically active, a number of similar compounds are under study. These include diethyldithiocarbamate (DIC), NPT 16416, thiabendazole, and thiazolobenzimidazole. More consistent activity and less toxicity makes these coupounds of interest.

Isoprinosine

This drug, a complex of p-acetoamidobenzoic acid, N,N-dimethyl-amino-2 propanol, and inosine (3:1 molar ratio), is licensed as an antiviral and immunostimulating agent in 74 countries, but not in the United States. It inhibits replication of several viruses, but high concentrations are required, and its maximal antiviral activity does not equal that effected by anti-metabolite antiviral compounds. The drug is nontoxic, and hyperuricemia has been reported as the only consistent side effect. It has been given to thousands of patients for treatment of viral disorders. Significant efficacy of a mild to moderate degree has been observed in well-controlled studies; reduction of symptoms, shortened disease duration, and decreased recurrences have been accomplished in subacute sclerosing panencephalitis (SSPE), herpes simplex Types 1 and 2, influenza, and rhinovirus infections.

Antiviral activity might explain these clinical results, but effects on the immune system are more likely. The drug induces lymphocyte differentiation comparable to thymic hormones and augments lymphocyte, macrophage, and NK cell functions. Activity of the drug has been more consistent than levamisole. Considerable data substantiate its augmentation of virus-specific cellular and humoral responses and of nonspecific immune responses such as mitogen and lymphokine responses.

Isoprinosine is active in several murine tumors and in autoimmune disease. It has promoted restoration of immune functions in cancer patients.

A number of structurally similar compounds have been studied. NPT 15392 (9-erythro-2-hydroxy-3-nonylhypoxanthine) shares the activities of isoprinosine at lower dosage. NPT 15392 induces differentiation and augments and modulates proliferative, helper, and suppressor functions of T cells. It also increases macrophage and NK cell activity. Side effects have been negligible; significant augmentation of antibody, NK cell, and cellular immune responses have been noted in mice. Murine tumor–, virus-, and chemotherapy-induced immunosuppression have been partially reversed by NPT 15392, correlating with increased survival or decreased metastasis formation. Trials in cancer patients have shown that the drug augments lymphocyte counts, active rosettes, and NK cells in some but not all patients. Clinical studies with this drug continue.

Muramyl Dipeptide

Muramyl dipeptide (MDP) is the smallest active component of the mycobacterial cell wall having adjuvant activity characteristic of complete Freund's adjuvant (CFA). Since it is water-soluble, it can be given by mouth, and a series of analogs have been made, particularly by French and Japanese investigators.

MDP has adjuvant potential when administered with antigen, and also has potential in protecting against challenge by virulent bacteria when given before and, to an extent, with the pathogen. MDP also induces fever and prostaglandin production by macrophages, both of which are prevented by inhibition of prostaglandin synthesis. The n-butyl ester derivative murabutide has both adjuvant and protective activity but does not induce fever. MDP promotes macrophage activation for tumoricidal and bactericidal activity and for secretion of enzymes and monokines. Combined with oil and antigen, MDP augments both humoral and cellular immunity. Though the major interest in MDP has been as an adjuvant with vaccines, it appears useful in cancer immunotherapy to prevent tumor recurrence and infections in which the macrophage plays a role in resistance. A complementary role might well be observed with lymphokines or isoprinosine. Murabutide has recently been introduced for toxicologic evaluation and clinical trials.

Azimexon

This orally active immunostimulating compound is under development for use in cancer. In vitro studies reveal direct action on both lymphocytes and macrophages, and in vivo, there is augmented cell-mediated immunity, T-cell–dependent humoral immunity, and NK cell activity, as well as expansion of the RE system with splenomegaly and leukocytosis. Its only significant side effect has been a dose-related toxic hemolytic anemia that may limit its clinical application to malignant diseases. The drug is more active than levamisole in increasing survival and longevity in cancerous animals when used as an adjuvant with irradiation and chemotherapy. Experimental use in human patients has effected improvement of a number of immune functions.

Bestatin

This low-molecular substance, extracted from *Streptomyces olivoreticuli*, is a nontoxic, orally active immunostimulator that probably acts on lymphocytes and macrophages. Increases in antibody production and restoration of immunologic function have been observed in tumor-bearing or chemotherapy-treated mice, together with some tumor growth inhibition. Toxicity in man has been negligible, and uncontrolled trials in small numbers of patients have been encouraging.

Tuftsin

Tuftsin represents residues 289 to 292 of the heavy chain of gamma globulin. It is liberated after cleavage and acts to stimulate tumoricidal or bactericidal activity of macrophages, neutrophils, and NK cells. It is a nontoxic peptide with effects apparently mediated in part by elevations of cellular cyclic GMP levels. Administration of tuftsin to mice activates macrophages for tumoricidal activity and increases antibody production and antibody-dependent cytotoxicity. Tuftsin prolonged survival in several murine tumors and, in aged mice, reduced the incidence of spontaneous neoplasms. It has not yet been used in humans.

Pyran Copolymers

Maleic anhydridedivinyl ether copolymers (MVE) have varying molecular weights; MVE-2 (15,500 daltons) is minimally toxic and has been well tolerated in animals while inducing RE expansion, its primary cell target appearing to be the macrophage. Interferon may be involved in macrophage activation, and it has been observed to increase lymphocyte numbers and functions and to potentiate delayed hypersensitivity. It has also been effective in virus and tumor challenge systems in mice. The mixed copolymers have been used in treating patients with cancer and have shown interferon induction, fever, chills, malaise, coagulation defects, leukopenia, and acute tubular necrosis of the kidney. Phase I trials with MVE-2 are in progress.

Pyrimidinoles

Interferon inducers are usually toxic, and a refractory state follows their administration. The 6-phenyl pyrimidoles are interesting in that they have antiviral and antitumor activity because they activate macrophages and NK cells. Clinical trials are currently in progress in the United States.

CONCLUSION

Figure 18–1 summarizes the effects of various immunotherapeutic agents on the immune system. These agents, which represent only a partial list of the biologicals and chemicals that have potential use in immunotherapy, have potential application

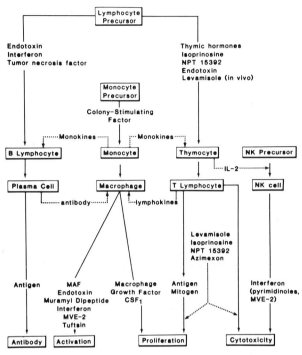

Figure 18–1. A summary of the effects of immunotherapeutic agents on the immune system.

in immune deficiency, infection, aging, and autoimmunity. No single agent can effect a cure, but an agent may be employed in combination with chemotherapy, surgery, or radiation to reduce recurrence and infection resulting from immunosuppression. It is already apparent that combinations of immunotherapeutic agents offer potentiating interactions that require further exploration. Additional prospective cancer treatments include tumor vaccines, in vitro expansion of tumor-responsive lymphocyte clones, and radionuclide or toxin-armed hybridoma antibodies specific for the tumor. The prospects of more successful therapy of cancer are encouraging as more potent techniques of immunorestoration and activation are developed. These will surely develop in relation to success in appropriately employing active and nontoxic agents and in learning their optimal use in combination. The use of single and multiple agents in other immunodeficiency states associated with infection, autoimmunity, and aging represents an encouraging therapy frontier.

Bibliography

Dean, J. H., Murray, M. J., and Ward, E. C.: Toxic modifications of the immune system. *In* Doull, J., Klaassen, C. D., and Amdur, M. D. (eds.): Casarett and Doull's Toxicology: The Basic Science of Poisons, 3rd ed. (in press).

Ehrke, M. J., and Mihich, E.: Immunoregulation by chemotherapeutic agents. *In* Hadden, J. W., and Szentivanyi, A. (eds.): The Reticuloendothelial System: A Comprehensive Treatise, Vol. V. New York, Plenum Publishing Corp., 1985.

Gibson, G. G., Hubbard, R., and Parke, D. V.: Immunotoxicology. London, Academic Press, 1983.

Hadden, J. W.: Immunomodulators in the immunotherapy of cancer and other diseases. Trends in Pharmacology 3:191–194, 1982.

Hadden, J. W., Chedid, L., Dukor, P., et al.: Advances in Immunopharmacology 2. Oxford, Pergamon Press, 1983.

Hersh, E. M., Chirigos, M. A., and Mastrangelo, M. J.: Augmenting Agents in Cancer Therapy. New York, Raven Press, 1981.

Rosenberg, S. A.: The changing approach to cancer surgery. Hosp. Pract. 20:105–107, 113, 116–117, 1985.

Rosenberg, S. A., Lotze, M. T., Muul, L. M., et al.: Observations on the systemic administration of autologous lymphokine-activated killer cells and recombinant interleukin-2 to patients with metastatic cancer. N. Engl. J. Med. 313:1485, 1985.

Spreafico, F., Alberti, A., Allegrucie, M., et al.: On the mode of action of immunodepressive agents. *In* Hadden, J. W., et al. (eds.): Advances in Immunopharmacology 2. Oxford, Pergamon Press, 1983, pp. 745–752.

Spreafico, F., and Anaclerio, A.: Immunosuppressive agents. *In* Hadden, J. W., et al. (eds.): Immunopharmacology 3. New York, Plenum Medical Book Co., 1977, pp. 245–278.

Webb, D. R., Jr., and Winkelstein, A.: Immunosuppression, immunopotentiation and anti-inflammatory drugs. *In* Stites, D. P., et al. (eds.): Basic and Clinical Immunology. Lange Medical Publications, Los Altos, CA, 1982, pp. 277–292.

19

Climate, Weather, Air Pollution, and Environmental Control

JOHN E. SALVAGGIO, M.D.,
and MANUEL LOPEZ, M.D.

Introduction	Photochemical Smog
Outdoor Environment	**Indoor Environment**
Climate	Home Environment
Humidity	Work Environment
Temperature	**Management**
Barometric Pressure	Environmental Control
Air Pollution	Climate Therapy
Industrial Smog	

INTRODUCTION

This chapter reviews the important effect of nonimmunologic environmental factors on the production and aggravation of allergic symptoms. The separate effect on the allergic patient of climate, meteorologic changes, air pollution, and home environment is difficult to define because of the complex interrelationships of these factors. The outdoor and indoor environments are analyzed separately, but their actions are intimately interrelated.

OUTDOOR ENVIRONMENT

Climate

Climate, the average course or condition of weather at a particular place, is the result of multiple meteorologic factors, including temperature, barometric pressure, wind velocity, and humidity. Climate affects allergic patients indirectly by influencing the growth of pollen-producing plants and molds. Meteorologic factors also affect the growth of plants and the release of pollen (and mold spores) into the air, thus markedly influencing their atmospheric concentration. Thermal inversions, which are characterized by air stagnation, cause marked increases of pollens and spores as well as of other pollutants, with deleterious health effects. Winds of low velocity favor accumulation of atmospheric pollutants, whereas those of high velocity disperse particulates and decrease their concentration. Assessment of the effects of single climatic factors on allergic symptoms is difficult because of the indirect effects of all climatic factors on the atmospheric concentration of multiple aeroallergens and inorganic particulates, each of which may affect allergic patients.

Humidity

An increase in the symptoms of allergic patients is frequently associated with changes in humidity. High humidity aggravates certain asthmatic patients, several studies having reported increased airway resistance in such patients exposed to high humidity. However, nonhumid heated air may dry respiratory mucosa and also exacerbate respiratory symptoms. Claims that low humidity aggravates respiratory symptoms and that home humidifiers are beneficial for patients with respiratory problems have not been validated. The use of humidifiers is complicated by the fact that cold-steam home humidifiers frequently become contaminated with fungi (especially yeasts and thermophilic actinomycetes) and other allergens that may exacerbate asthma or induce hypersensitivity pneumonitis.

Analysis of the available literature regarding the direct effect of humidity on allergic patients does not permit any conclusion. High humidity may be detrimental to some asthmatics but certainly not to all, and the effect of humidity may also result from such concomitant changes as increased atmospheric concentration of mold spores.

Temperature

The aggravating effect on some asthmatic patients of a sudden drop in temperature has been confirmed in the laboratory. The frequency of asthmatic attacks dramatically increases in many areas of the world with the influx of cold air at the beginning of winter. This may be due to a direct effect of cold air on the bronchial mucosa, to changes in atmospheric concentration of environmental allergens, or to irritants or other factors not yet identified.

The respiratory tract usually heats and humidifies inhaled cold air very efficiently even under extreme conditions. However, in some patients with such chronic respiratory problems as chronic bronchitis and asthma, there is an increase in symptoms on breathing cold air. Cold-induced increase of asthma has been thought to result from the stimulation of upper airway receptors, inducing reflex bronchoconstriction. Some studies have demonstrated that the combination of cold air and hyperpnea, whether produced by exercise or by isocapnic hyperventilation, markedly aggravates bronchoconstriction in asthmatics. These carefully controlled experiments demonstrated that the essential stimulus for this bronchoconstriction is heat loss from airway mucosa, the magnitude of which varies directly with the degree of hyperventilation and inversely with the temperature and water content of inspired air.

Barometric Pressure

Changes in barometric pressure may be associated with either an increase or a decrease in the frequency of asthma attacks. Several studies have reported that there is an increased incidence of asthma attacks associated with sudden drops in barometric pressure. However, a fourfold increase in the incidence of asthma in Philadelphia was observed during days of high barometric pressure. Major epidemics of so-called "New Orleans asthma" occurring during the late fall post-ragweed season were also clearly associated with rising barometric pressure (particularly when combined with decreasing temperature and relative humidity, and a minimal wind velocity).

Air Pollution

Air pollution is defined as an atmospheric accumulation of substances, usually man-made, to a degree that is injurious to humans, animals, or plants. Air pollution is usually identified with smoke from chimneys, factories or the exhaust of automobiles, but anything airborne can pollute the atmosphere. The pollutant may originate from natural sources such as forests, swamps, and desert dust; from man-made sources such as factories and residential chimneys; or from other point sources. Pollutants may also form by the atmospheric interaction of several agents with sunlight, heat, or water vapor. The total polluted air mass in a given populated area is highly unstable because of the continuous nature of atmospheric change.

Pollution is frequently referred to as smog, a combination of the words smoke and fog. There are two main types of smog, industrial and photochemical (Table 19–1). Industrial smog, which is the dominant type in large industrialized areas such as New York, Chicago, Tokyo, and London (the last being commonly referred to as "London Smog"), results from the combustion of solid or liquid fossil fuels. The second type, photochemical smog, accumulates in cities like Los Angeles and Denver, where there are a large number of automobiles and sufficient sunlight to permit photochemical reactions. This type of smog results from automobile exhaust emissions and is referred to as "Los Angeles Smog." Weather markedly affects the intensity of air pollution; the more important meteorologic factors that lead to accumulation of pollutants are temperature inversion, which limits vertical dispersion, and low wind velocity, which hinders horizontal dispersion.

Epidemiologic analysis leaves little doubt that air pollution aggravates respiratory illness. Sudden onset of prolonged episodes of increased air pollution, such as occurred in London in 1952, and Donora, Pennsylvania, in 1948, were associated with increased mortality and morbidity of patients with respiratory

Table 19–1. Smog Classification

Industrial Smog
Combustion of fossil fuels
Oxides of sulfur
Sulfuric acid
Particulate matter

Photochemical Smog
Automobile exhaust emission
Ozone
Nitrogen oxides
Hydrocarbons

Miscellaneous
Point sources pollutants

problems. A direct correlation between severity of asthma symptoms and levels of pollution has been noted in several studies, but the role of air pollution is difficult to quantitate because the degree of bronchial hyperreactivity, which is the hallmark of asthma, is notably variable. The bronchial response to inhaled histamine or methacholine, for example, increases for several weeks following viral infections. The threshold levels of air pollutants may thus become clinically important in asthmatic patients if bronchial reactivity increases following viral infections or after exposure to irritants or to occupational inhaled allergens. Secondly, and perhaps more important, some atmospheric pollutants may themselves induce bronchial reactivity, increasing the response of the patient to environmental allergens or to such nonspecific irritants as cold air. Ozone, sulfur dioxide, and oxides of nitrogen have all been demonstrated to increase bronchial reactivity. Epidemiologic studies must therefore consider the relationship between allergens, infectious agents, air pollutants, and meteorologic changes. The information derived from exposure to single agents under laboratory conditions cannot easily be duplicated in the field because of the complex environmental interrelationships.

Industrial Smog

The major components of industrial smog are sulfur oxides and other particulates whose source is the impurities in coal and oil fuels used in industrial processes, power generation, and heating of buildings.

Sulfur dioxide (SO_2) is the pollutant most frequently monitored to measure atmospheric pollution. Its atmospheric concentration averages 0.01 to 0.1 ppm, with an occasional peak to 1 to 1.5 ppm. During the London Smog episode of December, 1952, the concentration averaged 1.34 ppm over a 48-hour period.

Studies of the effect of sulfur dioxide on asthma have been contradictory. The discrepancy of the different studies on the effect of sulfur dioxide on airways resistance results from the different concentrations used and the variability of host reactivity. Approximately 10 percent of the "normal" population are "hyperreactors" responding with increased airways resistance to sulfur dioxide exposure. This may explain why only certain individuals in an exposed population will exhibit adverse effects during high pollution episodes. It has been shown that asthmatics exposed to SO_2 are at a higher risk than are healthy individuals. Asthmatics developed bronchospasm within a few minutes after exposure to sulfur dioxide at a level of 0.4 to 0.6 ppm during moderate to heavy exercise. Particulate pollutants can adversely affect the bronchial tree, either by acting as carriers for, or by potentiating the effects of, other pollutants. It is therefore difficult to separate the effects of inert particles from those of other air pollutants that originate from the same source and may have related actions.

Photochemical Smog

This type of smog characteristically occurs in cities with warm sunny weather and a large number of automobiles. The smog consists of hydrocarbons plus nitrogen oxides resulting from the interaction of emissions of automobile exhaust and stationary sources of combustion products that have reacted with oxygen and organic substances in the atmosphere, in the presence of sunlight. This interaction produces organic radicals that eventually degrade into carbon dioxide, carbon monoxide, water, and ozone. Ozone, the main component of photochemical oxidants, contributes up to 90 percent of the total oxidant level. Concentrations of ozone below 0.2 ppm are well tolerated by both healthy and asthmatic individuals, except during heavy exercise, when concentrations of 0.2 ppm can cause temporary respiratory irritation, particularly in asthmatics. Single exposures to ozone at concentrations between 0.2 and 0.8 ppm for 2 or 3 hours may induce mild degrees of airways narrowing, persisting for less than 24 hours, and an increase in airways reactivity. A significant increase in asthma attacks has been observed on days when the oxidant level in Pasadena, California, was 0.1 to 0.2 ppm, a concentration that causes eye irritation. Concentrations of 0.2 to 0.5 ppm reduce visual acuity, and levels of 0.3 to 1 ppm cause coughing, a choking sensation, and severe fatigue. Under the uniform air pollution index of the U.S. Environmental Protection Agency, 0.2 ppm ozone (1 hour average) has been established as the alert concentration.

The effects of air pollution on allergic patients can be summarized as follows:

1. Air pollution in concentrations found in urban areas can cause irritation of the respiratory tract and provoke bronchoconstriction.

2. There is a segment of the population that is more susceptible to bronchoconstriction by air pollutants, probably because of an abnormality of the autonomic nervous system.

3. Asthmatic patients as a group are more susceptible to

Table 19–2. Guidelines for Asthmatics During Periods of High Air Pollution*

Avoid unnecessary physical activity.

Avoid smoking and smoke-filled rooms.

Avoid exposure to dusts and other irritants, such as hair sprays, or other sprays, paint, exhaust fumes, smoke from any fire, or other fumes.

Avoid exposure to persons with colds or respiratory infections.

Try to stay indoors in a clean environment. Air conditioning may help. Charcoal filters and electrostatic precipitators may be helpful.

If it appears that the air pollution episode will persist or worsen, it is desirable to leave the polluted area until the episode subsides.

The physician should formulate specific instructions for each patient to follow in case of an air pollution alert. This should include the medication to use, how and when to call the physician, and when to go to a hospital.

The physician's special guidelines should be written and kept in a readily accessible place.

*From Weather and Air Pollution Committee, American Academy of Allergy and Immunology, 611 E. Wells St., Milwaukee, Wisconsin 53202.

the effects of air pollution and for this reason should take special precautions during high air pollution periods (see Table 19–2).

INDOOR ENVIRONMENT

There are few accurate data defining and quantitating the important indoor atmospheric components and their role in allergic diseases. A knowledge of the work environment is essential in evaluating a patient with allergic respiratory disease. Patients while at work may be exposed to gases, vapors, organic and inorganic dusts, and such other environmental components as air pollutants and smoke.

Home Environment

Allergic patients may be exposed at home to a variety of allergens, including dust, mites, animal danders, feathers, and molds. The home environment is also affected by such factors as air-conditioning and heating systems, humidifiers, and family habits and hobbies. Heavy cigarette smoking in a home and frequent use of insecticides, aerosols, and other sprays are sources of significant indoor pollution. Most of the components act as irritants rather than sensitizers, but allergic patients, especially asthmatics, are adversely affected by their inhalation.

Cigarette smoke is the most common indoor pollutant, and patients with rhinitis and/or asthma experience a variable increase in symptoms when exposed to tobacco smoke. Symptoms are often characterized by conjunctival irritation, increased nasal discharge and cough, and, in the asthmatic patient, by increased wheezing. Although the effect of passive or atmospheric cigarette smoke on the production of respiratory symptoms is unknown, the incidence of respiratory symptoms in children has been reported to increase in direct relation to their parents' smoking habits. Whether hyperreactivity to tobacco smoke is due to allergic mechanisms or is entirely irritative has yet to be resolved. Tobacco smoke has been reported to affect host defense mechanisms in man and experimental animals. Several studies have demonstrated that gas stoves contribute significantly to indoor nitrogen dioxide concentration. Other common sources of irritants at home include fireplaces, room deodorizers, furniture and floor waxes, and cooking odors.

Work Environment

The importance of occupational factors is being recognized in an increasing number of respiratory diseases, which include asthma and various interstitial fibrotic and granulomatous processes. Immunologic mechanisms are now recognized as being involved in the pathogenesis of many of these diseases, but nonimmunologic mechanisms also play an important role. Occupational asthma, for example, may involve not only a classic IgE-mediated allergic reaction but also a pharmacologic abnormality or an irritant effect. It is very important to review the work environment carefully in patients with allergic respiratory syndromes. A specific exposure at work may be the direct cause of the allergic problem or may contribute significantly to the patient's ongoing symptoms (Table 19–3).

MANAGEMENT

Environmental Control

An important component of the treatment of allergic respiratory diseases is the identification of environmental substances contributing to symptoms. Appropriate control measures may then be defined that will decrease the contact with the offending substances. Environmental control should be reasonable and based on the sensitivities of the patient as demonstrated by history and appropriate diagnostic studies. Patients allergic to

Table 19–3B. Industrial Materials Presumed to Be Allergic Pathogens

Material	Workers Affected/Industry/Source
Salts of nickel	Metal plating
Grain (including insect and related grain contaminants)	Farmers, grain elevator operators
Wood dusts	Wood mill workers, carpenters
Vegetable gums (acacia, karaya), natural resins	Printers
Ampicillin Spiramycin Piperazine Amprolium hydrochloride Antibiotic dusts	Medical pharmaceuticals
Diisocyanates (TDI, HDI, MDI) Pyrolysis products of polyvinyl chlorides Price labels and adhesives Soldering fluxes	Polyurethane, printers' adhesives Meat wrappers, electrical workers
Organic phosphorus	Farm workers
Cotton dust	Textiles, cottonseed oil
Formalin	Medical pharmaceuticals

Table 19–3B. Industrial Materials Presumed to Be Allergic Pathogens

Material	Workers Affected/Industry/Source
Salts of nickel	Metal plating
Grain (including insect and related grain contaminants)	Farmers, grain elevator operators
Wood dusts	Wood mill workers, carpenters
Vegetable gums (acacia, karaya), natural resins	Printers
Ampicillin Spiramycin Piperazine Amprolium hydrochloride Antibiotic dusts	Medical pharmaceuticals
Diisocyanates (TDI, HDI, MDI) Pyrolysis products of polyvinyl chlorides Price labels and adhesives Soldering fluxes	Polyurethane, printers' adhesives Meat wrappers, electrical workers
Organic phosphorus	Farm workers
Cotton dust	Textiles, cottonseed oil
Formalin	Medical pharmaceuticals

pollen, for example, should be made aware of the different pollen seasons and encouraged to decrease outdoor activities during the peak of the offending seasons. Indoor pollen levels may be reduced by closing windows and using central air-conditioning with electrostatic filters. Outdoor fungi grow on leaf surfaces, plant litter, and soil; spore concentrations vary with local cycles of plant growth. Mold-sensitive patients should avoid exposures to mulches, dry soil, compost piles, and leaf litter. Fungi may also grow indoors, in dark humid areas, and may contaminate humidifiers. Reduction of indoor mold spores requires careful control of areas capable of supporting fungus growth, e.g., foam rubber articles, shower curtains, plumbing fixtures, refrigerator trays and window moldings. A careful anti-dust program is essential for patients allergic to house dust and mites. The patient's bedroom should be made almost dust-free by covering pillows and mattresses with airtight plastic covers, eliminating carpets, and stripping the room of dust-collecting furniture. Animals should be removed from the environment if there is allergy to domestic animals. Exposure to such common irritants as cigarette smoke, room deodorizers, furniture polishes, floor waxes, and cooking odors should be minimized or eliminated.

The concentration of harmful agents in the workplace can usually be reduced by efficient environmental control and careful monitoring of antigens in the atmosphere. However, very sensitive individuals may not be relieved by optimal control measures, in which case job transfer may be necessary.

Climate Therapy

Moving to a different climate as a treatment for severe asthma has been advocated since ancient times. A dry climate with poor pollen-producing vegetation and low levels of air pollution is theoretically advantageous to a patient with allergic respiratory disease. However, the multiplicity of meteorologic and environmental factors influencing climate and the marked variability of the individual patient's response to those factors make it almost impossible to prescribe a favorable climate for a given patient. A change of climate is not necessarily beneficial, and a hypersensitivity may develop to newly encountered allergens. Most evidence for a favorable effect of climate change on asthma is anecdotal, and there is a paucity of well-controlled studies supporting this approach. Recommendation of a permanent climatic change for the allergic patient is seldom justified. When such change might be appropriate, a trial period of living in the new location to ascertain the benefits of such a move may help to make the decision.

Bibliography

Bethel, R., Epstein, J., Sheppard, O., et al.: Sulfur dioxide induced bronchocon-striction in freely breathing, exercising, asthmatic subjects. Am. Rev. Respir. Dis. 128:987, 1983.

Girsh, L. S., Shubin, E., Dick, C., et al.: A study on the epidemiology of asthma in children in Philadelphia: the relation of weather and air pollution to peak incidence of asthmatic attacks. J. Allergy 39:347, 1967.

Hackney, J. D., Thiede, F. C., Linn, W. S., et al.: Experimental studies on human health effects of air pollutants. IV. Short term physiological and clinical effects. Arch. Environ. Health 33:176, 1978.

Lopez, M., and Salvaggio, J.: Climate–weather–air pollution. In Middleton, E., Reed, C., and Ellis E. (eds.): Allergy Principles and Practice, Vol. 2. St. Louis, C. V. Mosby Co., 1983, Chap. 54.

McFadden, E. R., Jr., Ingram, R. H., Jr., Haynes, H. L., et al.: Predominant site of flow limitation and mechanisms of post-exertional asthma. J. Appl. Physiol. 42:746, 1977.

Salvaggio, J., Hassleblad, V., Seabury, J., et al.: New Orleans asthma. II. Relationship of climatologic and seasonal factors to outbreaks. J. Allergy 45:257, 1970.

Schoetelin, C. E., and Landau, E.: Air pollution and asthmatic attacks in the Los Angeles area. Public Health Rep. 76:545, 1961.

Slavin, R. G., Claman, L., Kailin, E. W., et al.: Guidelines for asthmatic patients during pollution episodes. J. Allergy Clin. Immunol. 55:222, 1975.

Symposium proceedings of occupational immunologic lung disease. J. Allergy Clin. Immunol. 70:1, 1982.

Tromp, S.: Influence of weather and climate on asthma and bronchitis. Rev. Allergy 22:1028, 1968.

20

Diagnostic Tests for Assessment of Immunity

DAVID T. ROWLANDS, JR., M.D.

Basic Principles of Immunologic Assays
  Lymphocyte Cell Surfaces
  Monoclonal Antibodies
  Radioimmunoassay (RIA); Enzyme-linked Immunosorbent Assay (ELISA)
  Fluorescence
Identification and Assay of T-Cell and B-Lymphocyte Subpopulations and Functions; Assay of Complement
  T Cells
    Assay of T-Cell Surface Characteristics
    Assay of T-Cell Functions
  B Cells

Assay of Surface Characteristics
Assay of B-Cell Functions; Detection of Antigens and Antibodies
Assay of Complement (CH_{50}, C3, C4)
Identification and Assay of Cells Other Than Lymphocytes
  Monocytes and Macrophages
  Eosinophils and Basophils
  Polymorphonuclear Leukocytes
Histocompatibility Testing
Skin Testing
  Immediate Hypersensitivity Tests
  Delayed Hypersensitivity Tests

BASIC PRINCIPLES OF IMMUNOLOGIC ASSAYS

During the last two decades, there has been a marked increase in the number, sensitivity, and specificity of clinically applicable diagnostic immunologic assays. This is the result of (1) enhanced understanding of lymphocyte cell surfaces, (2) the development of methods to produce monoclonal antibodies, (3) the elaboration of radioactive and enzyme-linked assays, and (4) the use of fluorescence technology.

Lymphocyte Cell Surfaces

Distinctive cell surface receptors and antigens characterize the subpopulations of lymphocytes (Fig. 20–1). Surfaces of T and B cells each have distinctive antigens that can be recognized with the aid of appropriate antisera; T cells also have surface receptors that bind sheep red blood cells; B cells have surface immunoglobulins, receptors for Fc portions of immunoglobulins, and receptors for complement components. Individual B cells generally have only one class of immunoglobulin on their surfaces; those with IgM may also have IgD receptors. Mature plasma cells are unusual B cells in that they have little, if any, cell surface immunoglobulin.

Monoclonal Antibodies

Until recently antisera were prepared by immunizing animals with appropriate antigens and purifying the antibody by adsorption to insolubilized antigen followed by elution of the antibody. The heterogeneity and variable specificity of such antibody depended on the quality of the initial antigen preparation and the adequacy of absorption of the antisera.

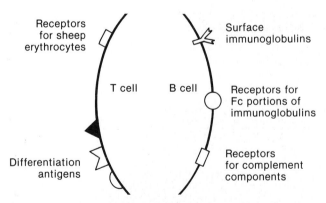

Figure 20–1. Variations of surface characteristics permit identification of lymphocyte subpopulations. Other cells (e.g., macrophages) may have similar cell surface features.

The methods of preparing monoclonal antibodies has provided antisera with great specificity. Rodents are first immunized with appropriate antigens (e.g., purified antigens or whole cells); antibody-forming cells are harvested from the splenic white pulp of the immunized animals and fused with non-secretory myeloma cells. Single fused cells are then tested for the antibodies they produce and are cloned and maintained in culture or as ascites tumors. Monoclonal antibodies obtained from culture supernates or ascites fluid are now commercially available for numerous antigens.

Radioimmunoassay (RIA); Enzyme-Linked Immunosorbent Assay (ELISA)

RIA utilizes antigen or antibody coupled to a radioactive isotope, while ELISA utilizes an antibody coupled to an enzyme. Both assays may be done directly or with a secondary antibody, and both methods are applicable at the tissue levels as well as in test tubes. They are of similar sensitivity, but ELISA methods have the advantage that they do not use radioactive reagents. This reduces the cost of equipment needed.

Fluorescence

Fluorescence-labeled antibody probes have been used to identify antigens in tissues, on cell surfaces, and even in nuclei. Recent adaptation of laser technology to this microscopic technique permits more precise and rapid recognition, enumeration, and isolation of cells labeled with fluorescent probes. Cell size, amount of nuclear chromatin, and reactivity with antibodies to cell surface antigens can be measured simultaneously with a computer-aided fluorescence-activated cell sorter. Such separation of cells by one or more cellular parameters is now widely adapted for qualitative and quantitative analyses of subpopulations of blood cells, particularly lymphocytes, in various diseases.

IDENTIFICATION AND ASSAY OF T-CELL AND B-LYMPHOCYTE SUBPOPULATIONS AND FUNCTIONS; ASSAY OF COMPLEMENT

Lymphocytes are heterogeneous in function and surface characteristics. T cells play major roles in cellular immunity (e.g., graft rejection) and in activating and modulating B cells. B cells synthesize antibodies.

T Cells

Assay of T-Cell Surface Characteristics

The several methods for enumerating T cells depend on surface characteristics. T cells form rosettes with sheep red blood cells (SRBC); to identify a T cell by this method, three or more SRBC should be found surrounding the lymphocyte. This method is adequate for enumeration of total T cells. It has the disadvantage that mononuclear cells must first be separated from whole blood by gradient centrifugation, and application of rosetting to tissue sections has had limited success.

The use of monoclonal antibodies to identify antigens on cell surfaces of T cells has significantly enhanced the resources available for study of these cells. Many T-cell antigens may be regarded as differentiation antigens. The nomenclature for these antigens varied with the investigator and later with the commercial supplier of antisera. Several of the antigens are generally considered to define functional subsets of lymphocytes—for example, helper (T_4) and suppressor (T_8) cells. These antigen-defined subsets may not be as functionally discrete as was previously thought; however, ratios of helper (T_4) to suppressor (T_8) antigen-defined cells have proved most useful in estimating activity in certain diseases, such as acquired immune deficiency syndrome (AIDS) and systemic lupus erythematosus (SLE). T_4 and T_8 cells can be measured by first tagging the T cells with fluorescein-labeled monoclonal antibodies. Enumeration of cells can then be accomplished by fluorescent microscopy or with a laser-activated cell counter. The cell counter permits the assays on whole blood as well as on separated cells, and analysis of small cell populations is possible with greater precision and ease. The monoclonal antibodies can also be used on tissues after labeling the antibodies with fluorescent dyes or enzymes. This has enhanced diagnosis of various diseases including tumors.

Assay of T-Cell Functions

Delayed Hypersensitivity Skin Tests. This is the most important and easily available method for clinical assessment of the status of cellular immune response. Failure to react to intradermal injections of selected antigens is a clinically useful indicator of anergy, i.e., diminished delayed hypersensitivity.

T-Cell Transformation. T-cell functions can be assayed in vitro by several readily available techniques. The most commonly used test is the response to plant lectins such as phytohemagglutinin (PHA). Lymphocytes are placed in culture with several different concentrations of PHA. Proliferation is estimated at 3 and at 7 days by either counting transformation of T cells into blast cells or by measuring uptake of radioactive thymidine by blast cells. The adequacy of response of the patient's lymphocytes is estimated by comparison with the response of lymphocytes from a normal population. Pokeweed mitogen, another plant lectin, stimulates both T cells and B cells and, in humans, is a thymus-dependent stimulant of B cells.

Lymphokine Assay. There are numerous lymphokines, of which only a few are of use in the clinical laboratory. One of these is migration inhibition factor (MIF). A simple assay of MIF is accomplished by placing mononuclear cells in a capillary tube, which is then placed in a petri dish containing agar. The cells normally migrate from the capillary tube and form a halo around the open end of the tube. However, if the patient has been sensitized and the appropriate antigen is added to the culture medium, MIF is produced by lymphocytes and macrophage migration is inhibited. Addition of exogenous MIF also retards migration. Reduction in the size of the halo is directly proportional to the MIF activity. Biologic assays to detect lymphokines are numerous but difficult to perform. The significance of these substances in infectious, immunologic, neoplastic, and other diseases is under active investigation.

B Cells

Assay of Surface Characteristics

Receptors for Immunoglobulins and for Complement. Cell surface immunoglobulins and receptors for specific fragments of immunoglobulins and for components of complement all have been used to enumerate B lymphocytes (see Fig. 20–1). Antibodies to heavy and light chains of immunoglobulins, when incubated with isolated mononuclear cells, recognize and bind to surface immunoglobulins of B cells. These cells can be counted using the fluorescent microscope or a fluorescence-activated cell counter if the antibody has been coupled with a fluorescent probe. Total numbers of B cells can be estimated by adding the numbers of cells reactive with anti-heavy chain serum. The assay is most often done by direct staining when a fluorescent microscope is used, but a "sandwich" technique, using unlabeled primary antibodies to the immunoglobulins and a secondary labeled antibody may be a better method when enumeration is done with the cell counter. In either case, it is desirable to preincubate cells overnight to rid them of immunoglobulins that adhere non-specifically to cell surfaces.

EAC Rosettes. The EAC (erythrocyte, amboceptor, complement) rosette identifies B cells by taking advantage of the presence of Fc or complement receptors on B cell surfaces. Addition of anti-SRBC antibody (amboceptor) to sheep erythrocytes in the absence of complement recognizes and complexes with Fc receptors. Addition of complement to this complex permits enumeration of cells with complement (C3b) receptors. Either SRBC complex is then incubated with human lymphocytes. Rosettes composed of three or more of either of the SRBC preparations around individual lymphocytes are counted as B cells.

Assay of B-Cell Functions; Detection of Antigens and Antibodies

Quantitation of Serum Immunoglobulins; Serum Electrophoresis. Electrophoretic separation of proteins is readily accomplished using any of several supporting media. The concentrations of the five principal protein peaks (albumin, α_1, α_2, β, and γ) can then be estimated based on their relative densities.

Immunodiffusion. Immunodiffusion detects a reaction between antibody and antigen by a precipitation reaction.

Double Diffusion in Agar (Ouchterlony) (Fig. 20–2). This technique is based on the principle that the diffusion of antigen and antibody through a semi-solid medium (agar) forms stable immune complexes which can be analyzed visually. The technique involves placing antigens (or sources of antigens) and antibodies in wells cut into an inert supporting gel. The visible line of precipitation that forms where the reagents are in equivalence permits a comparison of antigens for identity, partial identity (cross reactivity), or non-identity against a given selected antibody.

Single Radial Diffusion (Mancini) (Fig. 20–3). The double-immunodiffusion technique is qualitative and only semi-quantitative. The single technique introduced by Mancini in 1965 permits accurate quantitative determinations of antigens. The antigens are allowed to diffuse in gels containing dilute specific

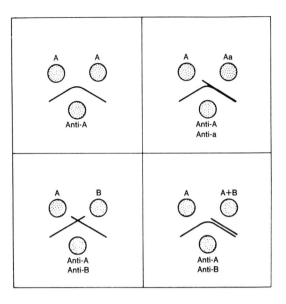

Figure 20–2. Ouchterlony double-gel diffusion in agar, showing precipitin patterns characteristic of identity (*top left*), reaction of non-identity (*bottom left*), and partial identity (*top right*). Complex pattern is also shown (*bottom right*). (From Bloch, K. J., and Salvaggio, J. E.: Use and interpretation of diagnostic laboratory tests. JAMA 248:2738, 1982. Copyright 1982, American Medical Association.)

antibodies. Wells are cut in the gel and the antigen samples, or dilutions of a standard, are applied to the wells. The resulting ring of precipitation surrounding various dilutions of antigen selected is proportional to the amount of antigen that has been placed into the well. The method is commonly used to quantitate IgG, IgA, IgM, IgD, C3, C4, and C1 esterase inhibitor, as well as other proteins.

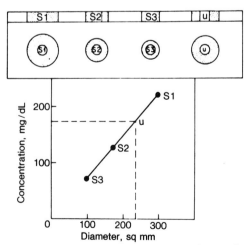

Figure 20–3. Three standard solutions of different antigen concentrations (S) and a sample of unknown concentration (u). After incubation for a sufficient time to allow equilibrium to be reached, the ring diameters were measured. The square of the diameter of the standard rings was plotted on the x axis, and the concentration of the antigen in the standard solution was plotted on the y axis, to obtain a standard curve. The concentration of the antigen in the test sample was then determined from the standard curve by finding the concentration of antigen corresponding to the square of the diameter of the ring formed by the test sample. Radial immunodiffusion quantities of this type are used to measure the concentration of serum immunoglobulins and complement proteins. (From Bloch, K. J., and Salvaggio, J. E.: Use and interpretation of diagnostic laboratory tests. JAMA 248:2738, 1982. Copyright 1982, American Medical Association.)

Immunoelectrophoresis (IEP). The technique of immunoelectrophoresis combines electrophoretic separation, diffusion, and immune precipitation of proteins (Fig. 20–4). A number of modifications of the original technique of Grabar and Williams have proved very helpful in the evaluation of immunological diseases.

Radioimmunoelectrophoresis (Radioimmunoassay [RIA]). RIA utilizes a purified antigen that is radioisotope-labeled and used to compete with unlabeled standard or unknown samples for a specific antibody. The method is much more sensitive than other methods of immunoelectrophoresis and its application has permitted assay of hormones, drugs, Australian antigen, and IgE.

Radioimmunosorbent Test (RIST). RIST is a modified RIA test of particular interest to the allergist because it accurately

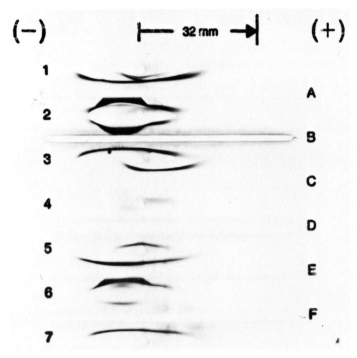

Figure 20–4. Immunoelectrophoresis with normal human serum in wells 1, 3, 5, and 7. The serum from a patient with multiple myeloma is in wells 2, 4, and 6. Antibodies to total immunoglobulins, IgG, IgA, and IgM, are in slots A, B, C, and D, respectively. Antibodies to kappa and lambda light chains are in slots E and F, respectively. The patient's IgG and kappa precipitates indicate the presence of an IgG-kappa monoclonal protein with an associated reduction in other immunoglobulins.

measures the usually small amounts of IgE that are present in serum or in body fluids. Anti-IgE antibodies are bound to an appropriate solid medium such as a paper disc. This preparation is then permitted to react with labeled [125]I IgE and an unknown serum. The whole mixture is washed after suitable incubation, and radioactivity is counted in a gamma counter. IgE in the unknown serum competes with radiolabeled IgE so that the greater the amount of IgE, the lower will be the binding of radioactive IgE. The IgE in the unknown serum is estimated by comparison with a standard curve that has been titrated at the same time.

Radioallergosorbent Test (RAST). RAST is designed to measure the amount of specific IgE directed toward specific antigens (such as from ragweed) (Fig. 20–5). The target antigens (e.g., ragweed antigen E) are bound to the discs. Serum containing

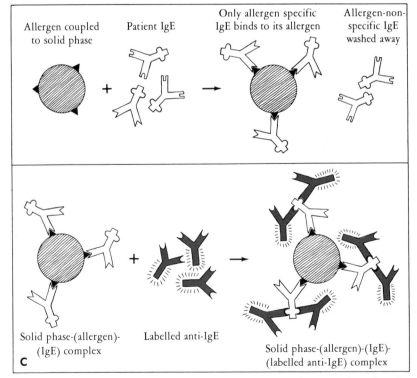

Figure 20–5. RAST (radioallergosorbent test). The target antigens are bound to the solid-phase disks. Serum containing antibody to these antigens reacts with antigens on the dish. The amount of bound specific IgE is then determined by adding radiolabeled anti-IgE and comparing binding of this to binding when nonallergic serum is used. (From Bellanti, J. A.: Immunologically mediated diseases. *In* Bellanti, J. A. [ed.]: Immunology III. Philadelphia, W. B. Saunders Co., 1985, p. 375.)

antibodies to these antigens is permitted to react with the antigens on the disc surface. The amount of bound IgE can then be determined by adding radiolabeled anti-IgE and comparing binding of this to binding when non-allergic serum is used.

Electroimmunodiffusion. The sensitivity of the technique of immunodiffusion in agar is increased considerably by the technique of electroimmunodiffusion. The probability of antigen and antibody meeting and the speed of development of a precipitant is greatly enhanced when the two are driven together electrically. The two variations of the technique described here have achieved wide usage.

One-dimensional Double Electroimmunodiffusion (Countercurrent Immunoelectrophoresis). This involves electrophoresis of antigen and antibody in opposite directions simultaneously from separate wells in a gel medium. The resultant precipitation takes place at a point between the two wells. It is possible to obtain visible precipitation within 30 minutes by this technique, which is at least 10 times more sensitive than the standard double-diffusion technique. This technique is only semiquantitative.

One-dimensional Single Electroimmunodiffusion (Rocket Electrophoresis or Laurell Technique). This technique is used principally to quantitate antigens other than immunoglobulins. It employs a specific antibody that is incorporated into a support medium from which the antibody does not diffuse. The antigen is then electrophoretically diffused into the antibody-containing agar. A pattern of immunoprecipitates forms that resembles a spike or rocket (hence the name). The length of the "rocket" is proportional to the quantity of antigen used. This method is a useful quantitative procedure, and several variations permit it to be used to quantitate serum immunoglobulins and complement components and to identify complex antigens.

Enzyme-Linked Immunosorbent Assay (ELISA). This technique attempts to circumvent both the expense and the inconvenience of radioisotope quantitation by linking various enzymes to either antigen or antibody as a label. The many variations of enzyme immunoassay are completely analogous to radioimmunoassays and to quantitative immunofluorescence. The difference lies in the use of an enzyme label. Frequently used enzymes include horseradish peroxidase, alkaline phosphatase, lysozyme, and glucose-6-phosphate dehydrogenase. However, almost any enzyme can be used as long as it is soluble, stable, and not present in biologic fluids in amounts that would interfere with serum determinations.

Assays of Agglutination and Agglutination Inhibition. The direct agglutination test is carried out with serially titrated antisera in twofold dilutions in the presence of a constant quantity of antigen. Tests are carried out in small test tubes or, more commonly, in micro titer plates with smaller amounts of reagents. The end point of the reaction is the greatest dilution of antiserum producing agglutinates.

Inhibition of agglutination of antigen-coated red blood cells is a highly sensitive and specific method for detecting small quantities of soluble antigens in blood or other tissue fluids. The technique depends upon the ability of soluble antigens to inhibit a standard antibody concentration from agglutinating sensitized erythrocytes.

Detection of Immune Complexes. Immune complexes have a pathogenic role in such diseases as rheumatoid arthritis, systemic lupus erythematosus, hypersensitivity pneumonitis, the Arthus reaction, some forms of glomerulonephritis, and vasculitis. Methods of detecting immune complexes are difficult. The methods take advantage of the high sedimentation rate, the ability to react with rheumatoid factor, and interactions of the complement system with immune complexes. Various methods use the ability of C1q to bind to immune complexes. Other methods use the Raji cell, which is a human lymphoblastoid cell with B-cell characteristics but without surface immunoglobulin.

Measurement of Autoantibodies

Antinuclear Antibody (ANA). This is a sensitive test for serum antibodies to one or more nuclear antigens. The assay is performed by overlaying sections of normal tissues with patients' sera and localizing the antibodies with fluorescein-labeled anti–human immunoglobulin antibodies. Under some assay conditions, nuclear antigens may be lost or greatly reduced, in which case titers of ANA do not help to establish the prognosis or to assess the clinical course of the patient. The incidence of positive ANA tests is age-dependent in otherwise normal subjects. Overall, fewer than 5 percent of normal individuals have a positive ANA test. The incidence of a positive ANA in healthy elderly subjects is < 10 percent.

Immunofluorescent patterns of ANA vary. The several ANA

Table 20–1. Nuclear Antigens

Antigens	Disease Association
Native DNA	SLE
Denatured DNA	SLE, many others
Sm	SLE
nRNP	MCTD
SS-A	Sjögren's syndrome
SS-B	Sjögren's syndrome
RAP	Rheumatoid arthritis with Sjögren's syndrome
Histones	Drug-induced lupus erythematosus
Centromere	PSS (CREST)

SLE = systemic lupus erythematosus; MCTD = mixed connective tissue disease; PSS = progressive systemic sclerosis (serum reactivity with centromeres is most prominent in the CREST variant of PSS); Sm = Smith antigen; nRNP = nuclear ribonucleoprotein; SS-A = Sjögren's syndrome–A; SS-B = Sjögren's syndrome–B; RAP = rheumatoid arthritis protein; CREST: see text.

fluorescent patterns are associated with particular diseases and various antinuclear antibodies are directed toward different parts of the nucleus (Table 20–1).

Antibodies in patients with systemic lupus erythematosus (SLE) usually react with both native and denatured DNA. There is an excellent correlation between the titers of antibodies to double-stranded DNA and the activity of SLE.

Extractable nuclear antigens (ENA) contain two distinct antigens. These are the Sm (Smith) and nRNP (nuclear ribonucleoprotein) antigens. Antibodies to Sm are highly specific for SLE but are found in only 30 percent of patients with SLE. Antibodies to nRNP, at titers of 1:10,000, are achieved in mixed connective tissue disease (MCTD). Other non-histone antigens such as SS-A (Sjögren's syndrome A) and SS-B (Sjögren's syndrome B) also help to make the diagnosis of SLE. Histone antigens, which are attracting increased attention, are now used principally to confirm the diagnosis of drug-induced lupus erythematosus.

Anti-mitochondrial Antibodies. Titers of anti-mitochondrial antibodies in excess of 1:160 confirm the diagnosis of primary biliary cirrhosis (PBC). Antibodies to centromere-associated proteins are found in patients with progressive systemic sclerosis and are most particularly associated with the CREST syndrome (calcinosis, Raynaud's syndrome, esophageal dysphagia, sclerodactylia, and telangiectasia).

Rheumatoid Factor. This is measured by mixing patients' sera with particles (e.g., erythrocytes, latex beads) coated with im-

Table 20–2. Rheumatoid Factor Activity

Activity in >50 Percent of Patients	Activity in <50 Percent of Patients
Rheumatoid arthritis	Tuberculosis
Bacterial endocarditis	Sarcoidosis
Sjögren's syndrome	Cirrhosis
Bronchitis	Myocardial infarction

munoglobulins and observing for agglutination. A positive reaction is usually due to activity of IgM antibodies against IgG autoantibody. Positive reactions may occur in a variety of diseases, some of which are cited in Table 20–2.

Assay of Complement (CH$_{50}$, C3, C4)

Total serum complement (CH$_{50}$) is estimated by determining the amount of serum needed to hemolyze 50 percent of predetermined numbers of sheep red blood cells previously sensitized by addition of a non-agglutinating concentration of anti–sheep erythrocyte antibody. The 50 percent hemolysis point is preferred because hemolysis follows a sigmoid curve, and 50 percent hemolysis falls in the center of the linear part of the curve where small changes in complement produce the most marked changes in degree of hemolysis (i.e., between 20 and 80 percent of hemolysis) (Fig. 20–6). Individual components of the complement system can be measured by antigen-antibody reactions or by the ability of a serum to replace a component known to be missing

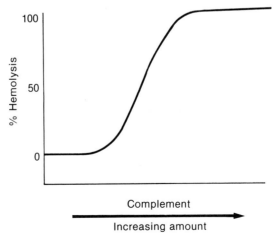

Figure 20–6. Complement mediate hemolysis. Complement is measured by comparing the amount of serum required to produce hemolysis of sheep red cells coated with subagglutinating amounts of antibodies to the red cells.

Table 20–3. Interpretation of C3 and C4 With Reduced CH_{50}

C3	C4	Possible Associations
N	N	Improper preservation or collection of serum; non-C3/C4 inborn errors
D	N	Acute glomerulonephritis, membranoproliferative glomerulo-nephritis, congenital C3 deficiency
N	D	Hereditary angioedema, congenital C4 deficiency
D	D	SLE, chronic active hepatitis, serum sickness

N = normal; D = decreased; SLE = systemic lupus erythematosus; Immune complex formation may be associated with decreased amounts of C3 and/or C4.

from another serum. C3 and C4 components are those most commonly measured in patients with a decrease in CH_{50}. Both the classical and the alternative pathways involve C3, whereas C4 is a necessary component of only the classical pathway. Determination of CH_{50}, C3, and C4 are quite adequate to assay the complement cascade in most patients. An exception is the absence of the terminal components of complement. Patients with this deficiency are susceptible to infections with gonococcus and meningococcus (see Chapter 3). Table 20–3 is a guide for the interpretation of changes in C3 and/or C4 when the CH_{50} is abnormal.

Hereditary angioedema (HAE) deserves special comment. In 85 percent of patients with HAE, the C1 esterase is deficient when measured immunochemically. A functional assay is needed to make the diagnosis in the remaining 15 percent of patients, and C4 is likely to be reduced in either case. C1q is decreased in the acquired form of the disease.

IDENTIFICATION AND ASSAY OF CELLS OTHER THAN LYMPHOCYTES

Monocytes and Macrophages

The monocytes and macrophages may present technical difficulty when enumerating B cells, since both monocytes and macrophages have Fc and C3b receptors. Morphologic identification of the monocyte/macrophage is often not satisfactory. Macrophages may be removed from other mononuclear cells by placing them in a magnetic field after ingestion of iron filings by the monocyte/macrophage cell population. However, the iron particles may injure cellular membranes of lymphocytes, which limits the use of this method. Alternatively, macrophages may be separated from other cells by their tendency to adhere to culture dishes.

Eosinophils and Basophils

Eosinophils and basophils can be counted by using conventional laboratory staining techniques. Determination of the absolute numbers of eosinophils present in the circulation is sometimes useful in evaluating patients with allergic diseases such as atopic eczema and allergic bronchopulmonary aspergillosis. Measurement of the amount of histamine released from basophils upon antigenic challenge is an index of immediate hypersensitivity but is still a cumbersome assay and remains an experimental tool. The intracutaneous injection of a non-specific histamine releaser (e.g., morphine) is a useful in vivo technique to assess the ability of cutaneous basophils to release chemical mediators.

Polymorphonuclear Leukocytes

The primary functions of neutrophils, or polymorphonuclear (PMN) leukocytes, are phagocytosis and killing of bacteria. Neutrophil phagocytosis, killing, and mobility can be assayed. A clinically useful assay for phagocytosis is a nitroblue tetrazolium (NBT) dye reduction test. When NBT is reduced after phagocytosis by the leukocyte, it can be quantitated. This is a useful test to determine the metabolic integrity of phagocytes and is an important diagnostic test in chronic granulomatous disease of children. Another useful phagocytosis assay is the microbicidal technique in which the ability of the leukocytes to kill ingested bacteria is determined. The ability of neutrophils and macrophages to undergo directional migration, known as chemotaxis, can also be measured in vitro using a Boyden chamber. This chamber consists of two compartments separated by a filter membrane through which leukocytes are attracted by the chemotactic factor.

HISTOCOMPATIBILITY TESTING

Two broad classes of histocompatibility antigens in humans (human leukocyte antigens [HLA]) have been recognized. Class I antigens are controlled at three loci and are recognized by serologic tests. Most of the available antisera used in such testing have, until now, been obtained from multiparous women sensitized to paternal antigens. These antisera are almost certain to be replaced by the use of much more specific monoclonal antibodies in future testing. The Class II (DR) antigens are evaluated with mixed lymphocyte cultures. The lymphocytes to be tested are placed in culture with stimulator cells of known DR type. If the test cells differ from the stimulator cells, they will proliferate.

Histocompatibility testing is of great significance in organ transplant patients. There is now an increasing interest, based on statistical correlations, in the relationships between some histocompatibility antigens and certain diseases (e.g., HLA-B27 and ankylosing spondylitis and Reiter's disease). (See Chapter 5.)

SKIN TESTING

Skin testing is the oldest and still the most valuable tool for the clinical allergist/immunologist.

Immediate Hypersensitivity Tests

The antigens to be tested are applied to the skin of the back or forearm, and the underlying skin is pricked or scratched. Positive tests appear within 20 minutes as raised, erythematous lesions, sometimes with pseudopods (wheal and flare reaction). Negative epicutaneous tests are followed by intracutaneous tests in which a small amount of a weak concentration of antigen is injected intradermally, enough to raise a small bleb, and interpreted in a similar manner to the epicutaneous test. A positive test, as with any test in medicine, must be correlated with the clinical history.

Delayed Hypersensitivity Tests

In vivo delayed hypersensitivity or cell-mediated immune tests can be done by either patch testing or intradermal injection of antigen. Patch testing is used to diagnose contact dermatitis. The test material is applied under an occlusive dressing, removed in 48 hours and interpreted. A typical contact eczema occurs at the site of the test material when the test is positive. Intradermal injections of antigens, as with *Candida albicans*, mumps, and trichophytin, are commonly done to determine whether the recall arm of the cell-mediated system is intact. Maximum reactions appear as raised, erythematous, indurated lesions within 48 to 72 hours after the injection.

Dinitrochlorobenzene (DNCB) is a chemical substance to which all normal individuals develop a contact sensitivity. It can be used to check the afferent as well as the efferent limb of the cell-mediated immune system.

Bibliography

Boyum, A.: Separation of blood leucocytes, granulocytes and lymphocytes. Tissue Antigens 4:269, 1974.

Grabar, P., and Burton, P.: Immuno-Electrophoretic Analysis: Application to Human Biological Fluids. London, Elsevier, 1964.

Lovincz, L. L., Soltani, K., and Bernstein, J. E.: Antinuclear antibodies. Int. J. Dermatol. 20:401, 1981.

Ludivico, C. L., Zweiman, B., Myers, A. B., et al.: Predictive value of anti-DNA antibody and selected laboratory studies in systemic lupus erythematosus. J. Rheum. 7:843, 1980.

Reinherz, E. L., and Schlossman, S. F.: The differentiation and function of human T lymphocytes. Cell 19:821, 1980.

Rowlands, D. T. Jr., Whiteside, T. L., and Daniel, R. P.: Cells of the immune system. In Henry, J. B. (ed.): Todd-Sanford-Davidsohn: Clinical Diagnosis and Management, 17th ed. Philadelphia, W. B. Saunders Co., 1984, pp. 822–847.

Swaak, A. J. G., Groenwold, J., Aarden, L. A., et al.: Prognostic value of anti-ds DNA in SLE. Ann. Rheum. Dis. 41:388, 1982.

Terhorst, C., Van Agthoven, A., Reinherz, E., et al.: Biochemical analysis of human T lymphocyte differentiation antigens T_4 and T_5. Science 209:520, 1980.

Index

Page numbers in *italic* type indicate illustrations; page numbers followed by t refer to tables.